THE DEAN DISORDERED

PECULIAR BODIES: STORIES AND HISTORIES
Carolyn Day, Chris Mounsey, and Wendy J. Turner, Editors

The Dean Disordered

Jonathan Swift and Humoral Medicine

PAUL WILLIAM CHILD

UNIVERSITY OF VIRGINIA PRESS
Charlottesville and London

The University of Virginia Press is situated on the traditional lands of the Monacan Nation, and the Commonwealth of Virginia was and is home to many other Indigenous people. We pay our respect to all of them, past and present. We also honor the enslaved African and African American people who built the University of Virginia, and we recognize their descendants. We commit to fostering voices from these communities through our publications and to deepening our collective understanding of their histories and contributions.

University of Virginia Press
© 2025 by the Rector and Visitors of the University of Virginia
All rights reserved
Printed in the United States of America on acid-free paper

First published 2025

9 8 7 6 5 4 3 2 1

ISBN 978-0-8139-5332-8 (hardback)
ISBN 978-0-8139-5333-5 (paperback)
ISBN 978-0-8139-5334-2 (ebook)

Library of Congress Cataloging-in-Publication Data is available for this title.

Cover art: Francis Bindon, portrait of Jonathan Swift, c.1735. (Crawford Art Gallery, CAG.2228)
Cover design: Joel W. Coggins

*To Chris, who always asks the right questions.
And to Susan, who gave me her greatest gift, time.*

When I received the honor and happiness of your last letter . . . I was afflicted with a pair of disorders that usually seize me once a year, and with which I have been acquainted from my youth, but it is only of late years that they have begun to come together, although I should have been better contented with one at a time—these are giddiness and deafness, which usually last a month; the first tormenting my body, and the other making me incapable of conversing.
—JONATHAN SWIFT TO MARY PENDARVES,
7 OCTOBER 1734

O poor old man! . . . [A]fter guardians had been appointed for [Swift], I went into his dining room, where he was walking, I said something to him very insignificant, I know not what; but, instead of making any kind of answer to it, he said, "Go, Go," pointing with his hand to the door, and immediately afterwards, raising his hand to his head, he said, "My best understanding," and so broke off abruptly, and walked away.
—DEANE SWIFT TO THE EARL OF ORRERY, 4 APRIL 1744

These are the last recorded words of the Reverend Dr. Jonathan Swift, Dean of St. Patrick's Cathedral, Dublin

CONTENTS

Preface	xi
Acknowledgments	xvii
1. Taking Swift Back	1
2. Stories of Illness and Retrospective Diagnosis	17
3. As Swift Would Have It	34
4. Help for the Humoral Body: Doctors and Friends	51
5. Disciplining the Humoral Body: Swift's Regimen	67
6. The Disordered Social Body and Humoral Identity	85
7. Swift in the Sick Role	101
8. Gulliver's Travels and Swift's Travails	124
9. Gulliver's Ordeals as Swift's Order	142
10. Voyages Out and Voyages Back: Navigating Madness	152
Conclusion	161
Appendix: Prescriptions for Swift from John Arbuthnot	177
Notes	181
Bibliography	245
Index	263

PREFACE

Jonathan Swift (1667-1745), the great Irish satirist and dean of St. Patrick's Cathedral, Dublin, was inarguably a chronically ill man. From his early twenties until his death in his seventy-eighth year, he suffered from a constellation of incurable disorders—"fitt[s] of Giddyness," "Noise in [his] Ears and Deafness."[1] These ailments aggravated him, frustrated his social life and political ambitions, at times terrified and disabled him. He feared that at any moment his vertigo would knock him to the ground. His deafness muffled his hearing and made conversation difficult, sometimes impossible. His tinnitus deafened and confused him. These disorders confounded his senses, perceptions, and understanding. Certainly, they also affected what he wrote and how he wrote it.

In the 1880s, Swift's disorders were diagnosed retrospectively as the symptoms of Ménière's disease, an inner ear disorder for which there is no known cause or cure.[2] With this diagnosis, said his biographers and critics, the mystery of his ailments had been solved at last. This clinical verdict has since then informed the readings of his life and works. However, despite the authority with which the clinic speaks—and despite the casual trust with which I myself once accepted this clinical opinion—I find a fundamental problem with the retrospective diagnosis. Swift's conception of his body and his understanding of his disorders were not the clinical ones of our own medicine but those of humoralism. In this older Hippocratic-Galenic conception, the body contained four vital humors: blood, phlegm, choler, and black bile. Disease was an imbalance of these humors. The challenge that Swift faced every day throughout his long life was how to impose order on a messy, disorderly body by rebalancing his humors.

Restoring Swift to his humoral body and his understanding of disease and treatment is the aim of this study. By historicizing Swift's body and illnesses, we free ourselves from what I see as constraints imposed by the modern clinical diagnosis. One is the absolute division between health and sickness that we make in our own lives. This tendency to see these two states as mutually exclusive conditions may explain, in part, why Swift's biographers and critics have given only passing attention to his disorders or have found difficulty in grappling with them. They worry, I suspect, that in seeing Swift as a chronically ill person, sickness will become the prism through which we view all of his life and accomplishments, that we will see Swift as a sick person whose life was punctuated by episodes of health. Returning him to his humoral body, I suggest, relieves some of this pressure by dissolving the distinction between sickness and health. In 1728, Swift himself wrote to his friend Thomas Sheridan, "I am in a middling Way, between Healthy and Sick, hardly ever without a little Giddiness or Deafness, and sometimes both; So much for that."[3] The "middling Way" of which he speaks is itself the humoral condition. As humoralism has it, neither health nor sickness, neither order nor disorder, is mutually exclusionary.

The clinical diagnosis also imposes a critical constraint upon Swift's works. Too often those who accept the modern conception of the body and disease make connect-the-dots correspondences between events in a work such as *Gulliver's Travels* and symptoms of Swift's disorders. So, for example, they see little Gulliver's dizziness as he stands upon the farmer's table in Brobdingnag as representation of the vertigo that symptomized Swift's Ménière's disease. True, perhaps. But by reducing Gulliver's experiences to clinical symptoms, these readers cannot appreciate as fully the *experience* of giddyness, what it felt like for Swift to be living every day in an imbalanced, fluid body that at any moment might topple over. Reconstructing Swift's own conception of his body and disorders frees us from the limitations of this programmatic approach and allows us to grasp more fully his lived experiences as a person disordered and his imaginative representations of those experiences.

With this I turn to Swift's persistent use of the word *disorders*, from which this study takes its title. In talking about his own physical distresses, Swift routinely used the words *disease, illness, sickness,* and *ailment,* usually without discriminating among them. But the term that he invoked most frequently in discussing his chronic sufferings was *disorders*: "For some weeks . . . I was very ill with my two inveterate Disorders, Giddyness & deafness"; "my disorders of deafness and giddiness increase daily"; "I have felt my head a little disordered."⁴ In the correspondence, Swift uses the word *disorder* or some variation thereof more than a hundred times to describe his ailments, the expression "out of order" an additional twenty-five. These words have particular resonance for his case. First, they emphasize that humoral imbalances threw Swift's constitutional equilibrium into chaos. Swift's particular humoral disorders were all the more unsettling because they not only made his body unstable but also confused his senses, which mediated between world without and world within. As he tottered uncertainly, so he worried about disordered cognitive functions—reasoning, judging, remembering. The disorders of body and mind explain, in part, the much-debated complexities of Swift's identity and imagination and what is sometimes called his "double vision" or "double consciousness."

Swift's persistent use of the word *disorders* has significant implications beyond his physical and psychological distresses as well. The disorders of his body were socially disruptive. They forced him into isolation. They frustrated his political ambitions. And they compelled him to redefine his social identity, making of a vigorous, athletic man a "Valetudinarian," of a ready conversationalist and performer in company a person "so disordered with a Noise in [his] Ears and Deafness" that he was "utterly unqualified for all Conversation or thinking."⁵ Finally, because the humoral body is permeable and coextensive with the world outside of it, Swift's return again and again to the word *disorder* helps us appreciate his particular anxieties about social and political order and what it meant to be a "disordered" person living in a "disordered" world.

Several years ago, I applied, unsuccessfully, for an NEH grant to support my study of Jonathan Swift and his health. One of the anonymous reviewers made charitable comment upon the proposal but suggested that, perhaps, there wasn't enough there to warrant a full book on the subject and that an article or two would do. One of my great surprises has been that there is, in fact, so *much* to talk about that what emerged over many years was a wobbly, hardly containable body of *everything* about Swift's health: his medical understanding and explanation of his own disorders; the stories that others have told about them; his sometimes desperate attempts to heal himself or at least manage his chronic disorders the best that he could; the impact of chronic disease and disability upon his social and political life; and the imaginative representations of his experiences as a chronically ill man in a work such as *Gulliver's Travels*. In trying to contain this sprawling study, I found that the subject common to all of these medical, biographical, and critical topics is containment itself. The running theme of all of these topics is that they have to do with Swift's efforts to control his unruly body. To that end, the chapters that follow all treat the same general topic, Swift's attempts to impose order upon a body and mind that had somehow to be governed. These chapters fall naturally into several clusters:

Chapters 1–3 treat narrative containment of the disorders, the stories that others told about the Dean sick and those that he told about himself. Chapter 1 serves as an introduction, making the argument that carries throughout the study, that to allow Swift to tell his own experiences as a sick person in his own terms, we must first restore him to the humoral body and to the understanding of disease that he himself knew. To that end, the chapter explains the humoralism that guided Swift's understanding of his own disorders and that proved persistent amid the emergence of new medical paradigms. Chapter 2 surveys the stories about Swift's illnesses that other people have told over many years. Early on, these were ways to explain his character, odd behaviors, apparent mental instability, and purported madness. With the ascendancy of the clinic in the nineteenth century, there were attempts to wrest the story of the Dean disordered away from this sort of character polemic and to diagnose Swift's diseases in clinical terms. This culminated in the diagnosis of his vertigo, deafness, and tinnitus as symptoms of Ménière's disease, a verdict that very few have questioned, even to our own day. Chapter 3 returns Swift to the humoral body that he *lived* and thus allows him to tell the story of his own disorders, as he understood them and as they conformed with medical understanding of the early modern world.

Chapters 4–5 treat physical containment of his disorders, Swift's attempts to cure or at least manage his disorderly body by keeping his chronic illnesses at bay. Here we see Swift within the medical culture of his day. He sought interventions from trained physicians, including doctor friends such as John Arbuthnot. Because there were not then strict lines between medical "professionals" and "lay" persons, however, Swift also took advice and medications from his friends, who spanned the social spectrum. In addition, he observed a strict regimen, regulating diet and exercise in particular.

Looking at Swift's exercising, which at times his own doctors thought excessive, is especially important, both as he turned to it in desperate efforts to relieve his ailments and as it tells us much about his temperament—he was a man of restless energies and ambitions who seemed terrified of sitting still.

Chapters 6–7 treat social containment of his disorders. As Arthur Frank's axiom has it, "What happens to my body happens to my life."[6] An important premise of my own study of Swift and his health is that we cannot abstract his physical ailments from any other circumstances of his life, his political and religious beliefs, his social identity, and his self-representations. Disease and life, life and disease. One cannot be disentangled from the other; neither can be defined discretely. Chapter 6 discusses the ways that Swift's chronic giddiness, deafness, and tinnitus affected both his social performance and his social identity, increasingly isolating him and keeping him from the company and conversation of friends. Often disabled and confined to the St. Patrick's deanery by his disorders, Swift bewailed the loss of the vigor by which he defined his own masculinity; he also felt the loss of authority in having to cede power to his domestic caretakers and servants. Even then, there were opportunities for reenvisioning himself in his illnesses. Chapter 7 discusses how Swift formed a sort of community with other sick persons, elevated himself socially in the world through representations of himself sick, and recast himself sexually. This reimagining of himself in the "sick role" was yet another way for Swift to impose order upon his disorders.

Chapters 8–10 treat representational containment of Swift's body and disorders. All of the self-reports of his illnesses and their disruptions to his daily life and ambitions involve self-representation, a way of putting his disorders off at a remove by framing them in words, images, and figures of speech. In many of these, Swift further objectifies and distances his experiences as a sick person by presenting them ironically. In his imaginative works, too, he tried to impose some order upon his disorders by setting them off from himself. This is especially true of *Gulliver's Travels*, in which we can read Gulliver's experiences as depictions of Swift's own. So rich are the opportunities for reading the *Travels* this way that I have divided this section into three parts. The first of these sees Gulliver's experiences as representations not merely of symptoms of a clinical disease but, more meaningfully, of the lived experiences of illness. The second chapter in this cluster turns to the problem of disordered identity. Gulliver, the Brobdingnagians determine, is lusus naturae, a thing of indeterminate identity. In Gulliver's indeterminacy, this chapter argues, Swift represents the uncertainties of what he himself was in a disordered, fluid body that was itself never quite fixed. The third chapter on Swift's imaginative representations of himself disordered engages the issue of his alleged madness in the *Travels*. His earliest biographers and critics found in the work evidence that Swift had lost his wits, especially in his savage portrait of humans as Yahoos; some still do find such evidence. This chapter suggests that if we place Swift in the context of humoralism, we can read the addled Struldbruggs and mad, misanthropic Gulliver not as Swift himself gone "idiot" or "lunatic" but as his horrified *representations* of the madness in which his unstable body, confused senses, and confounded faculties might eventuate.

The conclusion to this book places Swift and his disordered body and mind in larger cultural contexts and suggests that returning him to the medical milieu of humoralism helps explain the warring impulses of order and disorder in his life and works. The study ends by venturing some suggestions about how we can apply Swift's humoralism to reading works such as the "unspeakable" poems and to making some sense of writings that defy easy generic classification.

A note on cited texts: For all but a few fugitive pieces, I cite modern authoritative editions of Swift's writings, especially those in the recent Cambridge University Press edition of the works. I use David Woolley's edition of Swift's correspondence (completed in 2014), which has superseded the long-authoritative Harold Williams edition of 1963–65. Except in rare cases, I follow the spelling, capitalization, use of superscript, and punctuation practices of Swift's letters and the *Journal to Stella*, as established by the authoritative editions. So, for example, I reproduce Swift's dropped letters and abbreviated words, especially frequent in the slap-dash writing of the *Journal*, where he characteristically puts *th* for *the* and *y* for *you*. There, too, he often slips into the private "little language" that he shared with his old friends Esther Johnson (Stella) and Rebecca Dingley, using words like "im" for "is" and "disoddles" for "disorders."

ACKNOWLEDGMENTS

Among the most curious of private documents found after Jonathan Swift's death was a tally of those friends and acquaintances who had shown—or had failed to show—proper gratitude for his services: Swift had marked each name with the letter "g." (grateful) or "u." (ungrateful); there were also those deemed "doubtful" ("d.") and "indifferent partly grateful" ("i. partly g."). I am fortunate in that none of the many people who have supported me in this work are keepers of grudges. But because, like Swift, I place gratitude among the highest virtues, I hope that each of the following who have given advice, asked questions, and made resources available will remember me as "g."

Thanks, first, to two teachers and mentors without whom many years of research would never have borne fruit: Mary E. Fissell, whose steady guidance, astute suggestions, and tireless reading and rereading of this work in progress shaped my too-often-too-long prose into a readable book and whose scholarship serves always as the best model for . . . anyone's. As testimony to her generous spirit, I have seen this same statement of gratitude to her in more books and articles than I can remember. And to Christopher Fox, brilliant Swift scholar—and the kindest man I know. Discovering that I was at work on a project that he himself had already launched into, he quietly turned his attentions to other scholarship—and then sent me all of the resources that he had gathered, boxes and boxes of books and papers. He might say, modestly, that he was merely cleaning out his garage, but without these resources and his continued guidance and encouragements, this study would never have come into your hands.

My gratitude to friends and colleagues at Sam Houston State University, past and present, many of whom, often unknowingly, energized the work just by asking polite questions about its progress: Robert Donahoo, Rob Adams, Helena Halmari, Lee Courtney, Kimberly Bell, Carroll Nardone, April Shemak, Michael Demson, Audrey Murfin, Barbara Kaminska, Darci Hill, Tracy Bilsing, Linda Webster, Gene Young, Bill Bridges, Kandi Tayebi, Douglas Krienke, Ralph Pease, Scott Kaukonen, Nick Lantz, Drew Lopenzina, and Shane Graham. And to past-Chair Jacob Blevins, who provided timely advice, financial resources, and good cheer.

For other financial support, I am grateful to the Keough-Naughton Institute for Irish Studies at the University of Notre Dame, which funded travel to Dublin for research in primary documents. My thanks also for institutional support from Sam Houston State University's Office of Research and Sponsored Programs, which provided a timely sabbatical to complete work on the thesis from which this book germinated; College of Humanities and Social Sciences; and Department of English. And I am grateful especially to Ann Holder, former director of the Newton Gresham Library at Sam Houston State, who, against all odds and expectations, procured the Eighteenth Century Collections Online for a regional state university located in a small Texas town.

There are friends and students, too, who have provided encouragements and sometimes material resources: Kathy Cramer, best student and friend, whose interest and support never flagged; the ever-brilliant Jon Nelson; Penny Pitrucha; and Linda Crump, from far ago and long away. Thanks to friends in the graduate program at Johns Hopkins University who were in it with me: Michelle Silva, Nuno Oliveira, and especially Stewart Van Horn. And to James Buickerood, philosopher-scholar, whose friendship and brilliant thinking are all the more valuable to me because I enjoy them so late in life.

I am grateful, too, to colleagues in the larger community of scholars, who treasure still the life of the mind and who have provided encouragements, advice, and models of excellent scholarship along the way: Christopher Hamlin, Wayne Wild, David Shuttleton, Stephen Karian, Helen Deutsch, Carole Fabricant, Graham Mooney, Philip Wilson, and the late Roy Porter and William Ober, both of whom encouraged my study of eighteenth-century medicine many years ago in correspondence and conversation. Thanks also to Robert Geary, who introduced me to Swift in a first graduate course of forty years ago.

My family have encouraged and supported and have taken as much pride in my work as I have always taken in them: My mother, Julia O'Boyle

Child, and siblings Michael, Steve, and James Child, Anne Byron, and especially Mary Child, who offered valuable editorial advice. To my children, Jennifer and Tristan: While this work was growing slowly over many years, I hardly realized that they had grown into the best young woman and best young man that I know. To my granddaughter, Madeline, a smart, generous, and courageous soul who already does great things in this world. And to my wonderful in-laws, especially Autumn Child and Victor and Kimberly Andrews, who have always given unreserved encouragements.

There are also family and friends, now gone, whose memory inspirits this work: my late father, Col. Paul William Child Jr., soldier, scholar, teacher, athlete; if only I hadn't dawdled, he might have seen this work before he died. To the memory also of Col. Charles D. and Anna P. Herb; Tim Ruddle and Frederick Potter; and dearest dear old friend and running partner, Jerry Ruff, who has run on ahead before me.

Thanks to the anonymous external reviewers at the University of Virginia Press, whose expertise and thoughtful reading made all the difference in the version of this book that is now in your hands, and to Angie Hogan, Wren Morgan Myers, and the press's production staff, who collectively guided the work through from prospectus to publication.

And, finally, my gratitude to Professor Chris Buttram. The work germinated in conversations about our mutual scholarly interests years ago and grew in awkward adolescent fits and starts with her keen questions and gentle prodding. She read, reread, and made the wisest editorial suggestions from start to finish. Any of the best ideas and phrases in this book are hers.

THE DEAN DISORDERED

1
Taking Swift Back

This study began with a couple of apparently simple questions about the medical diagnosis of a famous man: From what disorders did Jonathan Swift suffer? And how did these illnesses affect what he wrote and how he wrote it? Throughout his seventy-eight years, Swift grumbled about various ailments—colds, piles, the ague, headaches, heartburn, barked shins—the sorts of ordinary maladies that most people get over in a short time. In his mid-forties, he suffered from a painful episode of shingles that lasted for several months. But it is the chronic disorders about which he complained incessantly—"giddyness," deafness, "Noise in [the] ears," and attendant nausea, anxieties, and cognitive lapses—that most compel medical, biographical, and critical interest. One reason is that, strung together over more than forty years of surviving correspondence, Swift's complaints about these ailments make a jeremiad of a gifted writer's progressive isolation and decline. Another is that because Swift suffered his diseases socially as well as physically, they are inseparable from all of the "identities" by which we know him: Dean, satirist, champion of Irish liberties, he was also a chronically ill man. Yet another reason is that he brings his disorders famously into autobiographical poems. "That old Vertigo in his Head," he wrote memorably in *Verses on the Death*, "Will never leave him, till he's dead." Elsewhere he is "Deaf, giddy, helpless, left alone."[1] Our understanding of his disorders illuminates the reading of his works, for in many of them—significantly, *Gulliver's Travels*—he represents the experiences of chronic illness.

Nonetheless, scholarly work has rarely given attention to Swift's experiences as a sick person. Until Allan Ingram's welcome 2022 study of Swift's and Alexander Pope's chronic illnesses and their attitudes toward the medical profession of their day, there was a single dedicated book-length study, published by Sir William Wilde in 1849.[2] Articles in medical journals, most by clinicians trying to solve a diagnostic riddle, what the Dean "really" suffered from, focus on symptoms and diagnosis but abstract the disorders from his life and works. Biographers characteristically treat Swift's illnesses in passing, seeing them as disturbances or annoyances that disrupted the busy social and productive literary life of an otherwise healthy man. As but one example, Irvin Ehrenpreis remarks that, "for all his talk of sickness," Swift "had remarkably good health," excepting his "familiar attacks of giddiness and deafness."[3] Gliding dismissively over that "talk of sickness," Ehrenpreis ignores Swift's understanding, imagining, and representing of himself ill. Curiously, until Ingram's recent work, only a few literary critics had considered how either the illnesses themselves or Swift's attitudes toward medicine of his day are represented imaginatively in his writing.[4] This lack of attention seems odd. Not many writers, after all, have compelled so much biographical and critical attention.

Here I suggest that two general narratives about Swift's chronic illnesses have discouraged new ways to think about them, each narrative trying to explain neatly the messy business of living day-to-day in a body—and life—disordered. The first of these is a tale about the sad decay of Swift's genius, the misdirection of his literary gifts, and his final slipping away into insanity. The chronic vertigo, deafness, tinnitus, and confounding of faculties, this story tells us, presaged the "total deprivation of his senses" at the end.[5] In fact, in 1742, after his cognitive abilities had markedly declined and his public behavior had become more eccentric, a Dublin Commission of Lunacy appointed to evaluate his condition judged Swift "unsound" of "mind and memory."[6] But too often, those who wrote about his chronic disorders, especially among his earliest biographers, tended to read them teleologically, important only as they ended inevitably in madness.[7] And so, declared Samuel Johnson, Swift's illnesses eventuated in "madness . . . compounded of rage and fatuity": "The disease of Swift was giddiness with deafness, which attacked him from time to time, began very early, pursued him through life, and at last sent him to the grave, deprived of reason."[8] Some, like his earliest critical "biographer," Lord Orrery, made a distinction between raging lunacy and a "state of idiotism" into which Orrery said Swift ultimately lapsed.[9] The narrative about his disorders is the same, however.

The chronic giddiness, deafness, and tinnitus led fatally, as in a Greek tragedy, to Swift's final madness. Even the earliest clinical diagnoses told the same story. Turning to the new authority of the clinic, Wilde attempted to rescue Swift's "character from some of the aspersions which [had] been cast upon it" by diagnosing his late-life dysphasia and dementia as symptoms of cerebral congestion, not lunacy. But his study, titled tellingly *The Closing Years of Dean Swift's Life*, gives little more attention than do the madness narratives to Swift's experiences in living with chronic illnesses for more than fifty years, to how they shaped his ambitions, his social identity, and his imaginative writings.[10]

A second narrative that constrains our understanding and appreciation of Swift's experiences as a sick person is the modern clinical diagnosis of the chronic disorders themselves.[11] In the early 1880s, the English psychiatrist John Bucknill diagnosed the Dean's "Giddyness," deafness, and "noise in [the] head" retrospectively as the symptoms of Ménière's disease, an idiopathic and incurable inner ear disorder "discovered" in 1861. Bucknill had thus made sense of the refractory physical ailments by framing them in the neat contours of the clinical diagnosis. In doing so, exulted one late nineteenth-century medical writer, he had "finally settled the point and determined the true character of Dean Swift's disease."[12] Swift's biographers and critics have since uniformly accepted Bucknill's diagnosis, often with a self-affirming presentism. His recent biographer Leo Damrosch declares, "It is often hard to tell, from symptoms reported by eighteenth-century sufferers, just what were the diseases that afflicted them. In Swift's case there can be no doubt, but no one then had the faintest idea of the truth."[13] Even the otherwise historically sensitive Ingram writes of the particular challenges of living with chronic disorders in an age "when the nature of those illnesses was as yet unrecognized and effective treatment therefore largely a matter of chance."[14] Given the epistemic, rhetorical, and cultural authority of the modern clinic, few medical writers, biographers, and literary critics have challenged the retrospective diagnosis, nor have they questioned the claim that it is indeed the "truth" of Swift's illnesses.

In considering how the study of Swift's disorders might enrich our understanding of his life and his imaginative writings, I find theoretical and methodological problems with the two prevailing narratives about his health. First, if we see his chronic disorders only as causes and precursors of inevitable madness, we reduce his lived experiences as a sick person to plot points in an aforewritten story. For example, John Hawkesworth declared ten years after Swift's death that his "fits of giddiness . . . became more frequent and more violent in proportion as he grew into years," until finally, in 1736, "he was seized with one of these fits, the effect of which was so dreadful" that "from this time his memory was perceived to decline, and his passions to pervert his understanding."[15] In this story of Swift's life, the chronic giddiness, deafness, tinnitus, anxieties, and cognitive confusions are all important only as they serve the narrative of those who would have him end in "rage and despair" or, more benignly, "a state of ideotism."[16]

This teleology not only elides nearly sixty years of lived experience as a sick person into a single end. It also encourages what I consider misdirected interpretations of his imaginative writings. With the madness narrative as critical lens, readers too often see the excremental female bodies in the so-called "scatological" verses, the grotesque Struldbruggs of *Gulliver's Travels,* and Gulliver's mad misanthropy as signs of Swift's own insanity or psychopathy. Swift himself worried that his disorders would end in utter loss of memory and "imbecility." But if we understand what Ingram calls aptly "the consciousness of experienced illness," what it felt like to live with vertigo that could strike him down at any moment and hearing disorders that confused and isolated him, we can see figures like the Struldbruggs and mad Gulliver as horrified *representations* rather than diagnostic signs.[17] The distinction is crucial. Imagining himself imbecilic or lunatic was an act of containment, a way of making sense of his physical and cognitive disorders by objectifying them and setting them off at a remove from himself. An acknowledgment that this was what he *feared* he would become.

The retrospective clinical diagnosis of Ménière's disease presents problems of a different sort. The first and more obvious is that Swift could not have been afflicted with a disease that did not exist until 1861, well over a century after his death. To borrow from Andrew Cunningham, people can suffer only from the sicknesses available to them.[18] Neither Prosper Ménière's disease nor Bucknill's diagnosis was available to Swift or his doctors. More generally, however, such a retrospective diagnosis commits the anachronism of submitting his reported symptoms to a different conception of the body, a different framework for understanding and explaining physiological processes, a different way of defining disease itself from those that Swift and his world understood.

The doctor of today might accept, broadly, the Galenic view of Swift's contemporaries Thomas Sydenham and Herman Boerhaave that disease is *functio laesa*, that which hinders or diminishes the natural and vital functions of daily life.[19] But while illness in the early modern world was, generally speaking, an imbalance or corruption of the fluid components of the body, the modern clinic defines disease in ontological terms, as an exogenous entity that invades or grafts itself onto our bodies and from which we then either recover or die. Even in thinking of chronic illness, we focus on the disease itself rather than on the individual who experiences the disease as a process of living and who struggles to make sense of and control it.[20] We speak of a person's "contracting," "having," or "surviving" rather than "living" a disorder.

Like the argument about Swift's inevitable madness, the clinical diagnosis in effect tells the story of his illnesses for him. In the modern medical encounter, the "clinical body," in contradistinction to the humoral body that the early modern world knew, is made a mute material object, subject to what Foucault called the "gaze," the detached and disinterested observation of the patient by the doctor.[21] Clinicians no longer acknowledge a subjective body, that is, the personal identity and lived experience of the patient, what it "feels" like to be sick. Instead, they impose upon the person their own way of seeing and their own narrative about the objectified body. The doctor's semiotics expropriates the patient's own authority to represent the experiences of being sick. With Swift, the retrospective diagnosis of Ménière's disease tells the story of his disorders for him, rather than allowing him to tell his own story. Enforcing a separation between the professional who knows and the layperson who does not, the clinic also presumes to understand and be able to treat the body better than the patient who lives in that body.

Like the medical writers and biographers who accept the retrospective diagnosis, those critics who read Swift's imaginative works in light of that diagnosis are limited not by imagination but by clinical fiat. To their credit, they do find in the works conscious representations of symptoms rather than signs by which we might diagnose the man himself. Gulliver's dizzying shifts of perspective and his dysfunctions of communication, for example, are Swift's expressions of his own vertigo, deafness, and tinnitus. But accepting and then interpreting the imaginative works in light of the retrospective diagnosis, these readers impose upon Swift a clinical body and then find depictions of a clinical disease: It is then the symptoms of Ménière's disease that Swift is representing, not the humoral imbalances by which he understood and explained his own illnesses. Reading his life and works through this clinical-cum-critical lens, they cannot fully appreciate how Swift himself creatively managed his humoral disorders and represented his lived experiences as a sick person. These representations go beyond mere symptomatology.

As Cunningham contends, instead of imposing our own understanding of the body and pathology on historical figures such as Swift, we must place "past disease firmly in the past, and [interpret] that past experience of disease in such a way that people of the present may empathise with that past experience, but not [turn] it into some early version of modern disease and hence of modern experience."[22] That is, if we are to allow Swift to tell the story of his own illnesses and are to appreciate more fully how he represented them imaginatively, as this study aims to do, we must begin by reconstructing as best we can the medical theories and practices by which he understood, explained, and treated them. This historicizing of his disorders demands first that we untangle his own medical understanding—that of humoralism—from the narratives that others have told about them. Swift lived not in the clinical body of Ménière and Bucknill but in a humoral body.

In returning Swift to his humoral body, I would not dismiss out of hand the argument that his chronic disorders eventuated in the "total deprivation of his senses." Swift himself saw connections between his physical distresses and his cognitive failings. "Infirmatyes hav[ing] quite broke me," he wrote to Pope in 1736, "I neither re[a]d, nor write; nor remember, nor converse."[23] A year later he groaned, "I have been many months the Shadow of the Shadow of the Shadow, of &c &c &c of D\ Sw—[:] Age, Giddyness, Deafness, loss of Memory, Rage and Rancour against Persons and Proceedings."[24] Likewise, I would not arbitrarily sweep away the retrospective diagnosis. Ménière's disease—its symptoms and its disabling physical and social disruptions—has value as *analogy* for Swift's chronic disorders. But we need to understand that the clinical narrative that we tell about our own disorders is but one sort of medical plot, a way of explaining how the body operates in sickness and health. The story that Swift told about his own body and illness was quite different. For Swift, disease was not a biomedical phenomenon indicated by laboratory findings and signs common to a disease "entity." It was not something independent of the body, a pathogenic bacterium or virus that had to be driven out. Nor was it cells multiplying at a runaway rate that had to be arrested and removed. Rather, disease was an imbalance of the fluid humors constituting his body. According to Swift's medical narrative, the disordered body could be put back into order only when humoral balances were restored.

In this book, I use the term *humoralism* broadly, to designate a comprehensive system of beliefs about the body and disease, and a set of medical practices that persisted from classical days until it was displaced at last in the nineteenth century by ascendant biomedical models of the body and germ theory. According to Hippocratic-Galenic principles, the fluid body was composed of four vital humors: blood, phlegm, yellow bile (choler), black bile (melan choler).[25] These constituent humors had qualities of heat and coldness as well as dryness and wetness. So, while choler was a hot, dry humor, phlegm was cold and wet. Black bile was cold and dry, while blood, the *humor* and not the liquid medium by which the humors were circulated, was warm and wet. Swift's contemporary John Moyle offered a classic explanation: "Now the Humid Part of the Body (or Mass of Blood) is made up of four different Humours; *Choler*, that answers the fiery Elements in Nature; and *Sanguis*, that represents the *Aereal*; and *Phlegma*, the Turgid Aquaous Part; and *Melancholy*, the more Grumous and Earthy Substance. While these Humours remain in that due Measure and Temper, that Nature assigned them, so long is the Body in Health."[26] The four cardinal humors were linked with organs of the body: blood with the liver, choler with the gall bladder, black bile with the spleen, and phlegm with the brain and lungs. In some refinements of the system, the four humors corresponded with the four elements (air, fire, earth, water), as in Moyle's model; the four seasons; the four ages of a person (infancy, youth, adulthood, and old age); and the four psychological "temperaments" (sanguine, choleric, melancholic, and phlegmatic). These correspondences manifest the interfusion of the individual body and mind, the larger natural world, and the cosmos itself.

A popular fallacy has it that the four humors existed in equal parts, one quarter each. In fact, every individual constitution (crasis) had its own natural balance. Invariably, one humor predominated, a constitutional emphasis that determined not only an individual's psychological temperament but also the person's predisposition toward certain disorders. So, while a disease like plague could originate as a "miasma" (polluted air) outside the body, a sanguine individual, in whom the humor blood predominated, was thought to be more susceptible to the disease; a person in whom choler predominated would be more resistant.[27] Because phlegm was thought to cause "cold" diseases, a person in whom that humor was out of balance would more likely suffer from congestive ailments like colds and pneumonia—and from the cephalic disorders like the giddiness, deafness, and tinnitus from which Swift himself suffered.

According to the humoral narrative that Swift tells about his own body, then, health was defined as a balance of humors (eucrasia) particular to the individual. Because the humors were fluid, however, they were always shifting and dynamic, subject to change over time, from year to year, from day to day, even from morning to evening. And, significantly to our understanding of Swift's particular disorders, the humoral body was permeable so that there were continual exchanges between one's inner body and the environment—of air and perspiration, food and drink, products taken in and products evacuated. These exchanges affected one's humoral balance. The challenge always was to maintain equilibrium as well as possible, of the humors in one's own body and of the humoral body in its environment.

By the same humoral logic, disease was a deficiency, plethora, or corruption of one or more humors (dyscrasia). "When *Plethory* abounds, or *Cacochymia* affects any one or more of them, then is the Body crasie," said the surgeon Moyle.[28] Any kind of internal disorder, therefore, from indigestion to vertigo to plague, was a humoral imbalance or corruption. The disordered body was "crasie."[29] In this way, humoral pathology was both simple and comprehensive: Every sick person suffered effectively from the same disorder—imbalanced or vitiated humors. Yet because each person's constitutional balance was skewed by nature and affected by habit, no two cases were the same. So Swift himself complained of his chronic deafness and giddyness, "I am sure there is not one Patient in my case through this whole Kingdom."[30] Although he sometimes thought himself exceptional, there is no perverse self-aggrandizement here. Swift's case was, in fact, unlike any other.

The trick was to figure out what particular humoral dysfunction one suffered from and then work to restore the natural balance. One might supply a deficiency with proper food and drink. But more commonly in humoral pathology, as the "English Hippocrates" Thomas Sydenham put it, disease was "caused by the Redundancy of the Morbific Matter which [Nature] cannot concoct [that is, process properly] and assimilate, by which the Patient is at last poison'd."[31] The body afflicted by a corrupt or overabundant humor, said Moyle, "Nature now endeavours to extrude what is Noxious, through the extern Parts."[32] Thus, for instance, humoralism explained the gout that laid up so many eighteenth-century gentlefolk. Popular cartoons might caricature the irascible, gouty squire with toes swaddled in bandages, yet the pain and burning in the toes presaged a favorable outcome. The gouty humor was working its way out of the body. In comic verse, Swift himself explained the prevailing theory about driving disease out through the extremities:

> As, if the gout should seize the head,
> Doctors pronounce the patient dead;
> But, if they can, by all their arts,
> Eject it to th'extreamest parts,
> They give the sick man joy, and praise
> The gout that will prolong his days.[33]

Suffering in his chronic disorders, Swift wished his own giddiness could be relieved by the gout. "I would compound for a light easy gout to be perfectly well in my head," he wrote in 1711.[34]

If one's constitution were hereditarily weak or enfeebled by dissolute habits or age and the body could not naturally expel an "ill humor," the patient might resort to medical interventions to prod or shock the body into driving out the foul matter—bleeding, vomits, purges, blisters, and sudorifics (which induced sweat). Failing by means of nature or medical art to extrude the poisonous humor, the person could die of a fatal congestion. Swift reports in the *Journal to Stella* that "lord Jersey died of the gout in his stomach, or apoplexy, or both."[35] And Queen Anne, he said in 1711, "is well, but I fear will be no long liver; for I am told she has sometimes the gout in her *bowels*."[36] Anne died at age forty-nine when "her constitutional gout flew to the brain," thought her doctors at first. Then said her physician John Radcliffe, "it was conjectured to be the gout in her stomach; and now it is thought to be the gout all over," everywhere, he sniped, "*excepting* the joints."[37] "Peccant" or "plethorick" humors that were not expelled could be fatal.[38]

It was the ability or inability of the individual body to expel the pathogenic humors and excrements that determined the simple but crucial nosological distinction in Swift's day between acute and chronic diseases. Acute diseases, said George Cheyne, are "*quick, sharp,* or *acute* Distempers, whose

Symptoms are more violent, their Duration shorter, and their Periods more *quick*, either of *sudden Death*, or a glorious *Victory* over the Disease."[39] In an acute disorder, the body would try to throw off the noxious humor through a fever, natural or induced, or through other means such as a skin eruption.[40] So Swift himself explained the painful shingles that he suffered for several months in 1712 while living in London.[41] Such "erysipelatous" disorders, the humoral explanation had it, were caused by an excess of choler, the "hot," "corrosive" humor. As it worked its way to the body's surface for natural excretion, so this "acrid" humor burned painfully. Swift wrote that the "Red still continues too, and most prodigious hott & inflamed." As painful as it was, the eruption of blisters on Swift's upper back—"great Red Spots," "little Pimples . . . grown white & full of corruption"—was the triumph of Swift's constitution, as it discharged the choler. He uttered with relief, "Th Doct[rs] say it would have ended in some violent Disease if it had not came out thus. I shall now recover fast."[42] Expelling the "Morbific Matter," the shingles eruptions precursed a favorable outcome. This was the victory of "Nature" over disease.

If the "peccant" or "plethorick" humor were not expelled by nature or medical art or did not end in a fatal congestion, it might settle in as a chronic disorder. "By Chronical Distempers," said the Edinburgh "Student in Physick" John Cook in 1730, "we mean, those that continue for several Months or Years . . . ; the Causes of all which proceed from the Depravity of some or all of the aforesaid constituent Parts of the Blood." While the root cause of all chronic disorders was thought to be the superfluity or vitiation of humors, they manifested as different diseases taxonomically, with a "vast Difference from the Place and Parts of the Body affected, and the Symptoms attending," because of persons' different constitutions. So, said Cook, the same humoral disorder would cause "a Leprosy in some Constitutions, which causes the Scurvy in others; and . . . the Gout in one, which occasions the Stone in another Body."[43] The chronic vertigo, deafness, and tinnitus that Swift himself could never shake throughout his adult life were cephalic disorders thought to be caused by an accumulation of phlegm.

Most humoral explanations of disease blamed corruptions or excesses of humors on improper "digestion." While digestion has some relation to our modern understanding of the means by which food is processed in the stomach for assimilation as nutrients or for expulsion as waste, the term in humoral physiology comprehends the larger physiological processes by which the aliments are broken down and transformed to humors to be "duly assimilated" throughout the "animal Œconomy" (or living system).[44] According to Galen, proper digestion depended upon the heat of the stomach. Having properly "cooked" the raw aliments, the healthy stomach would then separate out the component parts, as Thomas Cooper explained the process in the sixteenth century, into "the dregges or excrements of digestion made in the body: as fleume [phlegm], choler, melancholy" and the waste products "urine, sweate, snivell, spittle, milke, ordure."[45] The body would then expel the coarse "excrementitious Remainders" and convert the nutritious matter to chyme. Chyle, extracted from this chyme in the duodenum, would then be converted to humors in the liver for distribution throughout the body in the nutritive blood. If the stomach were too cold, as Swift thought his own was, it would not properly cook the aliments and, instead of producing pure "attenuated" humors, would leave incompletely digested crude matter like viscid phlegm, which would either throw the entire system out of balance or settle in various body parts.[46] Humoral imbalances could manifest as localized pathologies, even ulcers and tumors, when they "fermented" in a discrete part of the body.[47] Even so, humoralism more generally diagnosed and treated diseases of the whole body, even when they afflicted certain parts, as did Swift's own cephalic disorders.

In 1707, the physician Peter Paxton claimed that "the Doctrines of the great *Galen* concerning the four Humours, particular Facultys, *&c.* by the Discovery of the Circulation of the Blood, *&c.* has been sufficiently exploded."[48] Indeed by Swift's day, in the aggressive anti-Aristotelianism of the "scientific revolution," the Hippocratic-Galenic notion of the fluid body constituted of four distinct humors was ceding authority to mechanical, chemical, and corpuscular explanations of physiological processes and to an emerging neuropathology that saw disease as weak or irritable nerves rather than vitiated or superfluous humors.[49] These new notions of the body and pathology tracked a conceptual shift in the long eighteenth century, from humoralism to "solidism." While humoralism attributed sickness to imbalances of the fluid "complexion" of the body, solidism held that only the solid parts of the body—vessels, organs, glands, and bones—have vital properties and, therefore, are susceptible to disease.[50] Especially after William Harvey's discovery of the heart's role as a circulatory pump, health was defined, at least theoretically, not by the proper balance and quality of humors produced in the liver but by the tone, elasticity, and tensile strength of vessels that propelled their fluid cargoes.[51] For the iatromechanists, disease was no longer vitiated or excessive humors but obstructions in the pipes.[52] So, too, did the iatrochemists challenge humoralism. While the Galenists attributed proper digestion to heat, these chemists attributed it to gastric acids.[53] While humoralism defined disease as dyscrasia, a systemic imbalance, the iatrochemical disciples of Paracelsus defined disease locally, as "irritations" of specific organs. Similarly, Robert Boyle's eclectic "Corpuscular Philosophy," which conceived of the body as an aggregate of particulate matter, saw disease as the damage caused to specific body parts by the motions of "morbific particles." The proper "texture" of parts could be restored with chemical "specificks," remedies designed to act upon a particular body part or disease.[54]

Swift was well aware of these "new Schemes in Philosophy."[55] His own doctors William Cockburn, John Arbuthnot, and Richard Helsham numbered among the iatrophysicists, who saw the body as a machine, the workings of which could be explained by laws of hydrostatics and mechanics.[56] Like some other iatromechanists, though, Swift's intimate friend Arbuthnot worried about the reductive materialism lurking in his own mechanical view of the body: If this body is but a machine, however ingenious, what then inspirits it? In a late-life poem, he wondered if his identity were nothing more than a "Frame . . . [o]f moving Joints," a network of "branching Channel[s]" and "Pipes thro' which the circling Juices stray."[57] Swift anxiously but playfully imagined the same materialistic reductions of the new mechanical view of the body. In *A Tale of a Tub* and *A Discourse Concerning the Mechanical Operation of the Spirit*, he lampoons mechanistic explanations of vital functions by representing the frenzied transports of religious enthusiasts—"ejaculating the Soul"—as "purely an Effect of Artifice and *Mechanick Operation*."[58] Elsewhere, he depicts humans literally as machines. In *Gulliver's Travels*, the King of Brobdingnag, who "had been educated in the Study of Philosophy, and particularly Mathematics," conceives at first that Gulliver "might be a Piece of Clock-work . . . contrived by some ingenious Artist." Indignant always at being taken as mere material object—clever clockwork or Yahoo body—Gulliver protests, with increasing feebleness, that reason, with its functionary speech, elevates him above mere matter. Having been reduced to machine, he adds quickly that when the Great King hears him speak, he finds Gulliver "regular and rational." The King cannot "conceal his Astonishment."[59]

Swift was also well aware of the anti-humoralism of the iatrochemists such as Paracelsus, Sylvius, and van Helmont. In the *Essay upon Health and Long Life*—edited by Swift himself—Sir William Temple had written of the endeavors of Paracelsus, forefather of the iatrochemical school, "to overthrow the whole Scheme of *Galen*, and introduce a new one of His own, as well as the use of Chymical Medicines."[60] Indeed, in the materia medica of the pharmacopoeias and medical dictionaries in Swift's own library, "Galenicals" derived naturally from plants, animals, and minerals sat on the same pages with "Chymical Medicines" produced unnaturally by distillation, fermentation, and fire. Swift might nauseate the readers of *Gulliver's Travels* by cataloguing the repugnant ingredients of the vomits and clysters that the Galenists used to restore humoral balances.[61] But like Temple, he stood with the medicine of old. In the *Battel of the Books*, the venerable Hippocrates and "brave *Antient*" Galen drive back the modern mechanists and chemists: Harvey, with his "vast Body" of medical disciples, and Paracelsus, marshaling a "*Squadron of Stink-Pot-Flingers.*"[62]

Despite the challenges to the older belief that disease is an imbalance or corruption of the fluid humors, the term *humoralism* still best characterizes Swift's own understanding and representations of his disorders, for several reasons. One is the sheer tenacity with which the humoral system persisted as "vestigial doctrine," continuing to guide both the understanding of the body and the treatment of disease.[63] As Andrew Wear argues, while historians of science have "often and variously retold" the narrative that "the quantitative and objective world of the seventeenth century" displaced "the qualitative, subjective system of ancient and renaissance natural philosophy," the repositionings were "theoretical and ideological" rather than practical.[64] Because the discoveries of Harvey and the anti-Galenic medical alternatives of iatromechanists and iatrochemists brought "no one orthodoxy, and no certainty, about the physical order of things," says Noga Arikha, the "humours were not fully dismantled; nor did they become a mere antiquarian curiosity. New ideas did not necessarily cohere with the culture in which they emerged, and they did not necessarily result in innovative medical practices."[65]

Iatromechanists had reenvisioned the body as a "fine machine."[66] Their focus shifted from stomach as oven that cooked the aliments and liver that continuously new-made the blood, to heart as pump that circulated the same blood in a continuous round. Health depended not on the proper heat of the stomach but on the elasticity and tensile strength of the solid fibers of heart, vessels, and glands that propelled the fluids throughout the body. Iatrochemists, in turn, saw the body as a chemical laboratory. They might still regard the stomach as an important site of fluid production. But fermentations, acids, and alkalis, not Galenic heat, now legislated proper digestion. For all such reconceiving of the body and its processes, however, the story that the new medicines told was in its broad contours the same as the old humoral narrative, a distinction without much difference. Whether by mechanical action, chemical process, or Galenic heat, the fluids that circulated through the body had still to be properly processed. Otherwise, they would clog the vessels, irritate the nerves, or throw the system out of balance by accumulating where they should not. Perhaps, as in Swift's case, stuffing one's head and ears and occluding the senses or throwing off one's equilibrium in a giddiness. So even if an iatromechanist such as Cheyne looked to the elasticity and tonicity of solids, his popular regimen books, which sat on Swift's own shelves, insisted on proper diet to "mend the *Juices,* to cool, attenuat[e] and sweeten the circulating *Fluids.*"[67] In both popular and academic medicine, humoralism persisted as the chief narrative that people told about their bodies and their disorders.

The new medical theories also lagged far behind the older humoral *practices*. Theoretically, the superfluity of phlegm to which Swift ascribed his chronic illnesses or the choler that he blamed for the painful shingles could be measured mathematically. In trying to understand digestion, for example, the Italian iatrophysicist Sanctorius scrupulously weighed his own food and excrements for years. With the same aim of quantifying bodily processes, Cheyne guided readers of his popular books on fevers, the gout, and regimen through the mathematics of hydraulics pushing fluids through canals as they are constricted and dilated.[68] But, says Wear, "medicine in the end is practical."[69] Doctors were not doing the math at the bedside. New theories had hardly changed medical practices. And so, having written the obituary for the "Doctrines of the great *Galen* concerning the four Humours," Peter Paxton continued, "Notwithstanding such late Improvements in things, as regard both Philosophy and Physick, a multitude of Advantages have not hitherto been observ'd to proceed from them, either to fortify Mens Bodys against the Insults of Diseases, or to deliver them from the Dangers and Sufferings of such, when seiz'd with them."[70] Cheyne invoked Newton's theories of particulate attraction and cohesion and the laws of hydraulics to explain, at great length, the cause and progress of fevers. What cures did he then recommend? The old standbys of humoral medicine: liberal bleeding, vomiting, and sweating.[71]

Humoralism endured, then, in therapeutic interventions, with bloodletting and evacuations designed to let off humoral excesses. It also persisted in the regimens that were a fixture of both popular and learned medical culture of the day. These regimens aimed to maintain or restore one's constitutional balance by regulating the Galenic "non-naturals," the six environmental and hygienic variables by which the permeable body negotiated exchanges between inside and outside worlds: air, diet, sleep, exercise, evacuation and retention of excrement, and the passions. Day to day, Swift himself sought to control his own disorders by careful regulation of these non-naturals. But the focus on the non-naturals persisted in learned medical discourses also. Arbuthnot projected a whole series of regimen books, one devoted to each of the non-naturals. Before his death in 1735, he had finished *An Essay of Aliments* (1731) and *An Essay Concerning the Effects of Air on Human Bodies* (1733). In these works, he ostensibly takes an iatromechanical approach to health and illness. So, for example, the *Essay on Aliments* focuses on the mechanical (and chemical) processes of digestion, by which the stomach "concocts" various animal and vegetable foods and by which the resulting chyle is assimilated into the blood and distributed throughout the body for nutrition. He is concerned about both the assimilation of the chyle and the elasticity of the fibers, the mechanism by which the body receives its nutrition. Despite Arbuthnot's emphasis on the mechanical processes of the body, the humoral notion of maintaining one's constitutional balance remains the underlying premise here, as the full title of his book indicates: *An Essay Concerning the Nature of Aliments, and the Choice of Them, According to the Different Constitutions of Human Bodies*. The kindred Newtonian physician Cheyne similarly structured his best-selling *Essay of Health and Long Life* around the six non-naturals, as a means, he claimed, of achieving "some Order and Connexion."[72] He might have theorized the body in terms of particulate matter and motion, but he knew well that humoral notions of fluid balance and imbalance still suffused popular medicine.

Framing Swift's own disorders in humoralism thus returns us to the medical system by which he knew and explained his own ailments. Humoralism, as a holistic conception of the self, helps us recover Swift's own understanding of the connections between body and mind. His physical disorders—giddiness, deafness, and tinnitus—were disorders of the mind, too; they confused his senses and confounded his understanding. Because health and illness in the humoral system are defined qualitatively rather than quantitatively, seeing Swift's chronic disorders in the framework of humoralism also allows us to grasp the subjectivities of his illness, how he felt and experienced them.[73] Accordingly, this context gives us a ready vocabulary for discussing his illnesses as he himself knew them. By his day, the word *humors* itself was already being used in medical discourses to mean, generally, fluids that circulated in the body, in contradistinction to the solids through which they coursed.[74] But Swift ascribed his own chronic illnesses to more narrowly humoral processes: Because of a "cold stomach," phlegm was not properly thinned for fluid circulation throughout his body. It consequently accumulated in his head as a gluey "cephalick" disorder, occluding his senses and throwing off his equilibrium in terrifying vertiginous "Fitts." The language of humoralism, moreover, provides contexts for Swift's varied representations of his own illnesses in his correspondence and his imaginative writings. The fluid, permeable humoral body serves better historically as referent for the unstable sense of self that Swift imagines in works such as *Gulliver's Travels* than the mechanical, chemical, or corpuscular body does. Robert Boyle and other mechanists might see sickness as the breakdown of an "elaborate Engine" that is "out of order."[75] But for Swift's humoral body, disorder is much more than mere malfunction. It is chaos, instability, and uncertainty. Since the permeable body of the humoral system extends to the world outside, illness is not merely a failure of parts in the machine; it is coextensive with disorder in the world outside.

2

Stories of Illness and Retrospective Diagnosis

When we are sick, we try to make sense of our physical disorders and to cure or at least manage them the best we can. A first measure of exerting control over a disease is to recognize and name it as such. As Charles Rosenberg says, "Disease does not exist until we have agreed that it does, by perceiving, naming, and responding to it."[1] In this constructionist view, the very *perception* of the disease substantiates its existence. Then, with diagnosis comes an intelligible narrative about the etiology of the disease, its progress in our bodies, and outcome. This clinical narrative, the one the doctors tell us about our bodies, is itself an attempt to fit individual experience into a larger structure, to give it meaning beyond itself by seeing it as a disease entity shared by others with like symptoms. Thus an individual's singular experience becomes universalized.

In Swift's day, no less than in our own, the sick tried to make sense of their disorders—to impose some control upon them—by shaping them narratively. Some few who wrote about their own illnesses tried to see their bodies with cold, dispassionate objectivity. George Cheyne, himself a doctor and likely an acquaintance of Swift, reported of his own case in print, "I had a violent *humorous* Cough, and threw up great Quantities of gross viscid Flegm, which I knew to be the [food], not so sufficiently digested and attenuated, as to become thin enough to circulate freely through the small Vessels: but were thrown off, and despumated upon the larger *Emunctory* and open *Glands*."[2] Cheyne's unembarrassed description of the physical details of his disorders fits into a larger narrative about the body and so was a way for him to make sense of what might otherwise have seemed random and disconnected physical phenomena.

Such ostensibly objective self-descriptions were rare in Swift's day. More often, those who wrote about their illnesses saw in them the agency of Providence. Sickness was God's warning, physical experience that provoked spiritual reflection and mercifully allowed the survivor a second chance to undertake moral reform.[3] After a serious fever, Robinson Crusoe, whose experiences as a sick man are no less representative for their fictionality, reflects, "But now when I began to be sick, and a leisurely View of the Miseries of Death came to place itself before me; when my Spirits began to sink under the Burthen of a strong Distemper, and Nature was exhausted with the Violence of the Feaver; Conscience that had slept so long, begun to awake, and I began to reproach myself with my past Life, in which I had so evidently, by uncommon Wickedness, provok'd the Justice of God to lay me under uncommon Strokes, and to deal with me in so vindictive a Manner."[4] While Crusoe might call his ailment "Distemper" or "Feaver," in his Providential reading of his own physical experiences it is God's hand at work in the world. Even Cheyne, caught between the medicalized view of his own ailments and the subjectivity of his experiences as a man trying to find meaning for his individual sufferings, concludes his case self-study by ascribing to "an over-ruling *Providence*" the "meer *casual Hints*, far beyond the Reach of [his] *Penetration*," that directed him inevitably to both physical and spiritual health.[5] Thus "autopathography," Cheyne's story about the processes of his own body, becomes spiritual autobiography.[6] The reflecting sufferer reads the plot of his sickness teleologically, as directed toward the greater end of "God's plot." Such "mythic thinking," as Anne Hunsaker Hawkins calls it, not only universalizes and gives the individual experience greater meaning beyond itself but also imposes order upon disorder by shaping it narratively, typologically, and generically.[7]

In his correspondence, the *Journal to Stella*, and a scattering of other primary sources, Swift's own complaints about his chronic giddiness, deafness, tinnitus, loss of memory, and cognitive confusions span more than thirty years. He claimed to have suffered them for almost fifty. The first explicit reference to his vertigo comes in a note in his account book for November 1708: "From 6 to 16 often giddy G^d help me. so to 25th less."[8] After several similar entries over the next two months, he wrote from London to Archbishop King, his ecclesiastical superior in Dublin, "I should have acknowledged your Grace's Letter, if I had not been ever since persecuted with a cruel Distemper, a Giddiness in my Head, that would not suffer me to write or think of any Thing; and of which, I am now slowly recovering."[9] In September of 1710, we get a first reference to his hearing problems, however oblique, when he begrudgingly submits to Esther Johnson's (Stella's) and Rebecca Dingley's insistence that he seek medical help: "I don't think any lady's advice about my ear signifies twopence: however I will, in compliance to you, ask Dr. Cockburn. Radcliffe I know not, and Bernard I never see."[10] Between these early days and the final years of his life, Swift complained continually about his disorders, for the last time in a short letter of July 1740 to Martha Whiteway, his cousin and fiercely loyal late-life caregiver: "I have been very miserable all night, and to-day extremely deaf and full of pain. I am so stupid and confounded, that I cannot express the mortification I am under both in body and mind."[11] Swift was then seventy-two. Although he lived another five years, younger clergy took over his decanal affairs as he slipped into his dotage; but for a brief recommendation note of 1741, his letter to Mrs. Whiteway is the final surviving one that is characteristically his own.

As much as he complained about his ailments, Swift did not write a sustained, coherent autopathography in which he tried to make sense, comprehensively, of his sufferings. Few people of his day did. But for Swift, there seem to have been particular reasons for not writing this illness narrative. For one, notwithstanding the incessant complaints about his various ailments over a lifetime of correspondence, he claims to have found sick talk vain and self-indulgent. In Hints Towards an Essay on Conversation, he wrote, "Another general Fault in Conversation," among many, is that "those who affect to talk of themselves . . . will relate the Annals of their Diseases, with the several Symptoms and Circumstances of them."[12] As we shall consider later, he seems also to have been temperamentally disinclined to autobiography, even though autobiography—and autopathography—are *everywhere* in Swift. Finally, the chronic illnesses themselves would have frustrated autopathography's aim of imposing narrative order upon the disorders of the unruly body. In telling the story of the giddiness, deafness, tinnitus, and attendant physical and psychological woes that recurred episodically without warning and without any sense of how they would all come out, what shaping narrative arc could Swift have imposed upon them? And where could he have found narrative closure?

Because Swift never wrote a coherent account of his own illnesses, his biographers and medical writers have told it for him. It should not surprise us that they have written the story of his disorders as the culturally constructed medical, social, religious, and political narratives that have shaped their own thinking about the body and illness. The story of the stories about Swift's health that these writers have told is itself historically instructive.

During Swift's lifetime, after he had become famous as both writer and Irish patriot, newspapers worried anxiously about his health. "We hear from Dublin," reported the *Daily Post* in 1725, "that the Reverend Dean Swift is so well recovered of his late Illness, that he was arrived in that City from his Country Seat."[13] "Our worthy patriot the rev. Dean Swift lies dangerously ill," the *Grub Street Journal* informed its readers in 1737.[14] And an "Extract of a Letter from Dublin" in the London newspapers of 1741 announced that Swift "was lately taken with a sudden Illness, as he was going into the Deanery House, and fell down in a Fit, and continued speechless for a long Time" until "he recover'd, and continues in pretty good Health, to the general Joy of this City."[15] Such were the public's anxieties about Swift's health during his life.

After his death in 1745, contemporary memoirists and biographers traded in stories about Swift's disorders, sometimes to serve their own interests. The scandalous Lætitia Pilkington, for example, found an opportunity for self-promotion, congratulating herself that she was one of the few allowed to see Swift during his "Periodical fits of Deafness": "The Dean for the latter Part of his Life, contracted his Acquaintance into a very narrow Compass, for as he was frequently deaf, he thought this Infirmity made him troublesome, and therefore kept no Company but such as he cou'd be free with, as to bid them speak loud, or repeat what they had said. It was owing to this, that Mr. *Pilkington* and I frequently pass'd whole Days with him, while Numbers of our betters were excluded."[16] Pilkington prided herself on her access to the great man in his illness.

If Pilkington's discussion of Swift's health served her own narrative of self-vindication and social rise, others who wrote about the disorders, especially those who had known him in life, engaged a biographical polemic, using them to explain, attack, or vindicate his character. In the first full-fledged book on Swift's life and writings, Lord Orrery saw Swift's increasingly erratic behavior and final madness as the cumulative effects of his chronic giddiness and deafness. Orrery attributed the giddiness to reckless gluttonizing upon raw apples when Swift was a young man living with Sir William Temple: "When he had been about two years at *Moore Park*, he contracted a very long and dangerous illness, by eating an immoderate quantity of fruit. To this surfeit I have often heard him ascribe that giddiness in his head, which with intermissions sometimes of a longer, and sometimes of a shorter continuance," plagued him to the end.[17] As for Swift's deafness, Orrery ventures an iatromechanical explanation: "Possibly some internal pressure upon his brain might first have affected the auditory nerves," compressing them and thereby muffling his hearing or altogether preventing transmission of auditory sensation. Positing clear connections between the mind and the "fine machine" that was Swift's body, Orrery put the blame for his cognitive decay and final madness upon his hearing disorders and giddiness. The pressure upon the auditory nerves, "by degrees, might have encreased, so as entirely to stop up that fountain of ideas, which had before spread itself in the most diffusive, and surprising manner."[18] And his giddiness "pursued him till it seemed to compleat its conquest, by rendering him . . . [imbecile], a miserable spectacle, devoid of every appearance of human nature, except the outward form."[19] The decayed memory about which Swift himself often complained and the final madness that biographers and critics used to explain his eccentricities, his obsessions and rages, and the savagery of his satire in works such as *Gulliver's Travels*—according to Orrery, all find their cause in Swift's disordered body.

In the discussion of humoralism and madness that follows, I owe much to Orrery himself, who, in this earliest attempt to read Swift's works as a function of his singular character, made categorical distinctions between "lunacy" and "idiotism." These are the two taxonomic categories of madness by which Swift's own "derangement" was diagnosed by his earliest biographers and critics.[20] "Lunacy," says Orrery, "may in general be considered as arising from a depraved imagination; and must therefore be originally owing to a fault in the body, or the mind. We see instances every day, where, as in fevers, all the powers of sense and reason are utterly overturned by a raging madness: this frenzy conquers, or is conquered soon: but, from more slow and chronical causes, such obstructions may be formed, as gradually to produce various degrees of this disorder, and to remain invincible to the very last moments of life."[21] In Orrery's iatromechanical conception of the body and disease, the "obstructions" caused by the "more slow and chronical causes"—he does not specify what—foul and clog the vessels that mediate between senses and understanding, between passion and reason. The passions ungoverned, the lunatic raves and rages. In contrast, "a state of idiotism," Orrery continues, "is less deplorable, not less shocking, than that of [lunacy]. Idiots are afflicted with no turbulent passions: they are innocent and harmless, and often excite pity, but never occasion fear. . . . The absolute naturals owe their wretchedness to a wrong formation in their brain, or to accidents in their birth, or the dregs of fevers, and other violent distempers." He concludes that the "last was the case of the Dean of St. PATRICK'S."[22]

Orrery tracked Swift's chronic physical disorders to his pitiable end. The hearing impairments "stop[ped] up that fountain of ideas" that had supplied his genius; his giddiness eventuated in his final idiotism. But in these statements, Orrery elides the more complicated disease process by leaping over the "violent distemper"—that is, the lunacy—to which he attributed Swift's final, vacant imbecility. Elsewhere, he tells the story more fully. Because the causal connections between lunacy and idiotism are important to understanding Swift's representation of madness in the *Travels*, I quote at length:

> The total deprivation of his senses came upon him by degrees. In the year 1736, I remember him seized with a violent fit of giddiness. He was at that time writing a satirical poem, called *The Legion Club*, but he found the effects of his giddiness so dreadful, that he left the poem unfinished; and never afterwards attempted a composition of any length either in verse or prose. However, his conversation still remained the same; lively and severe; but his memory gradually grew worse and worse: and as that decreased, and was impaired, he appeared every day more fretful and impatient. From the year *thirty-nine* to the latter end of the year *forty-one*, his friends found his passions so violent and ungovernable, his memory so decayed, and his reason so depraved, that they took the utmost precautions to keep all strangers from approaching him: for, till then, he had not appeared totally incapable of conversation: but, early in the year *forty-two*, the small remains of his understanding became entirely confused, and the violence of his rage increased absolutely to a degree of madness. In this miserable state he seemed to be appointed as the first proper

inhabitant for his own hospital: especially as from an outrageous lunatic, he sunk afterwards into a quiet, speechless idiot; and dragged out the remainder of his life in that helpless situation.[23]

Orrery argues that the decay of memory and erosion of reason caused by Swift's bodily disorders confounded his understanding and fretted and inflamed his unregulated passions until he became lunatic. This lunacy flaming, as in a fever crisis, gradually burned out, leaving but the shell of the great man, docile, mute, imbecile.

Orrery's definitions of *lunacy* and *idiotism* coincide with popular categories of madness among literate people of Swift's own day, especially those who had read John Locke (whom Orrery himself cites). Locke had written that madness is "the disorderly jumbling *Ideas* together" and that "mad Men put wrong *Ideas* together, and so make wrong Propositions, but argue and reason right from them." "Idiots," on the other hand, "make very few or no Propositions, and reason scarce at all." Therein, he says, lies "the difference between Idiots and mad Men."[24] What makes Orrery's appropriation of Locke important for us is that he establishes the categories of idiotism and lunacy specifically in grappling with the critical question of how Swift's writings were a function of his character. Moreover, idiotism and lunacy are the categories of madness that Swift himself knew well. He routinely used them in his proposals for a madhouse in Dublin. Some ten years after publishing *Gulliver's Travels*, he wrote to Orrery himself, "I have now finished my will in form, wherein I have settled my whole Fortune on the City, in trust for building and maintaining an Hospital for Ideots and Lunaticks, by which I save the Expence of a Chaplain, and almost of a Physician."[25] Three years later, his letters having faded away to a whisper, he asks that his bookseller George Faulkner print a notice calling in debts so that he can afford "to build and endow an Hospital, in, or near this city, for the support of Lunaticks, Ideots, and those they call Incurables."[26] Given Swift's own reliance on the two categories, "ideotism" and "lunacy" become useful designations in discussing the much-debated representations of madness in the *Travels*, as a later chapter of this study does.

Some who succeeded Orrery in writing about Swift framed their discussions of his character and works in the same categories of idiotism and lunacy. Saddened like Orrery by the misdirection and frittering away of his rare literary genius at the end, the Dean's friend Patrick Delany attributed the savagery of his satiric temper to constitutional illness, which Swift had managed to keep at bay until 1723. In that year, says Delany, he "unhappily relapsed into the first infirmity of his constitution.... And from that time, became I dare not say, I dare not think, what."[27] But in this pitiable end, he added more compassionately, Swift had gone the way of all flesh: "To sum up all—he lived long an honour to the powers of the human mind: and died (as he had lived for some few later years) a sad monument of the infirmities incident to it in this house of clay."[28] Delany's sympathetic turn would not, however, exemplify most subsequent commentary on Swift's last years. The narrative about his having gone mad, stayed mad, died mad—this story came from attempts to explain his eccentricities, unsettling works, and misdirected genius, all of which vexed the understanding of his friends and early commentators. The unforgiving Samuel Johnson claimed that the chronic illnesses that relentlessly "pursued [the Dean] through life" sent him finally to his "grave, deprived of reason."[29] Drooling imbecile in his last days, said Johnson, "*Swift* expire[d] a Driv'ler and a Show"—that is, a pathetic spectacle.[30] Like Orrery, Johnson traced the progress of Swift's disorders from physical cause to lunacy and then to idiocy. Like the others on their way to a thesis about Swift's madness, he brushed aside the experiences of living day to day with chronic disorders of body and mind.

For at least a century after Swift's death, biographers and critics attributed the viciousness of his attacks upon humanity to lunacy. Some still connected the "depravities of his imagination" causally with his chronic disorders, as had Orrery. These ailments, they said, reached critical mass in the savagery of his satire. Edmund Gosse declared in 1889 that as Swift's "vertigo became chronic . . . so did his misanthropy." "It was with the horrible satisfaction of disease" that Swift rendered humans Yahoo. In this monstrous representation of us all, concluded Gosse, "there is something which suggests a brain not wholly under control."[31] And in his famous image of Swift as depraved misanthrope, William Makepeace Thackeray asked, "What fever was boiling in him, that he should see all the world bloodshot?"[32] He still associated Swift's "furious, raging, obscene" lunacy with his diseased body.

There were other attempts to map the narrative of madness onto Swift's body. In 1835, when his skull was disinterred during flooding in the basement of St. Patrick's, where he was buried, Dublin phrenologists who examined it found physical evidence to support the diagnosis of madness. The phrenological report tracked the same narrative of madness, from body to lunacy to idiotism, that Orrery and Johnson had told: "It would appear, from the depression on the anterior part of the head," the phrenologists concluded, "that the man must have been apparently an idiot. The bones of the skull must have undergone considerable change during the ten or twelve last years of his life, while in a state of lunacy."[33] Others sought physiognomic evidence of Swift's madness in his death mask and late-life portraits. Walter Scott saw in the death mask "the expression of [a] countenance . . . most unequivocally maniacal."[34] And in 1861 William Lecky read in Francis Bindon's painting of the seventy-three-year-old Dean signs that "every spark of intelligence had disappeared." At last, sighed Lecky, Swift "exchanged the sleep of idiocy for the sleep of death."[35] The apathetic "idiocy" of which Lecky speaks is the same imbecility that Orrery and Delany had seen in Swift's life. Lunatic or idiot, Swift had died deprived of the reason that had governed sanity and the understanding that had made him a genius.

The idea of Swift mad impelled people to write his biography from the outside in, as it were. Such psychoautobiographical approaches to his life and works found modern form in theories of a disembodied unconscious. Madness became psychopathy; insanity became personality disorder.[36] Notoriously, Freudian critics put Swift on the couch, read his correspondence and imaginative works as case notes, and concluded that he suffered from "coprophilia," "anal fixation," "an unusually severe castration complex," "psychosexual infantilism," "dread of a gigantic father," and, more comprehensively, "neuroses."[37] The chronic giddiness, deafness, and tinnitus, once thought to have driven Swift mad, had nothing to do with the aberrant personality disorders revealed in the repulsive female bodies of the "scatological" poems, Gulliver's obsessions with excrements and breasts, and his submission, again and again, to terrible father figures and "masters." T. G. Wilson, president of the Royal College of Surgeons in Ireland, wrote in 1958 that, beset as he was by debilitating chronic disorders, Swift "was not insane. But he was undoubtedly a psychopath, for his constant references to the bodily excreta amounted to a pathological obsession."[38] Wilson might rescue him from the charges that he was lunatic, but he still pathologizes his mental disorders by turning him over to the psychoanalysts.

Before the early nineteenth-century "birth of the clinic" that Foucault theorizes, there was little interest in explaining Swift's disorders in strictly biomedical terms or in solving a diagnostic riddle. Only in 1849, when the Irish ear, nose, and throat doctor William Wilde published a book-length study of the Dean's final illnesses, was there a shift in emphasis, from discussing his health in the framework of his character and behavior to reading the signs in an attempt to tender a clinical diagnosis. Wilde turned to the new authority of the clinic "in the hope of rescuing [Swift's] character from some of the aspersions which have been cast upon it."[39] He had in mind specifically the physician Thomas Beddoes, who had argued fifty years earlier that the "giddiness and coldness of stomach" that afflicted Swift throughout his life resulted from a "pitiable secret vice" (that is, masturbation) that had become habitual during his youth. The aberrant preoccupation with "things impure," said Beddoes, culminated in misanthropic madness.[40] Wilde protested that the expressive dysphasia and late-life dementia were not signs of "lunacy" but organic affections of cerebral congestion: "It may, we are free to confess, appear at first view an almost impossible task to write the history of Swift's case and *post mortem* examination upwards of a century after his death: nevertheless we have no hesitation in asserting that the following detail of symptoms, given chiefly in the words of the patient, afford us one of the best described, and certainly the very longest instance of cerebral disease which we have ever met with, extending as it does over a period of fifty-five years!"[41] In neither Swift's death mask nor "his expressions, nor the tone of his writing" nor "an examination of any of his acts" did Wilde "discover a single symptom of insanity, nor aught but the effects of physical disease, and the natural wearing and decay of a mind such as Swift's."[42] His defense of Swift is the same as Delaney's. The genius who had written *Gulliver's Travels*, the Irish patriot, and the scrupulous defender of Anglican episcopacy had gone the way of all flesh, declining intellectually in his final years but, says Wilde, by no means going mad. Wilde has reframed this defense as clinical narrative. In dislodging Swift's case from the "dyspeptic criticism" of Johnson and the dark aspersions of Beddoes, he wields the new authority of positivist science.[43]

There is clever irony in Wilde's representation of the attacks on Swift's character as "dyspeptic," with its suggestion of indigestion. Perhaps, the pun implies, the characterizations of Swift as lunatic arise from the fouled stomachs of Johnson, Scott, and Beddoes themselves. But the pun also draws on the old humoral connections between digestive processes and physical-cum-mental disorders. Even if the mechanical mincing and grinding of the iatrophysicists and gastric juices of the iatrochemists had displaced

Galenic heat in explaining digestive processes, the humoral notion that one's health is determined by proper digestion remained. As evidence of the enduring legacy of connections between stomach and disorders, physical and mental, we have Wilde's own diagnosis. Considering first that Swift "himself and his physicians" attributed his ailments "to some derangement of the stomach," Wilde concluded that Swift's "gastric attacks were, in early life at least, induced by irregularities of diet. It is also evident that they were attended with vertigo, deafness, sickness of stomach, pain in the head, diminution of muscular power, as shown in his tottering gait, and numbness or some slight loss of sensation in the upper extremities. That these in turn were symptomatic of some cerebral affection is manifest." Wilde maintains the humoral connection between impaired digestion and cerebration. How far Swift's "cerebral affection" "depended on, or was induced by gastric disease, it is now difficult to determine," said Wilde; "cases are, however, on record, which tend to show that all the early symptoms of the Dean's malady may be produced by affections of the stomach and alimentary canal. As Swift advanced in years his symptoms became more decidedly cerebral."[44] Wilde's clinical medicine, no less than the humoral medicine that had prevailed for more than twenty centuries, still suggested that the stomach could be the seat of an individual's physical and mental disorders.

In a brief note of 1881, the English physician J. Wickham Legg, intent like Wilde upon rescuing Swift's reputation, again from the defamations of Beddoes, suggested that the Dean presented clinically with the classic triad of symptoms indicating Ménière's disease: vertigo, progressive deafness, and tinnitus.[45] An incurable and progressively debilitating dysfunction of the inner ear membrane, known also as labyrinthine vertigo, the disorder had been identified only twenty years earlier by Prosper Ménière, a clinician of the Paris school and physician-in-chief to the Institute for Deaf-Mutes. In the *Gazette Médicale de Paris,* Ménière described the symptoms in one of his patients: "A healthy young man would experience suddenly, without apparent cause, vertigo, nausea, vomiting; a condition of indescribable distress drained his strength. . . . [L]ying on his back he could not open his eyes without seeing the objects around him whirling in space."[46] At first Ménière diagnosed this patient as suffering from cerebral congestion, as Wilde had Swift. But the young man did not respond to the standard interventions of bleeding and purging in such cases. And when the patient began to complain of both loud noises in his ears and coincident deafness,

Ménière concluded that the vertigo, tinnitus, and hearing loss were all signs of the same disease, an idiopathic disorder of the inner ear.[47]

Shortly after Legg ventured the diagnosis of Ménière's disease for Swift's own disorders, John Bucknill, a founding editor of *Brain*, elaborated upon this diagnosis.[48] Bringing the new authority of the clinic to rescue Swift from charges of lunacy, as had Wilde, Bucknill concluded that what those such as Johnson and Scott saw as "insanity" was, instead, dementia with accompanying aphasia, likely the result of a "localised left-side apoplexy or cerebral softening" in his seventy-fourth year.[49] He turned his attention then to the Dean's chronic illnesses. Having reviewed Swift's own statements about his collective disorders, he concluded that the diagnosis of Ménière's appeared "to conform in all important points with the life-long disease of the illustrious dean." A page later, he declared with greater authority, "This is certainly labyrinthine vertigo."[50] The clinical diagnosis made a coherent narrative of Swift's random reports and complaints.

Despite Legg's original suggestion, Bucknill is usually credited with solving the diagnostic riddle of Swift's symptoms, and his article is the locus classicus of the clinical explanation of the Dean's disorders. Moreover, he presents his diagnosis as the triumph of the clinic itself over the benighted claims of humoralism: Bucknill's article is as much an encomium on the modern clinic as it is an explanation of Swift's chronic disorders. "The knowledge of [Ménière's]," he rhapsodizes, "is one of the most recent triumphs of pathological research directed by physiological experiment."[51] Sixty years later, an anonymous writer in the *British Medical Journal* agreed that "Meniere's disease fits in with Swift's symptoms so well that there is no difficulty in accepting this diagnosis to the exclusion of such alternatives as otosclerosis and syphilitic labyrinthitis. Jonathan Swift's contemporaries understood his bodily ailments no more than they understood his 'fierce indignation which lacerated the heart.'"[52] As testimony to the ascendant authority of the clinic, medical writers, biographers, and literary critics have since the 1880s almost universally accepted Bucknill's retrospective diagnosis of Swift's chronic disorders.[53]

Over the last century, such clinical assessments of historical figures' ailments, including those of writers, have become an industry of sorts. Many of these, like William Ober's notorious *Boswell's Clap and Other Essays*

(1979) and John Ross's more recent *Shakespeare's Tremor and Orwell's Cough* (2012), have been written by clinicians. Their speculative diagnoses often engage spirited debates, not only in literary circles but also in the pages of medical periodicals such as the *Lancet* and the *British Medical Journal*: Did Jane Austen die of Addison's disease, lymphoma, or tuberculosis? Were Samuel Johnson's tics the result of Tourette syndrome or an obsessive-compulsive disorder? Was the Pott's disease that Alexander Pope was said to have suffered contracted from his wet nurse? Because of the tantalizing links between mental illness and creativity, diagnosing writers' mental illnesses has roused particular interest: Robert Burns, Virginia Woolf, Ernest Hemingway, and Sylvia Plath are but a few who have been diagnosed with clinical depression and mood disorders. Furthermore, retrospective diagnoses are continually written or rewritten to apply newly designated disorders. Hans Christian Andersen, Emily Dickinson, Lewis Carroll, James Joyce, and Swift himself have all lately been placed on the autism "spectrum." One recent writer has diagnosed Swift with Asperger syndrome.[54]

Retrospective diagnosis has certain appeals. For one, it may excite the interest of readers who seek potentially scandalous facts about important people. Did Shakespeare suffer from venereal disorders? Was Thomas Shadwell an opium addict? More constructive for some readers is the challenge of solving diagnostic riddles faced by those who would interpret clinical signs reported from the past. For literary critics, retrospective diagnoses also offer new ways of reading authors' imaginative works. For example, attributing John Milton's blindness to bilateral retinal detachment, a condition in which "subjective sensations of light persist even after the loss of sight," helps us appreciate the persistent images of light or even the fire without flame of the opening scene of *Paradise Lost* in hell.[55] Recognizing the disability and isolation that Flannery O'Connor suffered from lupus helps us understand the alienation and social psychopathy of a character like the Misfit in "A Good Man Is Hard to Find."

Piers Mitchell, who urges a "balanced approach" to historical and retrospective diagnoses, says that a "retrospective diagnosis can be a perfectly valid and reliable technique to apply to written sources from historic populations in order to gain a more nuanced view of health and disease in the past."[56] Indeed, the retrospective clinical diagnosis of Ménière's disease has biographical and critical value. But, I would argue, as *analogy*. Swift's own complaints fit neatly into the classic triad of symptoms with which the

Ménière's patient of our own day presents: vertigo, deafness, and tinnitus.[57] Like the Ménière's patient, Swift suffered from episodic objective vertigo, in which objects around him seemed to spin. "This morning, sitting in my bed, I had a fit of giddiness," he wrote in 1710. "The room turned round for about a minute, and then it went off, leaving me sickish, but not very."[58] Like the Ménière's patient, Swift suffered progressive hearing loss. Deafness is the most variable of Ménière's symptoms, but it usually begins in the left ear and, in at least a third of those afflicted, becomes bilateral and eventually permanent as the disease progresses. The patient typically loses hearing in the mid- to low-frequency range. In a letter to William Richardson of 1737, Swift talks of his earliest episodes of deafness, "before [he] was twenty. . . . Although it came but seldom, and lasted but a few days, yet [his] left ear hath never been well since." Now, these many years later, he says that "when the deafness comes on, [he] can hear with neither ear, except it be a woman with a treble, or a man with a counter tenor."[59] Like the Ménière's patient, Swift complained also of tinnitus, which further confused and impaired his hearing: "I have . . . been almost three weeks pursued with a Noise in my Ears and Deafness that makes me an unsociable Creature."[60] Even if episodes varied in length and severity, they became progressively persistent over the years; increasingly, they came together. "I have a constant Giddyness in my head, and what is more vexatious, as constant a Deafness," he wrote in his final decade.[61] For Ménière's patients, the disease process can be similar. And like Swift, Ménière's patients may complain of secondary afflictions—aural fullness and nausea—that sometimes accompany the vertigo, deafness, and tinnitus.

With the physical symptoms, the Ménière's patient also suffers continual anxieties. Although some afflicted with the disease describe an "aura" immediately before the onset of symptoms, there is the uncertainty of not knowing when the next attack will come, if a mere dizzy spell portends full-blown vertigo, and how long an episode will last. Often they hesitate to go out into the world, fearing the physical danger and embarrassments of falling.[62] Some Ménière's patients report short-term memory loss, confusion, and depression. Swift shared these anxieties and confusions. Like the Ménière's patient, he spoke of the "daily dread of Relapses," against which he readied his mind as best he could.[63] Increasingly, he avoided traveling and even going far from the St. Patrick's deanery in Dublin, writing that he could "never if possible be above an hour distant from home," lest he "be caught by a Deafness and Giddyness out of [his] own precincts."[64] He, too, feared memory loss and often felt confused and dispirited. Given all of the similarities of physical symptoms and psychological stresses, then, the retrospective diagnosis seems to explain Swift's disorders neatly. The Ménière's patient suffers physical afflictions similar to Swift's—vertigo, deafness, and tinnitus; often feels depression, dread, and vague terror about the unpredictable and debilitating return of these symptoms, as did Swift; and experiences social embarrassment, marginalization, stigmatization, and crises of social identity, as did Swift.[65] The Ménière's patient also has somehow to make sense of a chronic disorder for which there is no neat narrative closure.

Despite the interest and value of Bucknill's diagnosis of Swift, medical historians since at least the 1990s have challenged such diagnoses on both practical and theoretical grounds. First is the problem, methodological and arguably ethical, that the body that is the object of diagnosis cannot itself be examined. "A retrospectively diagnosing physician," says Axel Karenberg, "strongly violates the principles of the medical profession, because he gives his opinion on a patient he has never seen nor examined."[66] More significantly, some who challenge retrospective diagnosis see it as yet another example of "Whiggish" history that would impose an often self-congratulatory "presentist" interpretation upon the past.[67] By definition, retrospective diagnosis force-fits historical facts to the plot of the medical writer's and biographer's own culturally constructed narrative about the body and disease.

Given such problems, overlapping anachronisms come with diagnosing Swift's chronic disorders as Ménière's disease. Aside from the historical fact that the disorder did not exist as a "disease entity" until 1861, well over a century after Swift's death, Swift and his contemporaries would never have recognized either the body or the explanation of sickness that undergirds the clinical diagnosis of Ménière's disease. According to the standard clinical narrative, Ménière's symptoms result from endolymphatic hydrops, the accumulation of endolymph in the vestibular canals of the ears. This buildup of fluid irritates cilia in both the organ of Corti, causing fluctuations in hearing, and the vestibular cells, which then mistransmit signals to the brain, causing vertigo. True, the humoral narrative that Swift told about his own body also saw giddiness and deafness as the accumulation of fluid. But clinical anatomy and the biochemical model of disease differ greatly from, respectively, the body and explanation of illness that Swift knew. The organ of Corti, for example, was not discovered until 1851. And the exchanges of potassium and sodium described in the clinical plot about Ménière's disease were entirely unknown to Swift and his contemporaries. The fundamentally different conceptions of the body make Ménière's disease and humoral imbalances essentially different disorders. The retrospective diagnosis thus leads us to assumptions that we then ascribe, misguidedly, I argue, to Swift's body, his experiences, his social identity, and his imaginative writings.

For all of the clinical confidence with which those like Bucknill diagnosed Swift, this retrospective diagnosis fails in yet another way. While vesting its authority in positivist "fact," the Ménière's narrative is itself distressed by uncertainties, contested definitions of terms, and incoherencies. It remains ill-defined and perplexes easy nosological classification.[68] The disease is idiopathic, its origins finally unknown.[69] Because it presents so variously, it often baffles diagnosis.[70] It strikes intermittently, at irregular and unpredictable intervals. Some Ménière's patients suffer only one or two attacks in a lifetime; others suffer chronically and progressively. Treatments range widely, from surgery and the implantation of regulatory devices to dietary modifications and the administration of antisecretory drugs designed to relieve fluid pressure. The disease is incurable, however, so the most that doctors can hope is that such treatments will reduce the severity of symptoms. In view of the indeterminacies of the disorder for both patient and clinician, one twentieth-century authority declared that "Ménière's disease is one of the least understood disorders, by both doctors in general and specialists. It is variable in clinical presentation, imprecise in diagnosis, and because the effectiveness of treatment is doubtful, leaves the clinician disillusioned, depriving the patient of the potential cure that has become the rule."[71] The difficulties of defining Ménière's disease, identifying its pathogenesis, finding patterns of recurrence, and understanding its functional implications make the disorder mysterious to the clinician. The unpredictability of symptoms—when or whether they will strike again and how severely—leaves the identity of the Ménière's patient as a sick person uncertain.

One of the ironies of the retrospective diagnosis in Swift's case is that the diagnostic narrative by which the early modern age explained his disorders as humoral imbalance was more certain and coherent within its own logic than the modern clinical explanation. For Swift himself, there *was* no diagnostic riddle. The humoral explanation not only made perfect sense of his chronic giddiness, deafness, and tinnitus but, as we shall see, also guided his management of those disorders in ways that the clinical narrative does not do for the Ménière's patient. If the clinical plot is not wholly coherent or intelligible, Swift's humoral narrative was. Despite the clinical assertion that the "cause of his condition ... would never be known to him," Swift knew *exactly* what he suffered from: humoral imbalance.[72] He knew exactly what he had to do to treat it: restore humoral balance.

3

As Swift Would Have It

The story of an acute disorder, like the shingles from which Swift suffered in his mid-forties, has narrative closure. Reading Swift's account of this painful disease, especially in the *Journal to Stella*, we can follow the arc of the illness plot, as it moves from first pains to diagnosis and prognosis to crisis and then to recovery. It begins in late March of 1712 when Swift reports almost offhand to the "ladies," Stella and Dingley, "I have a Pain these 2 days exactly upon th Top of my left Shouldr, I fear it is something Rheumatick, it winches now and then."[1] A couple of days later, he is a sick man, so "extreamly ill" that he cannot leave his lodgings because the debilitating pain has "crept" from his "Should^r . . . to [his] neck and Collar bone."[2] A diagnosis follows. Having observed—and experienced—the symptoms and consulted with physicians, Swift announces, "The Disease is th Shingles."[3] Then the blisters on his upper back and neck, painful as they are, show the progress of the hot choler as it works its way through and out of the body in a sanative humoral process of excretion. "Great Red Spots" have erupted "in all those Places where my Pain was," he writes. "It would have ended in some violent Disease if it had not came out thus. I shall now recover fast. I have been in no danger of Life, but miserab^le Torture."[4] After three more months, the pain subsides to "itchings, & Scratchings, and small akings."[5] We hear nothing more of the shingles after mid-July. Having followed the court from London to Windsor, Swift has resumed his social rounds and become, as he represents himself, an important political player. He is a man recovered.

"The challenge for autobiographical narrative," says Thomas Couser, "is to achieve a closure of any sort."[6] As Laurence Sterne showed comically in

Tristram Shandy, the beleaguered autobiographer is always trying to catch up with his own circumstantiated life. The story of an acute illness, however, as it tracks the course of a person's disorder from onset to restored health, can claim the narrative closure of what Couser calls the "comic plot" of recovery.[7] Thus Swift could tell the story of his shingles from first pangs to cure. The humoral narrative of the body's pushing out the hot choler "through the extern Parts" was its structure.[8] In contrast, the story of his chronic illnesses, as it conveyed the experiences of his disordered body, could never find the same closure. Because his own giddiness and hearing disorders came in "Fitts" followed by easing of the symptoms, Swift at times spoke hopefully of "recovery." "I was in very ill health, and am since but slowly recovering," he wrote in 1721.[9] And again a couple of years later: "I have been above 7 weeks ill of my old Deafness and am but just recovered."[10] But as the episodes came more frequently, albeit still unpredictably, he eventually despaired of total cure. Having been deaf for two months without relief, he wrote to his friend Charles Ford in 1724, "I am afraid I shall never recover."[11] And almost ten years later, he lamented, "I am just recovered in some degree, of two cruell Indispositions of Giddyness and Deafness, after seven Months. I have got my hearing, but the other Evil hangs still about me; and I doubt will never quite leave me, till I leave it."[12] As I suggest later, Swift might imagine recovery in a work like *Gulliver's Travels*, but eventually he saw only the fatal arc of his disease. "I believe this Giddiness is the Disorder that will at last get the better of me," he wrote desperately to Thomas Sheridan in 1727.[13] In *Verses on the Death* is the grim comic prognosis "That old Vertigo in his Head, / Will never leave him, till he's dead."[14] For the sufferer of chronic disease and disability like Swift, says Couser, there is no reconciling the lived "experience of illness with the comic plot expected of autobiography"; "the culturally validated narrative of triumph over adversity may simply not be available."[15] What coherent explanation, then, could Swift himself use to make sense of, and thereby contain, an unstable, ever-fluid body that defied containment? Humoralism provided that very narrative.

Although Swift could not see the story of his giddiness, deafness, tinnitus, memory lapses, and other cognitive confusions through to its end in writing an autopathography, he did explain the onset of his chronic illnesses in a brief autobiographical fragment, written sometime around age sixty, and in letters to Henrietta Howard, Mary Pendarves, and William Richardson. A later chapter of this study gives greater attention to the autobiographical fragment, especially as it shows Swift's problems in determining his own identity. Here it is important as it documents his understanding of the cause of his disorders. In the fragment, he dates the first fit of giddiness to his earliest days at Moor Park with Sir William Temple, who had employed him as private secretary in 1689. Speaking of himself in the third person, Swift writes that "he happened before twenty years old, by a Surfeit of fruit to contract a giddyness and coldness of Stomach, that almost brought him to his Grave, and this disorder pursued him with Intermissions of two or thre[e] years to the end of his Life."[16] This is the same tale of physical ruin that Orrery "often heard him" tell.[17] In a well-known letter of 1727 to Henrietta Howard, he elaborates: "About two hours before you were born [ca. 1689], I got my Giddyness by eating a hundred golden pippins at a time, at Richmond, and when You were four years and a quarter old bating two days, having made a fine seat about twenty miles further in Surrey where I used to read and sleep, there I got my Deafness, and these two friends have visited me, one or oth[e]r, every year since, and being old acquaintance have now thought fit to come togeth[e]r."[18] Some eight years later, Swift told the same story to Mary Pendarves: "I got my giddiness by raw fruit when I was a lad in England, which I never could be wholly rid of, and it is now too late."[19] And in a letter of 1737 to William Richardson, Swift reported, "In England, before I was twenty, I got a cold which gave me a deafness that I could never clear myself of."[20]

Dating the respective onsets of his giddiness and deafness was one way for Swift to impose order on the disorders of his body. The problem is that the dates in his various explanations are inconsistent. In the letter to Howard, the dating of the first attack, when Swift would have been twenty-one, accords with his statement in the *Journal to Stella* of October 1712, "I have had my Giddiness 23 years by fits."[21] This date, though, is discrepant with that in the autobiographical fragment, in which he says that he contracted the disorder before he was twenty. Biographers and editors have attempted sometimes-strained explanations to resolve the apparent inconsistencies. In one extended discussion, Arthur Case agrees with Swift's nineteenth-century biographer John Forster that the giddiness first attacked Swift not when he was living with Temple but during one of his "boy-visits" to England, when, likely on break from college, he went to see his mother in

Leicester. He may have visited Temple's estate during one of these breaks, or he may have gorged himself in another nearby orchard.[22] Either way, we have an explanation for his having contracted his giddiness "before twenty years old." If, as Case argues, Mrs. Howard was born in 1687, some two years before Swift went to work with Temple, this, too, would solve the apparent contradiction of Swift's saying that he contracted the disorder in the year of her birth.[23] In the letters and the autobiographical fragment, written after Swift was sixty, we might forgive the discrepancies as lapses of memory. Even in his mid-forties, he complained to Stella and Dingley, "I have a worse memory than when I left y."[24] Having lived so long with his giddiness and deafness, he may have found it hard to distinguish the onset of ailments (which he could not have known at the time would pursue him to his end) from the episodes that followed. Yet it does seem odd that he would not be able to date with greater certainty an attack of an illness "that almost brought him to his Grave." The indeterminacy of dates reflects perhaps the uncertainty of the disorders themselves and of the fluid humoral body.

Notwithstanding the discrepancies in dating the onset of his chronic giddiness and deafness, Swift's explanation for why they struck him and why they continued to afflict him throughout his life conforms exactly with humoralism. A common humoral explanation of giddiness, as a "Cephalick disorder," saw a weak stomach as the culprit. The author of *The Family Physician*, published shortly after Swift's death, claimed that a "VERTIGO, *giddiness, or swimming in the head* . . . is either an original [that is, constitutional] disease, or proceeds from disorders of the stomach."[25] A contemporary "Physician," who warned of the potential "very dangerous Consequence" of vertigo, likewise blamed improper digestion of the humors: "It comes . . . chiefly from cold Humours and flatulent Vapours arising from the Stomach or other inferiour Parts, causing a continual Pain in the Head, Noise in the Ears, [and] Dulness of the Senses."[26] The author's simple iatromechanical explanation is that the fouled and superfluous humors, having accumulated in the head, put pressure on the brain and nerves, thus impairing healthy sense functions. The author then tells the story of a man who suffered from vertigo and who, when he died, was found to have water on the brain.[27]

If we are to accept the testimony of Swift's late-life attendants and those who witnessed his autopsy, the physician-author's explanation bears out in the Dean's own case. Patrick Delany blamed the "state of ideotism" to which Swift was finally reduced not on the accumulation of "black-bile" in the blood, "which physicians . . . describe to be its ordinary condition, in a state of lunacy," but to excessive cranial fluid, which "appeared clearly from the opening of his head, after his death."[28] The testimony for this finding comes from Dr. John Lyon, a canon of St. Patrick's who managed Swift's affairs late in life and likely witnessed his autopsy: "When the Dean was dead, Mr. WHITEWAY, an eminent Surgeon, nearly related to him, opened the Skull, and found much Water in the Brain."[29] The postmortem findings accord with the conventional belief that improperly digested humors had migrated to the head, where they accumulated, causing Swift's disorders. "Water in the Brain," no less than the choler of Swift's shingles, was humoral superfluity.

That Swift should persistently blame his overindulgence in apples for a chronic disorder that afflicted him for the rest of his life may seem odd to us. But the story conforms with humoral theory. Fruit was considered a "cold," "wet" aliment that, according to Galen, produced a "phlegmatic humour."[30] Gluttonizing on the cold, wet pippins, Swift might well have contracted the "coldness of Stomach" that permanently upset his system. His cold stomach could not properly concoct and attenuate the humors for healthy assimilation in the body. And so, by humoral logic, gluey phlegm (the cold, wet humor) clogged in Swift's head and caused his giddiness (and his hearing disorders).[31] That the fruit on which Swift overindulged should be raw was yet another explanation for his chronic giddiness. "All Apples are worst raw," said Thomas Muffett, whose popular *Healths Improvement* first appeared in 1655.[32] In a treatise of 1706 on the qualities and nutritive value of various foods, the French botanist Louis Lémery cautioned that, among the "*Ill effects*" of apples, which "contain much Phlegm," "they are not at all good for those who have a weak Stomach. Boil'd *Apples* are to be preferred before those that are raw, because they are of easier digestion."[33] In Swift's own humoral understanding, the superfluity of improperly digested humors explained his giddiness: Phlegm had congested in his head, disordering his equilibrium. "My head is pretty well," he reported in the *Journal to Stella*, "only a sudden turn any time makes me giddy for a moment, and sometimes it feels very stufft."[34] Swift's explanation for his vertigo plots the humoral narrative of disease.

Deafness, Swift's other most bothersome and socially embarrassing complaint, was defined broadly in one contemporary medical dictionary as "a Distemper of the Ear, which makes the Person incommoded with it, either not to hear at all, or to hear very imperfectly."[35] It was not, says historian of early modern medicine Ruben Verwaal, "a single and fixed physical state, but rather a flexible condition that could slowly or suddenly manifest itself, and just as easily disappear or remain permanent."[36] The fluidity of the condition, like the humors to which Swift ascribed it, explains the "recoveries" and "relapses" of which he often spoke. Temporary or permanent deafness could be traced to a variety of causes, including heredity, trauma, fevers (a "hot" cause), venereal disorders, even "Animals or extraneous bodies" that "insinuate themselves and lodge" in the passages of the ears.[37] In Swift's case, the humoral model of disease offered two explanations, both of them again related to imperfect "coction," that is, digestion of the humors. The first blamed a too-cold stomach. Because the aliments were not properly cooked, the concoction process failed to attenuate the humors fully. An accumulation of crude phlegm congested the ears and muffled hearing. The "too great a quantity of cold humours," said one writer, upset the humoral balance of the fluid environment of the ears and thus impaired the hearing.[38] The explanation accords with Swift's own complaints.

Because the humoral body was permeable with the world outside of it, many of Swift's day believed with his contemporary Peter Shaw that deafness could "proceed from the catching of cold."[39] The medical writers held that *cerumen aurium* (earwax) was among the "humors of different kinds separated from the mass of blood, circulating in an animal body."[40] One physician of the 1760s explained that the glands "deposited a deficient—too viscid a secretion—or constipation of the wax, from what is called catching cold."[41] Even if, by this writer's time, the word *humors* had come to mean bodily fluids more generally, earwax was thought to be a "phlegmatic" excrement.[42] Hearing impairment was still seen as a disruption of natural physiological functions caused by humoral imbalance. Like Swift, many people with hearing problems blamed this imbalance on catching cold. Samuel Pepys complained that he became "almost deaf" in one ear after he contracted a cold during a dalliance "with Mrs. Lane in the path of a draught."[43] In the middle of the eighteenth century, a certain Mary Smargins, the subject of an electrical experiment to restore her hearing, claimed to have become deaf "from a cold"; she was purportedly cured by the "warmth" of the electrical current.[44] And in Arbuthnot's *History of John Bull*, the character Frog makes "a shuffling Excuse" for breaking an appointment by professing that "he got a great Cold, that had struck him deaf of one Ear."[45] This may be a comic nod to his friend Swift.[46] Even late in life, the Dean always associated his hearing disabilities with cold. "If I were fit for any Company I would have waited on you," he wrote to Lord Orrery in the mid-1730s, "but am hindred by a certain return of deafness whenever I venture into the cold Air."[47] His understanding of deafness follows exactly from the logic of the humoral narrative.

A second explanation for Swift's deafness was an impairment of nervous function. At one point, Swift himself imputed both giddiness and deafness "to increasing years, and consequently a greater weakness in [his] nerves."[48] Elsewhere, in an elaborate verse apology to his friend Delany for not visiting with him, Swift blames his deafness on the sympathetic connection of "two Auditory Nerves," one going "to this, and one to t'other Ear." "When my Left Ear was deaf a Fortnight," he explains, "To t'other Ear I felt [the deafness] coming on."[49] Comically reductive, he does not explain the process by which one nerve communicates with the other. But mechanists who implicated the nerves blamed deafness on reciprocal relations between solid fibers and humors. "Perfect deafness . . . seldom happens," said the otherwise unknown "G. Bickerton" in 1719, except "when the auditory Nerve is grown stiff and immoveable or the Juice therein stagnates . . . by Reason of an Obstruction in the very Nerves, either by some gross Humour, or the nervous Juice render'd so glutinous that no Passage can be granted."[50] The "nervous Juice" here is the elusive "Animal or Sensitive Spirits," distilled in the brain in a final process of digestion; this was the fluid thought to carry sense impulses through the nerves and to manage sensation and movement.[51] (The familiar term "animal spirits" derives from *anima*, the vital principle or animating spirit.) If these animal spirits were not properly attenuated and were "glutinous," the transmission of sense information would be slowed.

Another mechanical explanation that blames deafness on impaired nervous function sees the cause not as sluggish or obstructed nervous juices within the tubal nerves but as an accumulation of ambient humors that constricts (pinches) the nerves from outside and retards the flow of the spirits. William Cockburn, Swift's own physician in London, explained deafness in this very way: Blood that had thickened because of "Coldness" would press upon "Contiguous Nerves," he said, "till at length by this continual stuffing the Nerve is so much compressed that it hinders the motion of animal

Spirits in those Canals, tho' their sides may not be quite squeezed together, and thereby will happen that a man may be thick of Hearing, or perfectly Deaf, he may be blind, lose his Taste, &c."[52] In his thesis about Swift's emergent madness, Orrery had speculated similarly that some "internal pressure upon his brain" might have compressed the auditory nerves and caused his deafness.[53] While Orrery tracked Swift's deafness to inevitable madness, however, Cockburn saw the possibility of recovery. The "Coldness being over" and heat returned either by natural physiological response or medical intervention, he wrote, the "Lentor" (viscidity) in the animal spirits is relieved, and hearing and other sense functions restored.[54] For Bickerton and Cockburn, the focus has shifted to the elasticity or laxity of the nervous fibers; they are no longer concerned with systemic humoral balance. Nevertheless, the culprit in their mechanical explanations of impaired nervous function is an improperly concocted humor. The humor in question, says Bickerton (in another context), is phlegm, which "obstruct[s] the Nerves, and hinder[s] the Influx of Animal Spirits."[55] This, indeed, is the very humor that Swift himself blamed for his disorders.

Swift's humoral explanations for how he contracted his giddiness and deafness do not account explicitly for the tinnitus of which he also complained frequently. In correspondence of the early 1720s, it is suddenly upon him. Like deafness, tinnitus could result from traumatic injury. More often, it, too, was explained as an obstruction caused either by cold or by improper concoction of the humors. Writing a decade before Swift's birth, the physician John Jonston claimed in a comprehensive treatise on diseases that "the Noise or Ringing of the Ears" can proceed from "*External Causes* exciting and raising up Vapors, to wit, the extream cold or over great heat of the Air, overmuch feeding and fulness either of food or Wine, from whence Crudities are heaped up together in the Head." There are also "*Internal Causes,*" said Jonston. The disorder may arise "from a *Humor Flegmatick* and cold, and then the Malady [begins] by little and little, & from less to greater; and returneth likewise at some certain seasons and by intervals; the noise or sound is cleerer and more distinct than ordinary."[56] In Jonston's humoral scheme, both external and internal causes of noises in the ears were linked with improper coction of phlegm.

Swift sometimes conjoined his deafness and tinnitus syntactically, as separate disorders. He complains, at the very time that he is writing the first two books of *Gulliver's Travels*, that he is "so disordered with a Noise in

[his] Ears and Deafness that [he is] utterly unqualifyed for all Conversation or thinking."⁵⁷ His deafness baffles his hearing; his tinnitus distracts his thinking. At other times, tinnitus *is* deafness. "I am plagued this month with a noise in my head, which deafens me; and some touches of Giddyness, my old disorders," he wrote to Lord Orrery in 1737.⁵⁸ Some medical writers of the day warned that tinnitus would lead to deafness. "A Tinnitus or Noise in the Ears is most frequently a chronick and very troublesome Distemper," wrote one authority. "It sometimes ends in an entire Deafness; it is seldom Cured, or if it be helped, it is apt to return again."⁵⁹ Usually, however, Swift himself makes no distinction between muffled hearing and noise in the ears. Both are physically, mentally, and socially troubling hearing impairments, collapsed under the comprehensive term *deafness*.

Taken separately or together, all three of Swift's persistent physical complaints—giddiness, deafness, and tinnitus—were considered "cephalick" disorders, with common blame in superfluous or peccant humors. Any one by itself was troubling. When the three came concurrently, they could presage dire consequences. A headache attended with vomiting, "deafness and watching, portends madness," declared Peter Shaw. "Being attended with noise in the ears, vertigo, deafness, and dullness of feeling in the hands, it threatens an apoplexy or epilepsy."⁶⁰ Arbuthnot agreed. Among the "immediate Forerunners of an Apoplexy," he said, "are commonly a Vertigo, Staggering, Loss of Memory," and "a Noise in the Ears," all afflictions about which Swift himself complained.⁶¹ Little wonder that the only certain narrative closure he could see for his chronic disorders was death itself, the foreboding that they "will at last get the better of me."⁶² In his fears that his chronic disorders would bring his death, we see yet another limitation of the retrospective clinical diagnosis: Ménière's disease is not fatal, despite its disorienting, at times terrifying symptoms and the hopelessness that sometimes attends them. Swift, though, could never know when his disorders would kill him.

If humoralism explains Swift's chronic physical disorders, it also explains the mutual disordering of his senses and cognitive faculties, which are more difficult to understand. In 1721, Swift wrote of a long-lasting fit of deafness, "which wholly disconcerts and confounds me to a degree that I can neither think nor speak nor Act as I used to do, nor mind the least Business even of my own."⁶³ Because of the "odious continual disorder in my Head," he confessed to Pope in 1736, "I neither re[a]d, nor write; nor remember, nor converse."⁶⁴ Reading, writing, and conversing, all were social performances by which Swift knew and negotiated the public world. Later, I discuss his cognitive impairments as social disability. But as a way of historicizing them in Swift's own fears of what was happening to him, we should first frame these disorders of mind within the humoral narrative. This begins by considering the importance of the senses in constructing order—"making *sense*" of the world and experience—and then mapping out the complex relations between the senses and the understanding.

Sentimentalizing Swift in his dotage, Orrery wrote of his late-life senility, "It is the more melancholy to me, as I have heard him often lament the particular misfortune incident to human nature, of an utter deprivation of senses many years before a deprivation of life. I have heard him describe persons in that condition, with a liveliness and a horror, that on this late occasion have recalled to me his very words."⁶⁵ Swift's cousin Deane, who knew him as well as anyone during his final years, insisted that, despite all of the stories of the "poor old man," he was not mad: "Sometimes he will not utter a syllable: at other times he will speak incoherent words: but he never yet, as far as I could hear, talked nonsense, or said a foolish thing."⁶⁶ In the debate over the final state of Swift's mind, which preoccupies so many early character studies, both Orrery and Deane Swift invoke the word *sense*—the "utter deprivation of senses" and "nonsense." In Swift's day, as in our own, people commonly remarked that a mad man was "out of his senses" or that he had "lost his wits." In this context, among its many denotations, the word *wits* meant both the five senses and faculties of mind like reason, understanding, and memory.⁶⁷ Senses and wits are both particularly germane to the topic of Swift's chronic giddiness and hearing impairments: Swift believed that his disordered senses disordered his cognitive functions.

Inasmuch as language imposes form on our lives by drawing referential boundaries for experiences and phenomena, the ways in which Swift and his contemporaries used the words *sense* and *senses* are themselves suggestive. Mad in love for him, Vanessa begged Swift, "Shew some tenderness for me or I shall lose my senses."⁶⁸ Swift reported to Knightley Chetwode in 1725, "I have recovered my hearing for some time, at least recovered it so as not to be troublesome to those I converse with, but I shall never be famous for acuteness in that Sense."⁶⁹ Not long after, he wrote that Stella resents a disfiguring "Tetter in her Chin . . . in a manner very unbecoming her good Sense, and the Philosophy" that he "hoped [he] had taught her."[70] And he complained in a letter of 1727 to Henrietta Howard that his distracting tinnitus caused him to "write nonsense."[71] In the surviving letters, spanning more than fifty years, Swift and his correspondents used *sense* and *senses* in almost every way: "the faculties of physical sensation" (that is, the five senses), perception (with its emphasis on consciousness), and reason or sanity. These meanings shade imperceptibly into one another.[72] So it was with the disorders of Swift's body and mind. The chronic giddiness, deafness, and noise, coming convergently and unpredictably as they often did, disordered his physical senses and the intellectual faculties by which he sorted through and "made sense of" the external world and of his own feeling body.

Returning Swift to his humoral body, we can appreciate more fully the connections between disordered senses and disordered mind, as he himself knew them. By Swift's day, as we have seen, the common assumption that madness in its various forms was caused directly by humoral imbalance—that a superfluity of yellow bile (choler) caused frenzy and mania or an excess of black bile caused melancholy—was giving way to an iatromechanical model of pathology that connected mental illness with the nerves. Even then, because of the role of the fluid animal spirits in transmitting sensation, the new model of the body as machine driven by hydraulics neatly conjoined with the humoral narrative. The superfine animal spirits shuttled sensations through the conduit nerves to and from the brain: data from senses to brain in response to external stimuli, and commands from brain to body that governed movement and response to sensation.[73] George Berkeley said that they were "the Messengers, which running to and fro in the Nerves, preserve a Communication between the Soul and outward Objects."[74] The "rational soul" of which Berkeley speaks, unique to mankind, governed "inward senses" like the imagination and memory, and it controlled speech. Above all, says Roy Porter, "it was the seat of the will and understanding, mind and consciousness, of reason itself."[75] These higher faculties resided in the brain.

Crucially, in transmitting the data of eyes, ears, and other "external senses" through the nerves to the brain, the animal spirits mediated between outside world and reason. In his *Physical Dictionary* (first published in 1684), Steven Blankaart says that sensation itself is the process whereby "the Motion impressed by the outward Objects upon the Fibres of the Nerves is convey'd, by the help of the Animal Spirits in the Nerves, to the common Sensory" in the brain. This "*Sensorium Commune,* or the Seat of common Sense, is that part of the Brain in which the Nerves from the Organs of all the Senses are terminated, which is in the beginning of the *Medulla Oblongata.*"[76] It was seen as a kind of clearinghouse for sense impressions, which were then conveyed to the interdependent intellectual faculties (such as understanding, judgment, and memory). These faculties "made sense of" those impressions. The understanding, or awareness, perceived the data. The judgment sorted through and put the data into ideational categories; as the critical faculty, it made decisions based upon the information that it received. The memory was the faculty of mind by which, said Locke, "we revive again in our Minds those *Ideas,* which after imprinting have disappeared, or have been as it were laid aside out of Sight." As a "Store-house of our *Ideas,*" he added, memory is important because it allows us to "make appear again, and be the Objects of our Thoughts," the ideas impressed upon our understanding by sense experiences, "without the help of those sensible Qualities, which first imprinted them there."[77] The imagination (fancy), too, received and was stirred by sense impressions; it had the power to create images from remembered sense experience. But it was incumbent upon the "higher faculties" such as judgment to govern the imagination by selection and proper association of ideas.[78] Madness, as Swift metaphorized it famously in *A Tale of a Tub,* ensues "when a Man's Fancy gets *astride* on his Reason, when Imagination is at Cuffs with the Senses, and common Understanding, as well as common Sense, is Kickt out of Doors."[79] The higher faculties were crucial to seeing "reality" as it was and to maintaining sanity. In negotiating exchanges between the world outside and these higher faculties, the animal spirits had to function perfectly.

While the emphasis of psychopathology shifted from stomach to brain and nerves in the seventeenth and eighteenth centuries, it was nevertheless framed still by the humoral narrative. As in the explanations for deafness, a congestion of humors could compress the nerves and retard the flow of animal spirits, or the "nervous humour[s]" themselves could become too viscous for proper transmission.[80] Obstructions, compression, fouling of the fluid spirits, all were humoral disorders that resulted from improper concoction. Crude phlegm might clog or compress the tubular nerves; failure of concoction to attenuate the superfine animal spirits would make them sluggish. This fouling or obstructing of the animal spirits that negotiated exchanges between the world outside and the understanding would confuse and distort the objective "reality" that the individual perceived. And so, by humoral logic, the disorders of Swift's dyscrasial body—the excessive phlegm that clogged his head, deafened him, and made him spin in nauseating vertigo—disordered his senses and understanding. This befuddling of his wits (in every sense of that word) may have inspired fantastical perceptions, sights and sounds and new perspectives that few others could have imagined. It also terrified and discouraged him.

The humoral conjunction of mind and body mediated by animal spirits helps explain Swift's own conviction that his chronic giddiness, deafness, and tinnitus; occluded senses; failing memory; and confused understanding were all, comprehensively, humoral disorders—vitiation, superfluity, or obstruction of the fluid humors that together determined the health of body and mind. This conjunction helps explain, as well, his complaints about his "decayd" memory and understanding in his final decade. "Spirits, I have none left; my memory is almost gone," he wrote to his old friend John Barber in 1737.[81] To Pope, his compatriot in suffering, he grieved, "I have entirely lost my memory, uncapable of conversation by a cruel deafness . . . and I despair of any cure."[82] Preoccupied with the waning of his faculties, Swift was said by Edward Young to have pointed to the "much withered, and decayed" "uppermost branches" of a tree, musing aloud, "I shall be like that tree. I shall die at the top."[83] The purported self-prophecy takes on new meaning if we consider the adage of his day that men, like trees, "die upwards." Gideon Harvey, physician to both Charles II and James II, specifically connected this "dying upward" with the senses when he described the final stages of mortality, as the senses shut down one by one. Feeling is the last to go, said Harvey, beginning in the toes, "wherefore its Custamarily said, a Man Dieth upwards, that is from below, being farthest from the Brain . . . so that in course the Brain must Die last."[84] Swift's remark about dying "at the top," reported years after his death by Young, may be apocryphal. But flipping Harvey's claim that the senses die last further indicates Swift's anxieties about disordered senses that confused and terrified him. Young's remark supported Lord Orrery's recollection that Swift dreaded most the "utter deprivation of senses." It also fed into the biographical narrative that he devolved into madness and ended "deprived of reason."

By Swift's day, some had repudiated the idea that the nerves were hollow tubes that carried fluid spirits. In 1705, George Cheyne declared that the nerves "are a bundle of fine, small slender *Pipes,* wherein the Animal Spirits are treasur'd up for the Expenses of Motion and *Sensation*"; the "subtil" (super-refined) "*Liquid Nervorum*" mediated between mind and matter.[85] Some thirty years later, he dismissed the notions of tubular nerves and fluid spirits as absurd. There is no evidence of "any Cavity in the Substance of the *Nerves,* or in the small Filaments into which they are divided," said Cheyne, and the very "Notion of *animal Spirits* is of the same Leaven with the *substantial Forms* of *Aristotle,* and the *celestial System* of *Ptolemy.*"[86] Nevertheless, knowing that most of his reading audience still cherished the idea of nervous fluid, he found the term serviceable, attributing muscular movement to the "Integrity and innate Action of the *Nerves,* or *animal Spirits* (if you please)."[87] This idea of fluid animal spirits lived on conceptually and linguistically in descriptions of persons' "moods." As Porter says memorably, the mechanical model of the animal spirits shuttling sensations through hollow nerves "pictured depression and disorientation as corporeal plumbing failures. If the tubes became clogged—if, for instance, 'heavy' diet and low habits were indulged—the fluids grew sluggish, causing 'heaviness' and 'lowness.'"[88] Returning the word *spirits* to its literal meaning within the explanatory narrative of humoral psychophysiology helps us appreciate Swift's own anxieties about his cognitive disorders and fears of madness. His frequent complaints that his deafness is an "importunate Ailment that quite disspirits" him or that his persistent giddiness "keeps [him] low in Spirits and humor" register the early modern belief that the disordered senses disordered the intellectual faculties.[89]

Swift's humoral explanation for the chronic giddiness, deafness, tinnitus, and cognitive failings gave him one means of imposing narrative order on the disruptions of body and mind. In the explanations of how he contracted these problems, Swift also situates them in a life's narrative of disappointed social ambitions and sad resignation to the reality in which he found himself. The story of his illnesses is generically the progress tale undone. To give his personal sufferings significance beyond themselves, Swift also invoked biblical and family typologies, likening himself to the fallen Adam and to his own heroic grandfather, Thomas Swift.

The autobiographical fragment in which Swift explained the onset of his giddiness was an attempt to write the story of his own life; it is also ostensibly a progress tale. He presents himself as a young man who had great promise but who, his father dead before his birth, is insecure in both social status and means. That he should be recognized for his abilities by Sir William Temple, one of the most esteemed men of his day, fits neatly into Swift's own myth of exceptionalism. Here is a man who will distinguish himself and establish his social identity by his talents and industry. At the same time that it celebrates Swift's merits, however, the fragment is also a tale of threatened and disappointed promise, which ends abruptly with his bitter memory of having been passed over for a position that he felt he deserved. As his disorder imperiled his health, so it imperiled his social ambitions. Debilitated at Moor Park by the "giddyness and coldness of Stomach" contracted by the "Surfeit of fruit," Swift "returned to Ireld by advice of Physicians, who weakly imagined that his native air might be of some use to recover his Health."[90] This is the progress tale frustrated, ironically with a return to the Ireland that he spent most of his life trying to escape; as such, it fits into the pattern of disappointed hopes that is a running theme in his adulthood. Disappointed now in his age, Swift tells the story of how he contracted the chronic giddiness and deafness that confine him to the deanery. It is at once humoral narrative and emblem of his sad resignation to living out his days in a "land of slaves."[91]

Swift's story about gorging on forbidden fruit is also obviously a lapsarian fable about having forfeited his health with an original sin.[92] That Swift should be tempted throughout his life to ruin his humoral health with fruit that he "durst not eat," and be moved always to "repent" his lapses when he did, establishes biblical typology.[93] Reading the story of Swift's reckless gluttony, says Carole Fabricant, "we cannot help thinking of another fruit whose consumption had catastrophic consequences and marked the beginning of man's sufferings in a fallen world."[94] The disorders of Swift's humoral body thus have clear significance in the disordered world outside of himself. In his own way, then, Swift universalized his individual experience with illness by mythologizing it as theodicy. But even here, there is ambivalent self-reimagining. In the letter to Henrietta Howard in which he specifies having ravened upon a hundred golden pippins at a single sitting, he casts himself young again, unrestrained, appetitive, prodigious, and sexual. This self-representation, however facetious or self-ironic, was a way of remaking himself imaginatively in his aging and illness.

In the story of his illnesses that he tells in the autobiographical fragment, Swift also establishes important connections between himself and his grandfather Thomas, the Royalist clergyman who was perhaps his only untarnished idol throughout his life. This Thomas, father to the father Swift himself never knew, was persecuted for his heroic guerilla resistance to Cromwell during the Commonwealth and deprived of his livings. But he died in 1658, before he could be properly rewarded for his services to the Stuarts: "He dyed about two Years before the return of King Charles the Second, who by the reccommendations of some Prelates had promised if ever God should restore him, that he would promote Mr Swift in the Church, and otherways reward his family for . . . his extraordinary Services and zeal, and persecutions in the royal cause. But Mr Swifts merit dyed with himself."[95] Swift tells us that his heroic grandfather had been disinherited by his own mother, "a capricious ill-natured and passionate woman," "for no greater crime than that of robbing an orchard when he was a boy."[96] Cast unceremoniously into the world without parents, Thomas "never enjoyed more than a hundred pounds a year" in his village living.[97] Swift himself was ambivalent in his attitudes toward the Stuarts. He nevertheless admired his grandfather for his fierce convictions and heroic self-sacrifice on their behalf. In tracing the cause of his chronic disorder to his own youthful surfeit upon fruit, he links himself to the orchard thief.[98] Thus he establishes his own heroic lineage. Because Swift himself was disappointed in his own hopes for a clerical "settlement in ENGLAND," after which he always "panted," says Deane Swift, there is also perhaps social ascendancy in linking himself typologically with Thomas.[99] Yet he also reimagines his own disappointments in this connection. Like the grandfather whose sacrifices were unrewarded, so Swift felt that his own merits would die with himself, alone and forgotten in Ireland.

The stories that Swift told about his illness were important ways to impose order upon the disorders of his body. The humoral explanation not only gave narrative form to his personal sufferings but also gave his experiences larger meaning beyond themselves. Even if he could grumble that his case was like no other in "this whole Kingdom," Swift's claims of having contracted his giddiness and deafness through humoral negligence fit his disorders into a common story about diseases.[100] Years later, he could write to his fellow "Valetudinarian" Pope that his deafness was but a "common illness."[101] As the humoral narrative made sense of the physical disorders, so, too, did Swift's invoking of the progress tale, biblical myth, and family typology. His story of his illnesses did not map out the Providential plot of those like Robinson Crusoe and George Cheyne. Nevertheless, likening himself in his illnesses to the apple thieves Adam and his own grandfather Thomas, Swift gave his individual experiences as a sick person greater cultural and personal significance. Both the story of mankind's fall and that of his grandfather's sufferings were open-ended narratives: Fallen mankind was unredeemed; his grandfather's sufferings were unrewarded.

And Swift's chronic illnesses were never cured.

4

Help for the Humoral Body

Doctors and Friends

In an acute disorder, a critical event like a fever or, as with Swift's shingles, a skin eruption, would determine outcome; in chronic disorders, the pathogenic humor would become "settled" in the system.[1] Yet this difference was not absolute: It is too simplistic to say that the patient either recovered or died from the acute distemper while the chronic disorder was there to stay. George Cheyne, for one, held that the sufferer of chronic disorders could also recover "in a great measure, and to some very tolerable Degree, by *proper Remedies,* and a due *Regimen.*" "[I]f due Care be had, to follow timeously [that is, in good time] the Advice of an *honest* and *experienced Physician,*" said Cheyne, "a *Period* certainly may be brought about to most *chronical Distempers.*"[2] As we have seen, Swift did speak at times of recovery, a restoration of "perfect Health."[3] But increasingly he had to acknowledge, "My head is never perfectly free from giddiness," even when it was sometimes "moderate."[4] While he imagined at times that he had "perfectly cured [his] deafness," he had finally to admit that he could never fully recover his hearing: "My fears of relapsing hang over me, and very much take down my mettle."[5] Although the humoral explanation of his chronic giddiness, deafness, and tinnitus did allow Swift to impose some rational order on the disorders of an ever-shifting and permeable body, the only narrative closure for diseases he thought incurable was death itself.[6] Having "pursued" him from his youth, these were the illnesses, he dreaded, that would "at last get the better of" him.[7] At times, he saw death as the only relief to his sufferings: "I continue very ill with my Giddiness and Deafness, of which I had two Days intermission, but since worse," he wrote to Thomas

Sheridan in 1727, "and I shall be perfectly content if God shall please to call me away at this Time."[8] In the meantime, he had to learn how to *live* with his disorders and to control them the best he could by restoring or maintaining humoral balances. This and the following chapter, in turn, discuss the two broad measures that Swift took to do so: the "*proper Remedies,* and a due *Regimen*" of Cheyne's recommendation above. Availing himself of the resources available to him, Swift accepted medical interventions and advice from not only the trained physicians but also his lay friends and acquaintances. Throughout his long adult life, he also tried to discipline his "crasie" body with a strict regimen that regulated the non-naturals.

In his afflictions, Swift turned to the medical counsel and treatment of trained physicians such as William Cockburn, John Arbuthnot, and Richard Helsham, even when he was skeptical of their abilities. "I agree with your notions of Physick and Physicians," he wrote to Charles Ford, "and have as little faith in them as in Mahomet or the Pope."[9] That he should continue to consult the doctors even when he doubted their powers at first seems baffling. But he still had hopes—and he had other medical resources as well. As Lucinda Beier puts it succinctly, "There was no consensus that licensed healers were the sole authorities in medical matters" during the early modern era.[10] At the same time that he swallowed Cockburn's pills and John Radcliffe's bitters and grumblingly suffered their ministrations, Swift took the advice and medicines of well-heeled friends such as Lady Orkney and Lady Kerry; exchanged medical advice with correspondents; and resorted to home "receipts" like garlic cloves steeped in honey, which he inserted into his ear at the suggestion of his tailor. There was no contradiction of terms here. Because laypersons and trained physicians shared the same conception of the body and saw disease as humoral imbalance, medicine was not the exclusive province of the doctor. A solicitous friend could arguably make the same claim to cure as Cockburn or Arbuthnot. Everyone shared the belief that the object of any medical intervention was to assist nature in restoring humoral equilibrium.

As we have seen earlier, the new experimental philosophy of Boyle and Willis, chemical doctrines of Sylvius and van Helmont, and clinical teachings of Boerhaave at (Gulliver's own) Leyden did not dislodge humoralism as an epistemology or a practical system of diagnosing and treating disease.

In part, humoralism owed its persistence to its simplicity. The basic principle that disease was humoral imbalance could be understood by anyone, the learned and the "vulgar," the medically trained and the medically illiterate. Because of this shared understanding of the body and disease, there was, as Nicholas Jewson says, "epistemological parity" in the encounter between doctor and patient, and health was the mutual undertaking of the two.[11] And while the professionalizing of medicine and ascendancy of the clinic in the nineteenth century put the understanding of the body and authority over it largely in the hands of the doctor, a number of historians since the 1980s have returned the patients themselves to the center of the early modern medical encounter. As Roy Porter, Mary Fissell, and others have shown, British persons of the long eighteenth century, of both sexes and across the wide range of social classes, knew a great deal about health and sickness.[12] They consumed vernacular medical literature, debated theory and practice in the pages of popular periodicals such as the *Gentleman's Magazine*, exchanged medical receipts, and often acted as de facto physicians to family and friends.[13] The pursuit of health, say Dorothy and Roy Porter, "was everyone's business."[14] Laypersons no less than trained doctors practiced medicine and produced medical knowledge.

While there is no evidence that Swift himself studied "Physick" systematically, he boasted great medical literacy. For a man whose intellectual temperament had been conditioned by a classical tradition, medicine was part of the common stock of knowledge, not the exclusive property of a profession. On the evidence of the sale catalogue of his library after his death, Swift owned some thirty medical texts or books of medical interest.[15] We cannot know for certain which books he read. Cheyne's popular *Essay on Regimen*, for example, appeared in 1740 as Swift was slipping into senility; other works, such as Francis Glisson's *Anatomia Hepatis* (Anatomy of the liver), are curiously narrow. But the books in Swift's library do represent a wide range of medical knowledge and genres. Among others are the classical texts of Celsus and Dioscorides; anatomies by Thomas Gibson and the aforementioned Glisson;[16] books on fever by James Primerose and Thomas Sydenham; Thomas Fuller's Latin *Pharmacopoeia*;[17] Noel Chomel's *Dictionary Oeconomique*, a family encyclopedia that included recipes for home medicines; two different editions of the classic *Regimen Sanitatis Salernitanum* and the more recent regimen books of Cheyne; and less orthodox works by those such as Paracelsus and William Salmon. Among the pamphlets (and perhaps unbound sheets) in his library, Swift left behind "three Bundles" of "Physical and Anatomical Tracts," whose titles we can only guess. We know that at one time he also owned a copy of Hippocrates's works in Greek and Latin. He presented volumes of Galen's *Opera Omnia* to his cousin Martha Whiteway's son, Theophilus Harrison, a medical student. And he spoke of having read Galen's "Notes on Hippocrates."[18] Aside from the works that he owned, he doubtless read numerous others, either in the libraries of medical friends like his Irish physician Helsham or in the library at Trinity College.

Swift also read widely among Sir William Temple's books during his time at Moor Park between 1689 and 1699.[19] He was said to have devoted ten hours a day to studying in Temple's library.[20] Given his mentor's own medical interests, the two likely engaged in extensive conversation about such matters. After Temple's death in 1699, Swift edited his *Essay upon Health and Long Life,* which endorsed the classical dictum of consulting nature in all medical matters. Moreover, as we know from his satiric send-ups of iatromechanists and iatrochemists, Swift was familiar as well with the medical developments of the "Moderns," likely acquired not only from his reading but also from his frequent conversations with doctors such as Arbuthnot and Cockburn in London and Helsham in Dublin. The breadth of his medical literacy served him well in his works, both as he lampooned the follies of medicine and as he used medical language to diagnose the body politic. Perhaps as important as thinking about how Swift's medical reading became source material is thinking about how his extensive knowledge of the body and of medicine impelled his fierce autonomy. Bristling always at the attempts of others to expropriate individual liberties, he resisted surrendering authority over his own body to a medical profession quickly staking out its economic, social, and "scientific" ground. The more that he knew, the greater authority over his own body he could claim.

The feelings of most patients toward doctors in early modern Britain, especially medically literate patients like Swift, wavered between faith and misgivings. An exchange between Swift and his friend William Pulteney exemplifies this ambivalence. Toward the end of 1736, Pulteney wrote, "I am now, God be thanked, tolerably well in health again, and have done with all Physick and Water: drinking; My Constitution must certainly be a pretty good one, for it has resisted the attacks of five eminent Physicians for five months together, & I am not a jot the worse for any of them."[21]

Swift responded, "I agree heartily in your Opinion of Physicians, I have esteemed many of them as learned ingenious men, but I never received the least benefit from their Advice or Prescriptions[.] And poor Dr Arbuthnot was the onely man of the Faculty who seemed to understand my case but could not remedy it."[22] The exchange between Pulteney and Swift gives us a glimpse into attitudes toward doctors and medical interventions: The doctor himself was regarded equivocally, granted increasing authority in some circles but eyed suspiciously in others, as a necessary evil in a fallen modern world.

In his treatise on health and long life, Temple wrote that the increasing number of diseases in the world resulted from self-indulgence and negligence, a new culture of luxury, and the crowding of cities. In England, he said, health has been found "rather on the Peak of *Darbyshire*, and the Heaths of *Staffordshire*, than the fertile Soils of other Counties, that abound more in People and in Riches."[23] "All the great Cities . . . are the Scenes of the most frequent and violent Plagues, as well as other Diseases," he held.[24] In Temple's Golden Age tale, it was the fall and alienation of men from nature that had forced "the Use, and indeed the Necessity of Physick in great Towns and very populous Countries; which, remoter and more barren or desolate Places are scarce acquainted with."[25] This postlapsarian narrative that new diseases were the wages of a fall into physical vices, self-indulgence, and indolence was common at all social levels. In his popular mid-eighteenth-century *The London Tradesman*, Robert Campbell agreed with Temple that as "Vice and Immorality gained Ground, as Luxury and Laziness prevailed, and Men became Slaves to their own Appetites, new Affections grew up in their depraved Natures, new Diseases, and till then unheard of Distempers, both chronick and acute, assaulted their vitiated Blood. . . . Then Physicians became necessary."[26] The coming of the doctor was a function of the fall.

According to the classical medical narrative that persisted in the practice of Swift's day, the doctor was apprentice to nature.[27] His job was to assist and encourage the body in righting or maintaining the humoral balance appointed to the patient *by* nature. The physician should resort to medical "art"—that is, more intrusive interventions—only when the disease was too strong for the ministrations and corrections of nature itself. Temple wrote that "the first Excellence of a Physician's Skill and Care is discovered, by resolving, whether it be best in the Case, to administer any Physick or none, to trust to Nature or to Art: And the next to give such Prescriptions, as if they do no Good, may be sure to do no Harm."[28] Ideally, then, the doctor must first determine whether to rely upon nature or art. This decision depended upon the "*Semiotical* Part of Physick," the ability to diagnose and then predict the course and outcome of a disorder by reading the signs.[29] Therein lay the doctor's expertise. Having observed the "great Red Spots," "little Pimples . . . grown white & full of corruption," and confluent blisters on Swift's upper back, his London doctors of 1712 could make a diagnosis: "The Disease is th Shingles."[30] By reading the signs, they were able to make a confident prediction about the outcome of the disorder: "Th Doct[rs] say it would have ended in some violent Disease if it had not came out thus. I shall now recover fast."[31] It was the physician's ability to predict outcomes with his "Doctrine of Signs" that made him useful.[32]

While the physician could claim medical authority with his semiotics, patients could make claim to understanding their own humoral constitutions as well as the doctor; after all, they would know empirically what disorders they were prone to and how their humoral balances might be disrupted by various foods, physical movements, patterns of sleep, and so forth. A man like Swift might make some claim to self-diagnosis or self-treatment. During his shingles episode, he himself first made a tentative diagnosis of his shoulder pains as "something Rheumatick."[33] While we think of rheumatic disorders as joint disease, a "rheum" in humoral medicine was, more generally, a "defluxion," that is, the "abnormal or excessive flow of ill-digested humors," and a "rheumatick" disorder the body's attempt to expel such viscous humors.[34] Swift's self-diagnosis accords with humoral medicine. It was Swift, too, who "advised te D[r] to use [the confluent skin eruptions] like a Blister," which the physician might otherwise have induced artificially to encourage expulsion of the superfluous and vitiated choler that had disrupted his humoral balance.[35] Given the experience of living in one's own body, any individual, but especially a medically literate man like Swift, might be irked at the notion that "the doctor knows best." As he suggested in his letter to Pulteney, the practical matter of providing relief was at issue when one relied on medical specialists. Even the best doctors could not always cure their patients. Lady Betty Germain, typical of many laypersons of her day, wrote to Swift, "I am always more frighted when my friends are sick . . . because theres neither Physick nor Physician that's good for any thing."[36] Despite their best intentions and their best interventions,

Swift's own physicians could not seem to do anything to relieve his chronic disorders.

Worse than this skepticism about the doctors' practical abilities was the fear among medical consumers that doctors would do harm. However unjust to men of great integrity such as Arbuthnot and Helsham, the alleged cupidity and fatal ineptitude of physicians were favorite themes of satirists and comic dramatists. A running quip was that the doctors kill with impunity. "When a Nation abounds in Physicians," Joseph Addison gibed, "it grows thin of People."[37] Swift himself routinely satirized medical practitioners as hoodwinking charlatans; Scholastic fools; excrement-bedaubing Bedlamites; and, worse, murderers who "swarm to shew their mortal skill, / And by their college-arts methodically kill."[38] His comic and satiric representations of the doctors aside, he worried about the serious consequences that their interventions could have upon the state. Alarmed by reports of Queen Anne's health in the summer of 1711, Swift wrote in the *Journal to Stella*, "You must understand I have a mind to do a small thing, only turn out all the queen's physicians; for in my conscience they will soon kill her among them."[39] This was more than grumpy skepticism about the doctors' abilities: The health of the nation itself depended upon Anne's health; so, too, did Swift's own hopes for political preferment and social elevation.[40]

Despite his skepticism about the doctors, Swift allowed them some credit for their diagnostic and prognostic abilities. There is no reason to doubt that Gulliver speaks for the author himself when he declares of physicians that "one great Excellency in this Tribe is their Skill at *Prognosticks*."[41] Swift granted that Arbuthnot, at least, "seemed to understand [his] case." And if he sometimes ignored his doctors' orders, he was no therapeutic nihilist. However much he complained at times, he swallowed their pills and suffered their vomits, evacuations, and blisters, all intended to take off superfluous humors and right his humoral balances, especially when his own attempts to keep them in check failed. During his days in London, he frequently consulted physicians such as "honest Dr. Cockburn," even when he pretended reluctance to do so.[42] Having written to Stella and Dingley that he would consult Cockburn about his impaired hearing only "in compliance to [them]," he followed a month later, "I saw Dr. Cockburn to-day, and he promises to send me the pills that did me good last year, and likewise has promised me an oil for my ear, that he has been making for that ailment for somebody else."⁴³ And then early in 1711: "I . . . take drops of Dr. Cockburn, and I have just done a box of pills."⁴⁴ During those years in London, Swift consulted other physicians as well—the celebrated Radcliffe, for example, who prescribed "some herb-snuff" for his giddiness.⁴⁵ And he socialized with others such as Arbuthnot, Samuel Garth, and John Freind, all of whom certainly gave him passing medical advice.

In his later correspondence, Swift frequently talks of consulting doctors for his chronic ailments. "I have been for a month past so disordered with my old giddyness that I have put myself into the hands of Deally and taking daily medicines," he wrote from Dublin to Charles Ford in 1733.⁴⁶ Several months later, he apologized to Ford for not having responded to an earlier letter: "For I have been some months in a bad dispirited way with Deafness, and giddyness, and Fluxes. . . . I have been twice severely vomited, to the utmost I could possibly bear, but without amendment. I believe my disorder is particular, and out of the Experience of our Physicians here. Doc^{tr} Helsham the best of them is very kind and visits me constantly. My Spirits are quite broke."⁴⁷ "For fear of another Attack," Swift took precautionary measures. "I must fence [against such an attack] by taking Vomits and other Medicines prescribed for me by some Physicians who happen to be my Friends," he wrote to John Blachford.⁴⁸ Elsewhere he admitted that he had "been forced to confine [himself] to the Precepts of [his] Physicians."⁴⁹ If medicine was among the other "professions" that Swift claimed famously to have "ever hated," he nevertheless consulted the doctors, took their advice, and endured their sometimes violent treatments.⁵⁰

In his *Essay upon Health and Long Life*, Temple frowned that "the usual Practice of Physick among us runs still the same Course, and turns in a manner wholly upon Evacuation, either by Bleeding, Vomits, or some sorts of Purgation; though it be not often agreed among Physicians, in what Cases or what Degrees any of these are necessary."⁵¹ Against such extreme interventions, Temple pleaded that "'tis very probable that Nature knows her own Wants and Times so well, and so easily finds Her own Relief that way, as to need little Assistance, and not well to receive the common Violences that are offered Her."⁵² Ideally, then, the healthy body would excrete the superfluous or vitiated humors through natural means—daily evacuations of waste, "insensible perspiration" in sleep, "sensible perspiration" in vigorous exercise. And other "excrements" such as the blood from piles, from which Swift occasionally suffered, were also seen as the body's natural response to humoral imbalances. "I am glad you got the Piles," he wrote to Sheridan, "because it is a Mark of Health, and a strong Constitution."[53] A healthy constitution was the first and most reliable defense against humoral disorders.

Despite the Galenic ideal that the body expel excessive or corrupt humors naturally, we hear more often in Swift's correspondence of induced, sometimes violent evacuations, the medical intervention of which Temple chiefly complained. Such evacuations were standard treatment for acute illness. During the shingles episode, Swift wrote that he "must purge & cl[y]st^r" to encourage the body to expel the corrupt humors; the natural extrusion of choler through pus was not enough.[54] Later, he reported to Knightley Chetwode that after suffering miserably for a fortnight with an ague, he was able at last to venture out into the world "after vomiting, swe[a]ting and Jesuit's Bark."[55] But most often in Swift's correspondence, we hear about evacuations as interventions for his *chronic* ailments. If, as Cheyne wrote, "most *chronical* Diseases proceed from *Repletion*, as appears from their being cured by *Evacuation*," Swift's resorting to such measures followed humoral logic.[56] Humoral balance thrown off by repletion, it made sense to restore it by forcing the excesses—of food, drink, blood, humors—out of the system.

In *Gulliver's Travels,* Swift inventories the emetics and purgatives in the medical arsenal in revolting detail. The "Fundamental" of physicians, Gulliver tells his Houyhnhnm "Master,"

> is, that all Diseases arise from *Repletion;* from whence they conclude, that a great *Evacuation* of the Body is necessary, either through the natural Passage, or upwards at the Mouth. Their next Business is, from Herbs, Minerals, Gums, Oyls, Shells, Salts, Juices, Sea-weed, Excrements, Barks of Trees, Serpents, Toads, Frogs, Spiders, dead Mens Flesh and Bones, Beasts and Fishes, to form a Composition for Smell and Taste the most abominable, nauseous and detestable, that they can possibly contrive, which the Stomach immediately rejects with Loathing: And this they call a *Vomit.* Or else from the same Storehouse, with some other poysonous Additions, they command us to take in at the Orifice, *above* or *below,* (just as the Physician then happens to be disposed) a Medicine equally annoying and disgustful to the Bowels; which relaxing the Belly, drives down all before it: And this they call a *Purge,* or a *Clyster.*

The logic of these "Artists," says Gulliver, is "that in all Diseases Nature is forced out of her Seat" and that they must, in turn, forcibly restore natural balances by violent interventions.[57] Although Swift might nauseate his readers with the foul ingredients of the vomits and clysters, he draws from the medical practice of his day. Minerals and gums (sap from trees and shrubs), oils and bark, even animal excrements, numbered among remedies listed "in the London Dispensatory approved by the Physicians," which Swift claims to have consulted in his own distresses.[58] Yet for all of the loathsomeness of the purgatives, Swift himself turned often enough to them for relief of his own humoral excesses. "I have been much out of order of late with th old giddyness in my Head," he writes in the *Journal to Stella*. "I took a vomit for it 2 days ago, and will take another about a day or two hence."[59] Many years later, during his final visit to England in 1727, he told Sheridan, "I am now Deafer than ever you knew me, and yet a little less, I think, than I was Yesterday; but which is worse, about four Days ago my Giddiness seized me, and I was so very ill, that Yesterday I took a hearty Vomit, and though I now totter, yet I think I am a Thought better; but what will be the Event, I know not."[60] Although the blisters and pills, clysters, sweating medicines, and expectorants were sometimes violent, such measures were thought necessary to restore the individual constitution to its natural humoral balance.

Swift spoke once of having seen physicians' commonplace books that served the doctors in ministering to their patients because "they are Collections of Facts or Cases."[61] No doctors' notes on *his* case survive, and, aside from his own incidental, sometimes amused comments about their diagnoses and treatments, there is little documentation of what his physicians thought about his disorders. However, we get a fairly good idea of medical opinions about his chronic ailments and of professional interventions by looking at two letters from Arbuthnot. The first of these, in December 1718, came after Swift, now in Ireland to stay, had suffered a fit of giddiness lasting several months. On May 3 of that year, he noted in his account books, without further explanation, a "—terrible Fall G^d knows what may be th Event. bettr twards th End."[62] And in his accounts for this time, he listed among "Extr^{ds}" (extraordinary expenses) specific outlays for medicines: "Phys^k. 1^s-6^d" and "Bitt^{rs} 1^s-6^d" on May 17 and "Phisick 7^d" on August 28.[63]

If Swift complained directly to Arbuthnot about his ailments at this particular time, no correspondence survives.[64] But we know that a confraternity of anxious mutual English and Irish friends had exchanged notes on his health. Arbuthnot begins the first letter,

> Dear Brother
>
> for so I had call'd yow before were it not for a certain Reverence I pay to Deans, I find yow wish both me & your self to live to be old & Rich. the second gos in course along with the first; but yow cannot give 7 (that is the tith of 70) good reasons for either glad at my heart should I be if Dr Helsham or I could do yow any good.[65]

We do not know if Arbuthnot had ever met Helsham, Swift's friend and personal physician in Dublin, but he presents himself rhetorically here as one who has both respect for his fellow doctor and a mutual concern for Swift's health.[66]

While Arbuthnot was universally represented as an amiable and modest man, there is nevertheless a subtle vying for authority in this case, as he addresses Helsham indirectly, through Swift. He suggests that, while Helsham "dos not want my advise in the Case," he himself has had recent success with another patient "in that Complaint of a Vertigo" by prescribing "Cinnabar of Antimony & Castor, made up into Bolus's with Confect of Alkermes." He adds, "Small quantitys of Tinctur Sacr: now & then, will do yow good." Cinnabar of antimony, composed of mercury, sulphur, and antimony sublimate, was used as both a "salivating Medicine," to "dissolve, and evacuate the *Mucous* and *Coagulation* of the *Lympha*, by Dividing and Cutting the Parts asunder," and as a diaphoretic, to induce perspiration.[67] This was a heavy-metal compound, typical of chemical cures from the Paracelsian materia medica. In prescribing it, however, Arbuthnot follows the humoral logic of dislodging and expelling the superfluous or peccant humours thought to cause Swift's giddiness. Castor, an "odoriferous animal-substance" taken from the beaver, was "looked upon as one of the capital nervine and antihysteric medicines."[68] And the tinctura sacra ("Tinctur Sacr") was a name applied to a variety of cordials and electuaries, most used as purgatives but also regarded as a "sovereign Preservative" against seasonal "Distempers that affect the Head."[69]

Arbuthnot's second letter, of November 1730, includes a much more extensive set of prescriptions and instructions for taking them. While Swift had not complained any more than usual of his chronic disorders in the months before this letter, he did plead sickness several times as the reason that he could not visit his English friends, including Arbuthnot. "Nothing could keep me from seeing you but the dread of my deafness returning," he wrote to Pope in May 1730.[70] Then to Oxford's son Edward Harley in August he explained, "Neither my present condition of health, or private fortune will suffer me to make larger Journyes."[71] It may be, then, that Arbuthnot wrote to give Swift some hope that he might visit England again. His letter begins,

> The passage in Mr popes Letter about your health dos not Alarum me both of us have had this distemper these 30 years. I have found that Steel the warm Gumms & the Bark all do good in it. therefor first take the Vomit A then every day the Quantity of a Nutmeg in a Morning of the Electury markd B with five spoonfulls of the Tinctur Mark'd D. take the Tinctur; but not the Elect in the afternoon yow may take one of the pills marked C at any time when yow are troubld with it or 30 of the drops markd E in any vehicle evn water. I had a servant of my owin that was cur'd merely with vomiting. Ther is another med[icine] not mentiond which you may trye the pull Rad [Val] sylvestris about a scruple of it twice a day.[72]

Arbuthnot then inserts a list of the five prescriptions for compounds specified as letters A–E, followed by a recipe for a bitter tonic drink. (A transcription and explication of Arbuthnot's prescription appear in an appendix to this study.) "Mr popes Letter" has been lost, so we do not know whether this was correspondence from Pope to Arbuthnot or, as David Woolley suggests, a letter from Swift to Pope, in which Swift gave news of his health, which Pope imparted to Arbuthnot in turn.[73] Because of Arbuthnot's own claim that he had shared the particular "distemper these 30 years," such a letter would clearly help us understand his diagnosis of Swift's particular disorders.[74]

While an early twentieth-century physician suggests that "these receipts may possibly be useful to some patient troubled with the Dean's complaint of giddiness,"[75] the medicines, all commonly found in the materia medica of the day, were prescribed so broadly for such a wide range of disorders that it is impossible to work backwards from prescriptions to discrete diagnosis. Swift liked to think of himself as exceptional, even in his illnesses. During his shingles episode, he wrote to Stella and Dingley, "In answer to y^r good opinion of my Disease, te D^r s sd they never saw any thing so odd of the kind; they were not properly Shingles, but Herpes miliaris, and 20 other hard names. I can never be sick like oth^r People, but always something out of th common way."[76] And we recall his comment to Ford, "There is not one Patient in my case through this whole Kingdom."[77] However, Arbuthnot's prescriptions follow a standard course of treatment for treating *any* kind of humoral imbalance: first expelling noxious matter, then strengthening digestion for proper assimilation of the humors, and finally relieving the pressure of accumulated fluids that might cause Swift's giddiness, deafness, and noise in the ears.[78] As the humoral explanation for Swift's chronic maladies provided an intelligible narrative for imposing order on his disorders, so Arbuthnot's prescriptions wrote a therapeutic narrative in kind. If by definition Swift's case was like no other because his constitution was like no other, he was, in his humoral body, very ordinary.

No response from Swift to Arbuthnot's prescriptions survives. Despite their close friendship, communications between the two lapsed for two full years. It finally picked up again in December 1732 when Pope and Arbuthnot wrote to commiserate with Swift about the death of their mutual friend John Gay. Arbuthnot took the occasion to prod Swift, "I have not had the pleasure of a line from you these two years. I wrote one about your health, to which I had no answer."[79] We do not know whether Swift found any relief from his friend's prescriptions; we do know from the correspondence with Pulteney of early spring 1736–37 that even the beloved Arbuthnot, who had himself died two years earlier, could never provide lasting help. Whatever relief the doctors could give, they could not cure Swift.

His skepticism about the physicians may have had one source in what he saw as their inability to provide practical help. But it likely also came from the still-tenuous claims to professional authority that the trained doctors of his day made. Corporate histories of British medical practice, dating as far back as Charles Goodall's 1684 history of the Royal College of Physicians of London, claim as a matter of institutional faith that medical practice in early modern Britain was a neat, hierarchically organized and dutifully regulated profession.[80] It is by now a commonplace of medical history that this was never the case. Rather, as especially Harold Cook, Margaret Pelling, and Charles Webster have shown, medicine was a sprawling, eclectic jumble of practices and practitioners vying for authority and custom.[81] The physician-fellows of the Royal Colleges of London, Edinburgh, and

Ireland were nominal arbiters of medical authority, but their practical powers were always dubious. There were apothecaries and surgeons, licensed by corporate statute and guilded, who often crossed professional boundaries, diagnosing and prescribing independently of the doctors. There were graduates of the foreign universities such as Leyden, often with progressive clinical skills, who never bothered with licenses, which they thought irrelevant. There were any number of other practitioners heaped together and vilified in the corporate histories as "empiricks" and "quacks." And there were the family members, friends, and casual acquaintances about whom we have spoken before, all of whom claimed medical authority by experience, family traditions, and their own, often extensive reading around in medical literature.[82] Swift himself wrote to Stella and Dingley in late 1710 of the victory of his own medical opinion in the case of his friend Sir Andrew Fountaine. Fountaine was gravely ill and had called in Swift "to have prayers, which you know is the last thing." The attending doctors, who were "all in despair about him," thought that Fountaine could not possibly survive much longer. Still, says Swift, "I believed he would live; for I found the seeds of life in him, which I observe seldom fail." That same evening the patient "was mightily recovered," and when Swift predicted that he would "do well," "the doctor approved [his] reasons." Fountaine recovered, albeit slowly, from what Swift reported was "some sort of bile."[83] He lived another forty-three years.

Swift might shore up form and ritual against disorder in the world, but he did not scruple over niceties of medical licensing or academic training when it came to his own health. Like most other sick persons of his day, he looked for relief from his sufferings wherever he could find it. So, while he submitted to the doctors, he also took both advice and medicines from friends and other medical "laity." At the same time that he was downing Cockburn's pills in London, he was also swallowing a medicinal drink given him by Lady Kerry: "I . . . take drops of Dr. Cockburn, and I have just done a box of pills, and to-day lady Kerry sent me some of her bitter drink, which I design to take twice a day: and hope I shall grow better."[84] Indeed, he reports a week later, his head "has been much better these last five or six days, since [he has] taken lady Kerry's bitter" (he gives no such credit to Cockburn's pills).[85] Within a week, he says that he is drinking "Dr. Radcliffe's bitter, and will continue it."[86] Not long after, he writes to Stella and Dingley, "I have left off lady Kerry's bitter, and got another box of pills."[87]

Swift's approach to health here is experimental; he is testing medicines in the laboratory of his own body. Taking them from various sources that he trusts, he does not make mutual exclusions between professional and lay medicine.

Solicitous of his health, well-to-do friends in London offered Swift ready advice and medicaments. Some of these were violent purges and lead-based ointments, not merely tamer "dyet" drinks and bitters. In the spring of 1713, he reported to Stella and Dingley, "L^{dy} Orkney is gone out of Town to day: and I could not see her for Lazyness; but writ to her. She has left me some Physick."[88] "For oo must understand . . . Ldy Orkney is my Physician," he half-joked.[89] The physick in question was a strong purgative electuary, "Hiera picra 2 spoonfull, devilish Stuff." Taken "over night," it "works [him] next day" so that he is "forced to go home" after some brief business at court.[90]

Even Queen Anne herself was enlisted in the program to remedy Swift. When his giddiness sidelined him from social activities in September 1712, his particular friend, the royal favorite Abigail Masham, "made th Queen send to Kensington for some of her preserved Ginger for [him]."[91] Many years later, Swift was still taking the advice and medicines of his friends among the upper orders. In 1724 he asked that Ford convey his "most humble Acknoledgments to M. d. V. [Viscountess Bolingbroke] for her Receit": "I will certainly make use of [it], because I think there is more Virtue in her Influence, than in the Medicine it self."[92] I consider later how the concerns of the well-to-do for his health figured prominently in the ways that Swift reimagined himself socially in his illnesses. For now, it is enough to know that these were among the many nonprofessionals from whom he took medical advice.

Swift never hesitated to take suggestions from his acquaintances among the middle and lower orders as well. Having run out of the popular liniment Hungary water for rubbing into his painful shoulder during his shingles episode, he resorted to "Spirits of wine, w^{ch} [his] Landlady" told him was "very good."[93] For his chronic disorders, he likewise accepted the advice of those from all social orders. In the spring of 1722, he thought that he had found a cure at last for his intermittent deafness: "I thank God for some time past I am pretty well recovered, and am able to hear my Friends without danger of putting them into Consumptions. My Remedy was given me by my Tayler, who had been four years deaf, and cured himself as I have done, by a Clove of Garlic steeped in honey and put into his Ear, for wch I gave him half a Crown after it had cost me 5 or 6 Pounds in Drugs and Doctors to no purpose."[94] While the tailor's recommendation sounds like homespun lore, the garlic-honey cure for impaired hearing appears routinely in both folk medicine and learned physic of Swift's day. Among others who advised the remedy was John Wesley. In his book of natural healing, *Primitive Physick*, he urged those suffering "DEAFNESS with *Head-ach* and *Buzzing* in the *Head*," "Peel a Clove of *Garlick*; dip it in *Honey*, and put it into your Ear at Night with a little black Wool. Lie with that Ear uppermost. Put the same in the other Ear the next Night. Do this, if need be, eight or ten days."[95] Learned physicians also endorsed the use of both garlic and honey for deafness, even late into the century. In the authoritative *Edinburgh New Dispensatory*, William Lewis noted that "some have recommended, in certain cases of deafness, the introduction of a single clove, wrapt in thin muslin or gauze, into the meatus auditorus."[96] Honey, like garlic, "is very penetrating and deterging," said the apothecary John Quincy, "and is therefore good in all Obstructions, especially from viscid and tough Humours [like concretions of earwax].... [T]here is no Disorder from *Phlegm*, or any thing which is the Produce of a cold Constitution, which it is not of service in."[97] The lesson is that despite any imagined divide between the "empiricism" of folk medicine and the "reason" of learned medicine, the cures were often the same, even if framed in different epistemologies.[98] A sufferer such as Swift, looking for relief from any quarter, would not have quibbled over who had intellectual authority.

5

Disciplining the Humoral Body

Swift's Regimen

In the hands of Galenic practitioners of the kind that Temple celebrated, medical intervention was never intended as an independent means of cure. Rather, it was expedient to the greater goal of restoring natural humoral balances, preferably by prodding the system gently to right itself but, if need be, by shocking the stubborn body into submission or dislodging recalcitrant settled disorders. However, because chronic disorders like Swift's were attributable, finally, to a humoral constitution weakened by heredity or disease, or ruined by dissolute habits, they could rarely be fully cured. Any recovery, cautioned Cheyne, demanded "long Time, much Care, and great Caution, unwearied Patience and Perseverance, and so long a Course of *Self-denial*, as few People are willing to undergo."[1] Even for the most disciplined patients, some chronic diseases are "such, either by having gone *too far*, or by being *Hereditary*, and interwoven into the *Principles of Life*, as never to be totally overcome."[2] Cheyne, who made a business of writing regimen books, advised that the unfortunate sufferers of chronic disorders try their utmost to maintain or restore balance in their own bodies. Individuals might swallow the medicines and submit to the treatments of medical practitioners and solicitous friends, but because they presumably knew their own constitutions better than anyone else, self-governance in matters of humoral health was a practical imperative.

In the letter to Swift about having survived the assaults of "five eminent Physicians for five months together," William Pulteney vowed that he was done with the doctors: "For the future I will preserve my self by your advice, and follow your Rules, of rising early, eating little, drinking less, and riding daily. I hope this Regimen will long be of use to both of us, and that we may live to meet again."[3] Swift congratulated him and presented himself comically as doctor: "To conquer five Physicians all eminent in their Way was a victory that Alexander and Cesar could never pretend to. I desire that my Prescription of living may be published, which you design to follow, for the benefit of Mankind."[4] If Swift's own strict course of diet and exercise seemed at times medical zealotry, however, his "Prescription of living" was hardly a proprietary secret that might be published "for the Benefit of Mankind." As early as the fourth century BCE, Hippocratic writers had urged that patients follow a systematic plan of eating, drinking, and exercising to maintain or restore humoral balances. Centuries later, Galen had codified regimen as a central article of "hygiene"—the pursuit of health.[5] The *Regimen Sanitatis Salernitanum*, dating to the twelfth or thirteenth century and appearing in a number of English translations in the sixteenth and seventeenth centuries, had systematized Galenic rules for maintaining humoral balances.[6] And in the long eighteenth century, regimen books addressed *ad populum* battened upon a new breed of medically literate men and women and a culture of self-determinism in matters of health. Cheyne's *An Essay of Health and Long Life* (1724) had been through eleven London "editions" (reissues) by mid-century; his *The English Malady* (1733), which touted a "milk-seed" diet, went through six reissues in its first two years. Aside from two different early seventeenth-century editions of the *Regimen Sanitatis Salernitanum*, Swift himself owned copies of both *The English Malady* and Cheyne's later *An Essay on Regimen*.[7]

In trying to restore humoral balances appointed by nature, the individual was advised especially by popular regimen books to regulate the six earlier-mentioned non-naturals: air, diet, sleep, exercise, evacuation and retention of excrements, and the passions.[8] Because the designation "non-naturals" seems odd in the context of restoring *natural* balances, Cheyne speculated that "they are so called, possibly because that in their preternatural State they are eminently injurious to human *Constitutions;* or more *probably,* because tho' they be necessary to the Subsistence of *Man,* yet in respect of *him,* they may be considered as *external,* or different from the *internal* Causes that produce *Diseases.*"[9] In their advice to individuals who would govern these variables, regimen authors typically devoted a separate section to each of the six health factors. The medieval *Regimen Sanitatis Salernitanum* that Swift owned is organized around the non-naturals. Cheyne,

Arbuthnot, and many other regimen writers of the long eighteenth century continued to organize their own books around the same non-naturals. Discussion of these qualities in the established genre of the regimen book thus served a structural purpose as well as a medical one.

The popularity of medical self-help books tells us that Swift's own devotion to regimen was nothing unusual for his time.[10] In observing a strict regimen that aimed to regulate the non-naturals, Swift was like so many others of the day who tried to manage their chronic illnesses. Like them, he conformed to beliefs about hygiene that had persisted since the days of Hippocrates and Galen. But he also found in regimen those habits that suited his own temperament and inclinations: physical discipline, performative rituals, and the enforcement of order in the world. With regimen, Swift sought to rule over the anarchic body. That he should rely increasingly, even obsessively, upon exercise in imposing his will upon that body tells us as much about his character as it does about his understanding of his constitution and of disease. Walking, running, riding, rowing, and swimming might shake loose the improperly digested phlegm that clogged his senses and dizzied him; perspiration might carry it out of the body. Strenuous physical exertion, though, was also the natural occupation of a person who seems always to have been in motion, a man who could not sit still. That he ignored the advice of his physicians, who worried that he exercised too much, also says much about Swift's personality. His flouting of the doctors' warnings was an act of defiance against their attempts to appropriate authority over his body. "Fig for your Physician and his advice, madam Dd [Dingley]," he had written in the *Journal to Stella*; "if I grow worse, I will; otherwise I will trust to temperance and exercise."[11]

In a letter of 1736, Thomas Sheridan entreated Swift to preserve his life by following a strict regimen:

> I would have written last post, but I had such a violent head ach, that I could no more think than a cabbage. And now all the business I have is to make you a paper visit, only to ask you, how you do? You may think me impertinent for the question; but when I tell you, that I have not above three friends, you will not wonder that I should be afraid of losing one of them; and therefore I must give you some rules of regimen.

1. Walk little and moderately.
2. Ride slow and often.
3. Keep your temper even with my friend Mrs. Whiteway.
4. Do not strain your voice.
5. Fret not at your servants blunders.
6. Take a chearful glass.
7. Study as little as possible.
8. Find out a merry fellow, and be much with him.

Get these precepts by heart, and observe them strictly, and my life for yours we shall see better times in the next century.[12]

Even without benefit of Sheridan's good-humored advice, the evidence of Swift's attempts to maintain or restore humoral balances by regulating the non-naturals is everywhere in his correspondence. In the *Journal to Stella*, Swift writes, "I never impute any illness or health I have to good or ill weather, but to want of exercise, or ill air, or something I have eaten, or hard study, or sitting up; and so I fence against those as well as I can: but who a deuce can help the weather?"[13] The statement could well serve as an epigraph for discussing Swift's lifelong observance of a regimen in pursuit of health. Not only does he explicitly associate four of the non-naturals with his own health—exercise, air, diet, and sleep—but he also invokes here the self-responsibility that moralizes humoral medicine: The individual must calibrate the balances of his own permeable body in the environment and cannot blame the environment itself ("good or ill weather," for example) for his ill health.

Swift's own concerns with regulating the non-naturals were deeply inscribed in his daily life. These were often interdependent. Proper food and drink determined sleep; sleep promoted evacuation of "insensible perspiration"; exercise aided digestion and encouraged proper evacuations; and exercise also brought Swift out into the open air. It is difficult, therefore, to extract his attention to the non-naturals individually from the more comprehensive regimen that he observed. Attempting to do so is nevertheless instructive. Situating Swift's attention to the non-naturals in both the theory and practical advice of regimen authors shows how his own daily habits conformed with the classical humoral medicine that persisted well beyond the new discoveries of the experimental philosophy. It gives us a better sense of the experiences of living with chronic illnesses, in a daily war of will and body. Putting each of the non-naturals in comparative relief with the others that he struggled to regulate tells us much about his character, too, especially his sometimes bizarre self-contradictions, restless nature, and stubborn resistance to authority.

Swift, we find, turned increasingly to diet and exercise in his attempts to alleviate his chronic disorders. Yet attention to the other non-naturals—air, rest, evacuations and retentions, and the passions—is also scattered throughout his correspondence. He was well aware, for example, of the importance of clean air to his health; predictably, this is often associated with the country. "I never wanted so much a little country air, being plagued with perpetual Colds & twenty Aylments," he wrote to Knightley Chetwode from Dublin in 1714.[14] On the prospect of a tour of the countryside in 1719, he claimed that he was "going to try a more lazy Remedy of Irish Country Air."[15] Writing to Sheridan during his final visit to England, in 1727, Swift reported, "I continue very ill with my Giddiness and Deafness. . . . I have mentioned the Case as well as I knew it, to a Physician who is my Friend; and I find his Methods were the same, Air, and Exercise, and at last Asses-Milk."[16] In his early biography, Deane Swift wrote of his cousin that in "his character as Dean of St. Patrick's, he was perfectly regular and exemplary" in attending services every morning. But his "physicians, long before his death," worried about the dampness of the cathedral air during winter and "pressed him" to avoid going every single morning. Characteristically stubborn, Swift "continued his old practice for a great while, in spight of their remonstrances, until he found by repeated colds and experience, that he could bear it no longer."[17] The advice of his doctors and Swift's own hard experience conform with humoral theory. Because the body was permeable in its environment, the individual had to take care not to expose himself to ambient air that might poison the system or disrupt the humoral balance. Especially for a man who attributed his chronic disorders to the accumulation of phlegm, sallying out into cold, wet air was ill-advised.

Swift also knew the value of getting proper sleep for managing his disorders. "I remember old Culpepper's maxim," he wrote to Stella and Dingley: "Would you have a settled *head,* You must early go to bed: I tell you and I tell't again, You must be in bed at ten."[18] Lack of sleep might disrupt his daily activities: "This day has gone all wrong, by sitting up so late last night."[19] It might also upset the appetite and digestion so crucial to humoral health. His sleeping schedule thrown badly off one day, after a midday nap to "mend [his] night's sleep," Swift "sent for a bit of mutton and pot of ale from the next cook's shop, and had no stomach."[20] In 1716, he wrote to Thomas Walls, "I sate up till four this morning writing Dispatches. . . . and am now in no Condition to write, being quite disorderd with scribbling over a dozen Letters at a Heat, and want of sleep, which I shall endeavour to make up after I have answered some Parts of y^r Lettr."[21] Years later, he complained to Alexander Pope, "My state of health is not to boast of; my giddiness is more or less too constant. . . . I sleep ill, and have a poor appetite."[22] Like his aim of taking in pure air for health, Swift's aim of getting proper sleep also conformed with humoral theory. The physician Richard Brookes wrote that it "is not possible for those to preserve their Health, who do not go to sleep in a regular Manner; for Sleep repairs the Spirits, which are dissipated by watching; and consequently it restores the Strength of those who are weak, indisposed, or labour much; it likewise promotes Perspiration, contributes greatly to Digestion, and more to Nutrition."[23] Sleep not only restored the body but also encouraged the excretion of excess humors.

While Swift talked often of taking vomits, sudorifics, and various purgatives, we usually cannot tell if these were special interventions during times of particular distress or routine medicines taken to regulate evacuations in his daily regimen. Swift's account books, which occasionally note medical expenses, do not help much here, as they do not show regular outlays for purges and clysters. Most of the purges and clysters about which Swift does speak seem to have been not a routine part of his daily regimen but medical interventions that he suffered during his fits of chronic giddiness and deafness. We do not, in fact, know how Swift's concerns about retentions and evacuations figured into his daily regimen. But evacuations were closely tied to sleep, diet, and exercise. During sleep, "insensible perspiration," the imperceptible excretion of moisture as vapor, took off excess humors. The Italian iatrophysicist Sanctorius, whose book of aphorisms about the non-naturals numbered among the volumes in Swift's library, claimed that "at least, three Pound of Excrement" was eliminated through insensible perspiration every night.[24] Obviously, a diet proper to one's particular constitution would also affect regular evacuation of excrements. In exercise, too, especially the vigorous kind that Swift undertook, "sensible Discharges" took off noxious and superfluous humors.[25]

Perhaps the most slippery of the non-naturals were the "Passions" or "Affections of the Mind"—emotions like "Joy, Sorrow, Anger, Love, Hate,

Envy, Hope and Despair"—which were thought to affect the body as much as somatic disorders.[26] Medical writers warned that any excess of passion, a pleasant one no less than a pernicious one, would upset the humoral balance. "You see, Sir," wrote a "Physician in London" to his friend, "with what Efficacy the Affections of the Mind work upon the Body; therefore it is as necessary for Health to hold a Mean and Moderation in them, as in the five other forenamed [non-naturals]."[27] Aware of the tax that immoderate passions levied against his health, the oft-outraged Swift himself spoke occasionally of trying to regulate his own. Although he had "as much Provocation to it as any man alive," he pointedly tried to avoid "th Spleen," that protean disorder that was variously a medical condition—an excess of humors that manifested as anger or depression—and a simple feeling or expression of pique, ill humor, or testiness.[28] Swift tried as well to regulate his political passions: "A Man without Passions might find very strong Amusements," he said of the Whig-Tory "Scituation." "But I find the turn of Blood at 50 disposes me strongly to Fears, and therefore I think as little of Publick Affairs as I can."[29] Swift might claim to restrain his political passions, but he was a man of famously volatile emotions, embattled against the world, who vented his rage and outrage at political opponents and human folly, even if refracting them through irony and comic misdirection helped him to manage those passions. Acquaintances like Pilkington presented him as mercurial and irascible, given to unpredictable fits of pique, even cruelty. Patrick Delany attributed the eventual "decay in his understanding" to "that sourness of temper which his disappointments first created in him: and the indulgence of his passions perpetually increased."[30] Swift himself wrote, "Our Passions are like Convulsion Fits, which tho' they make us stronger for the Time, leave us the weaker ever after."[31] Even acknowledging this, he continued to snarl into his final years in "Rage and Rancour against Persons and Proceedings."[32] To avoid humoral disaster, the Dean had to control his passions as he did any of the other non-naturals.

While Swift understood that regulating air, rest, evacuation and retention of excrements, and the passions was important to his health, his attention to the non-naturals focused mostly on diet and exercise, likely for several reasons. First was the simple logic of humoral digestion. If most disease could be traced to the imperfect attenuation of the humors, regulating both the types and the quantities of food and drink was obviously important. Swift had, after all, attributed the overthrow of his very constitution to his reckless gluttonizing on cold, wet fruit. Exercise, too, was crucial to health, since vigorous movement broke down the fluids and made "a great deal of Perspirable Matter . . . ready for Expulsion."[33] Sweat then took off excess humors that might otherwise accumulate in the body. Second, of all the non-naturals, diet and exercise are the most easily quantifiable. The satirist who knew so well the psychology of projectors and statisticians also kept his own meticulous household accounts, exhaustively inventoried dressing rooms in his poems, and even tallied grievances and debts of gratitude. Swift might not weigh his daily intake and excrements or calculate the volume of his perspiration obsessively, as did Sanctorius.[34] Yet some general accounting of (and for) the amount of wine that he drank or the number of miles that he rode and walked structured his daily life. Finally, the exercise that was the preoccupation of his regimen—walking, riding, running, rowing—was both a way to contain a restless nature and a performance of his masculinity. There were times of isolation and dejection when he had to admit sadly that he had become a "Valetudinarian." These, however, were poised always against self-representations of bluff, hardy, athletic vigor. His obsessive exercising was affirmation of sexual vitality, even into his final years.

In a letter to Pope, George Lyttelton joked that while "the immortal Doctor Cheyney" would "live at least two centuries by being a Real and practical Philosopher," Swift, as a "Gluttonous Pretender" to the philosophy of a strict regimen, would "die of Eating and Drinking at [merely] fourscore."[35] If Swift worried at times that he was growing fat, he never resorted to the radical milk-seed diet by which the behemoth Cheyne reduced his weight from thirty-two stone (448 pounds) to a still-formidable three hundred pounds.[36] Still, in trying to manage his own humoral body, Swift followed a regimen of moderation in food and drink throughout his adult life. "I ate nothing but herrings," he reported of one dinner with the Vanhomrighs in London: "You must know I hardly ever eat above one thing, and that the plainest ordinary meat at table; I love it best, and believe it wholesomest."[37] Especially during fits of giddiness, he ate foods thought to be easily digestible. "My head is not in order, and yet it is not absolutely ill, but giddyish," he wrote to Stella and Dingley in January 1710–11. "I am very temperate, and eat of the easiest meats as I am directed."[38] Later that spring, he reflected upon a recent fit, "My head . . . is better; but to be giddyish three or four days together mortified me." Having vowed to "be very regular in eating little and the gentlest meats," he could say at day's end, "God be thanked, I am much better than I was, though something of a totterer. I ate but little to-day, and of the gentlest meat. I refused ham and pigeons, pease-soup, stewed beef, cold salmon, because they were too strong."[39] "All victuals are equal to my affections," Swift wrote later in life, "yet I dare not meddle with strong meats."[40] Managing the sick body meant eating food that his cold stomach could properly digest, to avoid the humoral crudities that would clog the system.[41]

During the shingles episode, Swift wrote that he lived on a liquid diet: "I eat nothing but Water gruell."[42] And suffering a painful midlife visitation of strangulated hemorrhoids, he recounted, "I fell into a cruel Disorder that kept me in Torture for a Week. . . . the Learned call it the Hæmorrhoides internæ which with the attendance of Strangury, loss of Blood, water-gruel and no sleep require more of the Stoick than I am Master of, to support it."[43] The thin, cool diet of water gruel in these acute disorders encouraged the expulsion of the hot, acrid humors. Because of the importance of digestion to maintaining humoral balance, suiting the quantity and type of food and drink to one's constitution and condition was as important in *chronic* disorders. Cheyne exhorted the chronic sufferer to follow "a strict Regimen of a *thin, fluid,* spare and lean Diet."[44] Swift followed this advice in trying to manage his giddiness, deafness, and tinnitus: "I thank God, [I] am much better in my head. . . . My breakfast is milk porridge: I don't love it, faith, I hate it, but 'tis cheap and wholesome."[45] Famously parsimonious, Swift had a medical rationalization for eating frugally. Household economy aside, his thin diet conformed with humoral logic. In eating the "gentlest" meats, Swift was implicitly following the authorities' prescription that the diet for a man in his condition be "of a light and easy Digestion" and so more easily assimilable into the body.[46] His recourse to water gruel and milk porridge for both acute and chronic diseases followed the logic that an "attenuating" diet would prevent or thin any "Viscidities," accumulated humors, or concretions in the body so that they could be expelled as excrements.

In his correspondence, Swift and his friends often discussed what they drank as a matter of health.[47] The relative value of various kinds of milk was of particular interest. John Barber, who frequently exchanged notes on health with Swift, wrote of his asthma in 1738, "I impute my being so much better to my drinking constantly the asses milk, which is the best specifick we have. I wish to God you would try it, I am sure it would do you much good."⁴⁸ Indeed doctors of the day widely recommended ass's milk, which is, said one writer on gout, "of all the thinnest, next to human."⁴⁹ In other words, observing the principle of matching like with like in nature, it could more easily be attenuated during digestion in the human body. Extending this humoral doctrine to its logical end, some suggested drinking woman's milk. The celebrated Dutch physician Gerard van Swieten wrote, about mid-century, "Of the several kinds of milk, the best of all . . . is human milk, as being most analogous to our nature, and is therefore always to be preferred to that of all other animals."⁵⁰ In the simple logic of humoralism, human milk was most natural to humans and, therefore, most easily assimilable. Accordingly, Lord Bathurst urged that Swift himself drink a woman's milk, claiming that it would both "cool" the Dean's fiery satiric temper, which had savaged the ironmonger Wood in *The Drapier's Letters*, and relieve his giddiness. Bathurst suggested that Swift "contrive some way or other" to have as his only servant "one sound wholesome wench" who "shou'd have milk": "I can assure yᵘ it is the opinion of some of the best Phisitians that womans milk is the wholesomest food in the world."⁵¹ How Bathurst would have Swift "contrive" that his servant "shou'd have milk" we can only guess. Swift responded with a wink to Bathurst's sexual innuendo: "My old Presbyterian Tory house keeper . . . will not suffer a femal[e] in the house who is younger than her self, under pretence that if it were otherwise, my men and the maids together would multiply my family too much." Nevertheless, he added, "I have gotten into your direction about milk, onely with the addition of a little rice, sugar and nutmeg, in which I hope you will be so good as to indulge me."⁵² He seems to have respected the humoral logic behind drinking human milk enough to advise that Pope do so in his infirmities: "I am glad you are got into Asses milk. It is a remedy I have a great opinion of, and wish you had taken it sooner"; "My old Presbyterian House keeper tells me, that if you could bring your Stomach to woman's Milk, it would be far better then Asses."⁵³ There is nothing to suggest here that he is not being serious.

Wine was Swift's preferred drink, even when he claimed to dislike it. "I drink less than usual," he wrote to Pope in 1733, "but to drink so little as you or my Lord Bol—is not to be expected; and yet I do not love wine, but take it purely as a medicine."⁵⁴ The next year, he reported to Arbuthnot, "I drink a bottle of French wine myself every day, though I love it not; but it is the onely thing that keeps me out of pain."⁵⁵ Swift might claim not to love wine, but he routinely drank a bottle daily. "I drink a pint and half of wine every day," he wrote to Pope, "the pint at noon, & the half at night."[56] And to Barber: "My chief support is French wine, which although not equal to yours, I drink a bottle to my self every day."[57] Afflicted with "cold" disorders, Swift believed that wine warmed his stomach and thereby aided digestion. "Wine is good for me," he wrote again to Barber. "I drink a Bottle to my own share every day, to bring some heat into my Stomach."[58] He frequently folded reports of wine-drinking into discussions of his health: "My disorders, with the help of years, make wine absolutely necessary to support me."[59] Drinking wine, he believed, preserved his very life. "I am sorry it should cost you two pence to have account of my health, which is not worth a penny," he wrote to a fellow clergyman in 1735, "yet I struggle, and ride, and walk, and am temperate, and drink wine on purpose to delay, or make abortive, those schemes proposed for a successor."[60] Prolonging his life by drinking wine, he smirked, would frustrate the ambitions of any younger clergyman eyeing his position as Dean of St. Patrick's.

In matters of food and drink, said Temple, "all Excess is to be avoided, especially in the common Use of Wine: Whereof, the first Glass may pass for Health, the second for good Humour, the third for our Friends; But the fourth is for our Enemies," presumably because that fourth, immoderate glass will hasten one's demise.[61] Following Temple's advice, Swift always aimed at temperance in drinking and in his other habits. "I am now resolved to drink ten times less than before," he vowed to Stella and Dingley in 1711.[62] Perhaps with his own reckless gorging upon apples in mind, he clucked at the immoderate habits of others. "I am griev'd to hear that my Lord Bolingbroke's ill health forc'd him to the Bath," Swift wrote to Pope. "Tell me, is not Temperance a necessary virtue for great men, since it is the parent of Ease and Liberty?"[63] He enjoined Charles Ford, often the target of his pleas for moderation, "I beg you will force your nature as much as possible upon temperance and exercise, I mean temperance in a physicall sense."[64] Years later, he wrote to Ford, "I was and am more temperate than You. I do not value long life; but, while it continueth, I endeavor to make it tolerable by Temperance."[65] Temperance was both moral restraint and humoral prudence.

Swift's lifelong love-hate relationship with fruit brings into sharp relief the contest between appetite and regimen for rule of the body. We know of his conviction that his youthful gluttonizing on raw apples had caused his initial attack of giddiness. Although Swift loved fruit, he vowed to avoid it. "I envy people maunching and maunching peaches and grapes, and I not daring to eat a bit," he wrote to Stella and Dingley.[66] And to Thomas Sheridan many years later: "I will be very Temperate; and in the midst of Peaches, Figs, Nectarins, and Mulberries, I touch not a bit."[67] With his lapses came relapses of the chronic disorders. "I eat some Kentish cherries t'other day, and I repent it already," he confessed. "I have felt my head a little disordered."[68] Reporting later that he had "been much out of order of late with th old giddyness in [his] Head," Swift wrote to the ladies, "I have eat mighty little Fruit, yet I impute my disorder to that little, and shall henceforth wholly forbear it."[69] Many years later, he still blamed his ailments on his weakness for fruit. "I have been this ten Days inclining to my old Disease of Giddiness, a little Tottering," he wrote to Sheridan in 1727. "Cyder and Champagne and Fruit have been the Cause."[70] In these confessions and resolutions, scattered throughout many years of correspondence, is an anguished battle between appetite and self-denial.

Swift, of course, would never have seen his own daily labor to maintain humoral balances by minding what he ate and drank as an abstract battle between will and desire playing out in the contested site of his body, or his denial of fruit as emblematic of what Carol Houlihan Flynn has called his "fascinated revulsion towards the physical."[71] Nor, despite his preoccupation with maintaining order in the world, would he have seen his regimen as a means of containing unruly matter itself. Even if the humoral explanation of his disease helped Swift make sense of his individual sufferings and the therapeutic regimen was a measure of imposing order on a disordered body, he did not see himself and his experiences as a sick man in terms of a grand cultural metanarrative. For Swift, regimen was functional and commonsensical. Afflicted with chronic, episodic bouts of giddiness, deafness, and tinnitus, he took what practical steps he could to restore humoral balances and relieve those disorders.

Swift might make claims to temperance in diet and drink. But both friends and doctors worried, especially in his later years, that he had become obsessive in his exercising. Certainly, he worked to regulate the other non-naturals in "fencing" against his chronic disorders. It was exercise, however, that became the preoccupation of his lifelong regimen. Walking, running, riding, rowing, even swimming (a rare spectacle in his day)—these were habits that kept him always in motion, from his early adulthood to the very end of his life, even after he had slipped into senility. Despite the chronic infirmities that afflicted Swift from his twenties, he was athletic and vigorous. Deane Swift says of him, "His constitution was strong, and his limbs were active." And he was unusually agile and robust: "Upon his own feet he ran like a buck from one place to another. Gates, styles, and quicksets, he no more valued than if they had been so many straws."[72] During his time with Sir William Temple between 1689 and 1699, Swift "spent ten hours a day . . . in hard study." But every two hours he would break for exercise, running "up a hill that was near Sir W. TEMPLE'S, and back again to his study; this exercise he performed in about six minutes: backwards and forwards it was about half a mile."[73] If this image of Swift in motion seems amusing, later accounts that he trotted horse-like are even more so. "The Dean walked, or rather trolled, as hard as ever he could drive," recalled Lætitia Pilkington. "I could not help smiling at his odd Gait, for I thought to myself, he had written so much in Praise of Horses, that he was resolved to imitate them as nearly as he could."[74] Perhaps this is merely Pilkington's comic representation of yet another of his eccentricities; perhaps Swift was purposefully trying to amuse his spectators or vex their expectations. The image is nevertheless suggestive. At the same time that Swift exercised for health, he was also aware of physical performance. As we see in letters to friends, he often represented himself as physical performer, riding, walking, moving always with masculine vigor.

Swift, who stood at a then-average five feet, five inches, worried about gaining weight during his earlier years; his exercising as a younger man may have been motivated in part by a desire to shed pounds. In early 1711, he reported to Stella and Dingley from London of his walks with his friend Matthew Prior, "This walking is a strange remedy; Mr. Prior walks, to make himself fat, and I to bring myself down."[75] Increasingly, he exercised to manage his chronic disorders. He wrote often about his walking in the *Journal to Stella*: "I walked gravely home this evening; and so I design to walk and walk till I am well: I fancy myself a little better already."[76] And again: "I had good walking to-day in the city, and take all opportunities of it on purpose for my health."[77] To his ecclesiastical superior Archbishop King, he wrote in 1721, "My Lord, I row after Health like a Waterman, and ride after it like a Post-boy, and find some little Success."[78] When the Irish weather prevented him from exercising outdoors, Swift roamed the halls of the deanery. "I seldom walk less than four miles, sometimes six, eight, ten, or more, never beyond my own limits," he wrote to Barber in later years. "Or, if it rains, I walk as much through the house, up and down stairs."[79] So vigorous was Swift in bounding up and down the steps of his residence for exercise that Pilkington worried that he would hurt himself: "The Dean then ran up the Great-Stairs, down one Pair of Back-Stairs, up another, in so violent a Manner, that I could not help expressing my Uneasiness to the good Gentlewoman [his long-time housekeeper, Mrs. Brent], lest he should fall, and be hurted; she said, 'It was a customary Exercise with him, when the Weather did not permit him to walk abroad.'"[80] Swift might seem eccentric in his overexercising; he nevertheless believed that it was one of the few ways to alleviate the pain, loss of equilibrium, and anguish that came with his chronic afflictions. Having been "quite broke" with "years and Infirmatyes," he wrote wretchedly to Pope in 1736, "All I have left is to walk, and ride."[81] His best creative years behind him, increasingly obscure as a political figure, and despairing of any other powers, Swift still moved through the world as best he could.

"I walk . . . as much as I can: because sweating is good," Swift said bluntly in 1712.[82] Physical motion, the authorities all agreed, "helps to break the Perspirable Matter smaller, and thereby render it more capable of passing thro' straighter Pores."[83] The ever-pragmatic Thomas Sydenham said that in "Chronical Diseases" "there is nothing that contributes so effectively to the Digestion of the Humours, and to the strengthening of the Blood and Parts of the Body, as *Exercise.*"[84] Exercise assisted nature in thinning the humors, opening the pores by heating the body, and expelling excess or vitiated matter through sweat. It is, said Steven Blankaart in his popular *Physical Dictionary,* "a most powerful, and prevalent thing to preserve Health, being that which purges, and drives away the superfluous Humours of the Body."[85] "If some of the Advantages accruing from Exercise, were to be procur'd by any one Medicine, nothing in the World would be in more Esteem," said Francis Fuller in *Medicina Gymnastica.*[86] Swift himself echoed those sentiments: "I continue in an ugly State of Health by the disorder in my Head, which Blister upon Blister and Pills upon Pills will not remove, and this whole Kingdom [Ireland] will not afford me the medicine of an unfoundred trotting Horse."[87] Exercise must succeed when medical interventions failed.

Among other self-injunctions in "When I come to be old," which Swift wrote before he was thirty, is the warning to himself "not to be too free of advise nor trouble any but those that desire it."[88] Yet with evangelical zeal, he urged his friends to exercise for their health, invariably using himself as a model. "What shall we do for poor Ppt?" he wrote to Stella from London in 1711. "Walking has done me so much good, that I cannot but prescribe it often to poor Ppt"; "use exercise and walk, spend pattens and spare potions, wear out clogs and waste claret."[89] (That is, spend money on walking shoes, not on medicines.) Swift scolded his ailing friend Anne Long, "Your Illness is the Effect of too little Exercise. I fence against the same Distemper you complain of, by perpetually walking when the Weath^r will permit me."[90] His certainty that exercise helped to restore or maintain health emboldened him even to remark of Queen Anne, "The Queen is in very good Health, but doth not use as much Exercise as she ought."[91] In the same sense of social leveling through shared health concerns, he wrote to Edward Harley, the Second Earl of Oxford, "The good account you are pleased to give me of my Lady Oxford's health, hath removed a great load from my shoulders; for I was ever in pain about her Ladyships want of appetite: and could often hardly forbear acting the Physician, by prescribing my onely remedy, which I take twice a day in fair weather, and once in fowl; I mean Exercise, which although it be the cheapest of all drugs, yet you great people are seldom rich enough to purchase."[92] Swift's worries about the health of particular friends led him to nag them again and again to exercise. If we are to believe their responses, his friends, high and low, took his advice. Pulteney, we have seen, promised to follow Swift's rules for sleeping, eating, drinking, and exercising. Lady Betty Germain submitted to Swift in 1731, "To show how stricktly I obey your orders I came from the Dutchess of Dorsets Country House to my own, where I have ridd and Walked as often as the Weather permitted me."[93] Similarly, others reported better health by following Swift's lead. "I remember your prescription," wrote John Gay, "& I do ride upon the Downs, and at present I have no Asthma."[94] In this case, both exercise and country air worked interdependently to bring relief.

Temple cautioned that "the best Cares or Provisions for Life and Health . . . consist in the discreet and temperate Government of Diet and Exercise: In both which," he added, "all Excess is to be avoided."[95] Despite this injunction, Swift exercised with what in his own day was seen as increasing obsession. In later years, his devotion to this *medicina gymnastica* worried his friends and physicians. In his suggestions about regimen, we recall, Sheridan advised that Swift "Walk little and moderately" and "Ride slow and often."[96] Though his friend Ford allowed that riding was supposed "to be good for a giddy head," he wrote to Swift, "I have often wished that you would be more moderate in your walks" because "the violent sweats you put yourself into, are apt to give colds, and, I doubt, occasion much of your other disorder," that is, the deafness attributed to cold.[97] Swift's doctors worried, too, in part because he had lost too much weight in his walking and riding. "Doctor HELSHAM and Doctor GRATTAN, frequently admonished him of his.... incessant and intemperate exercise," Delany recounted. In keeping with humoral theory, Delany himself acknowledged that "the constant and free discharges by perspiration from exercise, kept him clear of coughs and rheums, and other offensive infirmities of old age. But he carried this contention, (as he was apt to do every other) too far."[98] This concern about excessive or too-violent exercise was shared uniformly by medical authorities, from the days of Hippocrates and Galen to Swift's own. "Ancient Physicians, who were sagacious Observers, have been apprized of some ill Effects that followed the *Violence*, or a *continuing* too long in the Exercise they had recommended," wrote Swift's London doctor Cockburn.[99] Rather than encouraging proper digestion, as it should, warned the Newtonian physician Nicholas Robinson, excessive exercise "greatly impairs the Constitution, and is apt to overstrain the Solids, and on a full Stomach is still worse; for then it raises Flushings, and, instead of a good Digestion, causes Flatulencies, and a *Languor* upon the Nerves and Spirits."[100] In exercise, as in all things non-natural, balance begets balance.

Why, we should ask, did exercise become the preoccupation of Swift's health measures, even when his doctors, indeed all of the medical wisdom, warned against immoderation? Because, Swift himself said, he had wagered the labor—and dangers—of exercise against its benefits. Under this conviction, he made a desperate and uncertain bargain with time in his efforts to control his intractable body. I "battle with [my] disorders ... by riding and walking," he wrote to Pope in 1731, "at which however I repine, and would not do it meerly to lengthen life, because it would be ill husbandry, for I should save time by sitting still, though I should dye seven Years sooner; but the dread of pain and torture makes me toyl to preserve health from hand to mouth as much as a laborer to support life."[101] Here again the socially aspirant Swift casts himself as a toiling laborer, working strenuously to restore humoral balance.

His arduous exercise also suited his habits and temperament. Even in his final years, against the terror of stasis, Swift walked the halls and stairs of the deanery for hours. But his refusal to moderate his exercise was also a function of his fierce autonomy. Delany wrote that the Dean "paid no sort of regard to [his doctors'] monitions" that he cut back on his exercise.[102] This refusal to moderate his regimen may have been the resistance of a man whose long experience with his own body had taught him that the physicians' interventions and advice brought little relief. His disregard of the doctors' warnings, though, was as much an act of disobedience by a man who always chafed at being told what to do, a willful movement of the body in defiance of the physicians'—or anyone else's—attempts to wield authority over his contested body.

In his defiant independence, Swift was often alone. As we see in the next chapter, he became increasingly isolated socially because of the chronic giddiness that made his body unstable and the progressive deafness and tinnitus that embarrassed his ability to communicate with others. Despite sharing his enthusiasm for exercise with his friends, Swift seemed more and more alone, and lonely, in the pursuit of health as well. "I go where I was never before," he wrote during one of his long rambles through the Irish countryside, "without one companion, and among people where I know no creature; and all this is to get a little exercise for curing an ill head."[103] Forced into a smaller world by his chronic disorders, he said wretchedly to Chetwode, "I live wholly within my self; most people have dropt me, and I have nothing to do, but fence against the evils of age and sickness as much as I can, by riding and walking."[104] His increasingly lonely and increasingly obsessive exercising continued even into his final senility. "The Dean's understanding . . . quite gone" by 1742, his cousin Martha Whiteway reported that he "walked ten hours a day" through the halls of the deanery.[105] What had once been exercise taken in pursuit of humoral health had become an obsessive habit, which contributed to the popular notion of Swift in his final years as a mad, haunted genius.

In considering the practical measures to which Swift resorted in trying to manage his disordered body, we may glean important lessons. One is that the experience of living in the humoral body required constant vigilance and governance. Patients like Swift could never be passive. They might find a cure for an acute disorder such as shingles as the superfluous or peccant humor was driven out of the body. But this cure was not the killing off or driving out of an exogenous pathogen; rather, it was the righting of the humoral balance natural to the individual constitution. This balance would shift from year to year as the body aged, from month to month as the seasons changed, from day to day or morning to evening as one ate and drank, breathed in the ambient air, slept, indulged or restrained the passions. Chronic disorders, said Cheyne, might be cured by some extreme act of will and vigilance. More likely, however, the chronic sufferer would have to find some way to live with them. He would resort to the evacuants, sudorifics, and vomits and the surgical interventions like bleedings and blisters in hopes not of curing himself but of balancing the humors. Additionally, he would try to keep the humors in check with regimen. For Swift, these measures were a medical—and moral—responsibility.

Another lesson is that Swift's own devotion to regimen, as immoderate as it sometimes seemed to doctors and friends, conformed with canonical humoral principles. Swift could laugh at the excesses or follies of the doctors or describe the foul processes of the humoral body in the "scatological" poems or a work like *Gulliver's Travels*. Nonetheless, he accepted the "Fundamental" humoral precept "that all Diseases arise from *Repletion*" and that the individual was responsible for restoring or maintaining humoral balance.[106] In his final years, he believed that he had nothing else left to keep this balance but exercise; it was, he sighed, "all I have to trust to, though not in regard to Life but to Health."[107] Even then, the fact that he favored exercise over other means of managing the non-naturals tells us much about his temperament, habits, and image of himself as a vigorous, athletic man. It is also emblematic of the discipline that he tried to impose upon his unruly body. Perhaps, as his lapsarian tale of gorging on apples suggests, he thought that the flesh needed to be punished. The greater possibility is that he saw his regimen as the way, however severe at times, to discipline and impose order upon an "unteachable" Yahoo body by putting it to hard labor. Otherwise, it would brim over into humoral chaos. In this way, as I propose in the final chapter of this study, his attempts to keep his disorderly body in check were a counterpart to his concerns for political, religious, and social order in the larger world.

6

The Disordered Social Body and Humoral Identity

Describing illness is itself a powerful means of containing the disorders of the body. Language objectifies and puts experiences into order, making them available for rational scrutiny. Thus Swift's humoral narrative about his illnesses was an important way for him to make sense of them. But the language of pain or, for that matter, any physical sensation or state of mind, is inevitably self-referential, so expressing the subjectivities of sickness—what it *felt* like to be giddy and deaf, distracted by a roaring in his ears and fearing the decay of his intellectual faculties—challenged even the Dean's formidable verbal abilities. Occasionally Swift resorted to narrative. We recall, for instance, his recounting to Stella and Dingley that in a fit of vertigo his room seemed to spin round for a full minute. Much later in life, he "was seised with so cruel a fit of that giddyness" while riding outside of Dublin that he "was forced to lie down on a bed in an empty house for two hours before [he] was in a condition to ride" home.[1] When narrative failed, Swift turned to metaphor. In his giddiness he walked "like a drunken Man."[2] His tinnitus churned with "the Noise of seven Watermills" and roared like "a hundred oceans."[3] Even then, the self-experience of his physical sufferings was mediated always by language that was never quite sufficient.

In describing the psychological experiences of suffering from physical disorders that attacked without warning, Swift faced the same limitations. What vocabulary does one have for expressing the terrors and confusions of living "disordered"? In one of the earliest surviving records of his giddiness, in December 1708, Swift reported a "bad fitt at Mrs Bartons 24. bettr, but—dread a Fitt. *2ᵈ Month* better still to *the End*."⁴ This note is all the more revelatory because it comes in a private account book; it is one of the few statements of illness in which there is no studied self-representation for the sake of others. Yet in letters to friends throughout the years that followed, Swift used the same language of simmering fear. He frequently described the "dread of pain and torture" that could surprise him at any moment.⁵ He was "seldom in a tolerable humor by the frequent returns or dreads of Deafness," he said in 1729.⁶ To his friend Thomas Sheridan he wrote a few years later, "Some sudden turns are every day threatning me with a giddy Fit."⁷ This talk of dread and terror, though, is little more helpful in conveying the singular experience of illness than the language that Swift used in trying to describe his bodily sufferings.

Unable to express adequately (or even to understand fully) the subjectivities of illness, Swift referred instead to the language of social experience. Increasingly, the body disordered was his social identity disordered, the story of his disordered body a social narrative. Forced to withdraw from the world during "Fitts" of illness, he could not attend to church duties, entertain company, or travel to see friends. He spoke of the embarrassments of giddy tottering in public and of the "unconversable" deafness and tinnitus that made conversation impossible with any but those persons with "treble and Counter-tenor Voices."⁸ The man who thought himself exceptional found himself inconsequential; often the idioms of disappointed ambitions and sickness were the same. The neglect and ingratitude of those who had left him forgotten and unthanked in Ireland, the isolation and confinement in his chronic illnesses—Swift frequently spoke of these in one breath.⁹ The man who aspired to rank and influence was helpless in his disabilities and dependent upon others when he could not do things for himself. The man who prided himself on his masculinity and athletic vigor felt weak, effete, and impotent; he complained that the ladies had "forsaken" him in his illnesses. The man who saw his correspondence as conversation found even that social mode disordered by his failing faculties. Worse, the man so preoccupied with maintaining order in the world against the anarchies of "Party-mad[ness]" and crazed religious enthusiasm was terrified that his own disorders would eventuate in the "utter deprivation of senses many years before a deprivation of life."¹⁰ His disorders, he feared, would irrevocably cut him off at last from society.

The social narrative of Swift as an ill man did not begin with his life in Ireland after 1714. In 1712, the shingles episode took him off the London political stage for several months and cut him off from the company of polite society and those men of power in whom he placed his hopes for preferment. Because "the Pain has left my Should^r and crept to my neck and Collar bone," he wrote to Stella and Dingley, "I was not able to go to Church or Court to day."[11] As a clergyman and political player, Swift found his professional and social identity in church and court; illness has disordered this identity. Even earlier, as we have seen, the first attacks of chronic illness interrupted his political and social ascent. At the very moment when his future seemed brightening in the employ of Sir William Temple, his giddiness sent him back "to Ireld by advice of his Physicians."[12] This was the progress tale frustrated by his physical disorders. His "banishment" to Ireland in 1714, however, brought a distinct turn in the way that Swift saw his physical disorders as social disorders.

While Swift claimed to be "hindred by perfect Lazyness, and Listlessness, and anneantissement" after first going into his Irish "exile" in the summer of 1714, he engaged his new clerical duties energetically and conscientiously.[13] Still, these were days of dark despondency, adjustment, and political danger. Associated with those who were agitating for the return of the Stuarts to the English throne, Swift was suspected of Jacobite sympathies by the new Whig authorities. His letters were seized, and he was alerted that he was under surveillance: "I had warning given me to beware of a fellow that stood by while some of us were talking—It seems there is a Trade going of carrying stories to the Gov[ernmen]t."[14] The Tory friends in England in whom he had entrusted hopes for his own social elevation—Oxford, Bolingbroke, Arbuthnot, Matthew Prior—had all lost their positions. Charles Ford had been arrested, and the Whigs were gathering charges against Oxford and Bolingbroke. Swift had heard talk that he himself would "be examined upon these Impeachments."[15] At one time he imagined himself "at Court again," before waking to the grim reality of his situation: "I recollected I was in Irel^d, that the Queen was dead, the Ministry changed, and I was onely the poor Dean of St. Patrick's."[16] Swift was also trying to keep the importunate Esther Vanhomrigh—Vanessa—at bay. Having fallen passionately in love with him during his years in London, she had followed him to Ireland in November of 1714, despite his attempts to discourage her. Not long after, ostensibly concerned about "the Tattle of this nasty Town [Dublin]," he appealed to her discretion: "That was the Reason why I said to you long ago that I would see you seldom when you were in Irel^d."[17] For all of these pressures, public and private, we hear little about his health. Swift complains about "perpetual Colds & twenty Aylments"; reports on an injury to his thigh while riding; and writes the melancholy poem "In Sickness," which is a complaint more about his banishment to Ireland, where his "State of Health none care to learn," than about illness per se.[18] But for nearly four years, at least in his surviving correspondence, there are no explicit complaints about his giddiness or deafness.[19] In fact, Swift managed his "health well enough" by riding often and regulating his diet.[20]

Then in his account book for May of 1718, Swift noted without explanation the "terrible Fall" that he had taken.[21] Although he did not specify whether this fall was caused by a severe attack of giddiness or a tumble from his horse (of which he sometimes complained), entries in his account books may help clarify matters. Over the next few months, there were outlays for "physick" and bitters, "internal" medicines, which Swift had not listed for some time. In November he reported to Knightley Chetwode that he had been unable to correspond earlier because he had "been hindred from writing by the illness of [his] head, and eyes, which still afflict[ed] [him]."[22] Then, in December of 1718, Arbuthnot sent the first of two letters prescribing medicines for the "Complaint of a Vertigo."[23] The following year, Swift began to complain regularly of his giddiness and deafness. "I have been long pursued with one or two Disorders, which though not very painfull, are so incommodious, that they quite disconcert me," he wrote to Prior in January 1719–20. "Since I begun this Letter I have been so pursued with a giddy Head that I could not finish it."[24] The "cruell" giddiness, deafness, and tinnitus that "pursued [him] from [his] Youth" stalked him relentlessly from this time until the end of his days.[25]

For Swift, it was not only the sudden, vertiginous spinning of the world around him but also the inability to control his performative body that was so disconcerting. He who tried to enforce order through ritual and forms dared not attend to his clerical duties at St. Patrick's or even venture beyond the safety of the deanery walls during episodes of vertigo. In 1735, he wrote to John Barber that he could not risk going to church, for fear that "a Fit of Giddyness" would seize him as he stood in the pulpit.[26] Two years later, Swift sighed to the same "dear old Friend," "I have not been out of Doors further than my Garden, for severall Months."[27] He who slipped seamlessly in and out of character in company and conversation now "tottered" embarrassedly as he walked and sometimes had to leave guests for bed without warning. Such situations had been occurring for years. Swift wrote to Ford in 1720 that a sudden fit of giddiness made him deputize one of the Grattan brothers to stand in for him as host: "Three Days ago having invited severall Gentlemen to dinner, I was so attacked with a fitt of Giddyness for 5 Hours, that I was forced to constitute a Grattan to be my Deputy and do the Honors of the House while I lay miserable on my Bed."[28] How desperate the disorders of his body must have been for him to cede control of conversation and company to another.

Swift's hearing disorders did not affect his physical mobility or send him to bed, but they restricted him no less than his giddiness. And they were even more socially disabling. "Frequent Fits of Deafness," Swift wrote in the early 1720s, "hath confined me . . . to my Deanry-House and Garden."[29] In another letter of this time, he groaned, "Noise in my Ears and Deafness . . . makes me an unsociable Creature, hating to see others, or be seen by my best Friends, and wholly confined to my Chamber."[30] "I never stir out, or suffer any to see me but Trebbles and countertennors, and those as seldom as possible," he wrote to Chetwode in January 1721–22.[31] Unable to shine brilliantly among the men of learning and influence by whom he defined himself socially, he progressively had to exchange their wit and conversation for the voices of those he could actually hear. Even if his bad ears made them scream to be heard. In 1738, he wrote to Orrery, "I continue my Deafness with some Increase, and shall soon tear the Lungs of poor Mrs Whiteway."[32]

Discussing Swift's Dublin life in the late 1730s, Irvin Ehrenpreis speaks of the "continued vitality of [his] social pattern even at this time."[33] However, in his illnesses, Swift often represented himself as an increasingly isolated and friendless man in a contracted sphere of company and influence. Writing to Mary Pendarves during an episode of giddiness in January 1735–36, he mourned, "I confine myself entirely to a domestic life. I am visited seldom, but visit much seldomer. I dine alone . . . having few acquaintances, and those lessening daily."[34] Yet when well-intentioned friends did visit, he groused, no doubt with some pleasure, about their solicitudes: "I am vexed when my visiters come with the compliment usual here, Mr. Dean, I hope you are very well."[35]

Having long cherished hopes of preferment and political power, Swift now found his scope of influence restricted by the very body that he tried so desperately to govern. He made extended visits to Irish friends whose homes allowed him *some* measure of control: Sir Arthur and Lady Anne Acheson, who tolerated him good-naturedly at their Market Hill estate for months at a time, and Sheridan, whose home in squalid Quilca, in County Cavan, was less savory, his wife less welcoming (Swift dubbed her "Diabollisam").[36] In 1725, Swift stayed with the Sheridans for five months, to escape company during a long onset of deafness. "Your Lordship['s] Letter," he wrote to the Second Earl of Oxford, "was sent to me where I now am, and have been four months in a little obscure Irish Cabbin about forty miles from Dublin, whither I fled to avoyd Company in frequent Returns of Deafness."[37] His claims of avoiding company were not entirely genuine: With him at the Sheridans were Stella and Dingley.[38] But these were the intimates who would nurse him and accommodate his disabilities.[39] He did not have to worry that deafness would stymie or embarrass the public performance that was his currency on the stage of public affairs.

With the increasing length and unpredictability of the paroxysms of vertigo and deafness in Dublin, Swift kept to the domestic space and "Monastick life" of the deanery of St. Patrick's.[40] After his final trip to England in 1727, during which he was much confined to his hosts' homes because of his disorders, he abandoned future travel plans. There was excited talk in 1731 of visiting John Gay and his patrons, the Duke and Duchess of Queensberry. It came to nothing. By January of 1735–36, he was writing to Mary Pendarves, who had urged him to travel to Bath to take the waters, that he "had neither health nor leisure for such a journy; those times [were] past" with him.[41] Soon the dread of a sudden attack of giddiness kept him from traveling far even in Ireland. He wrote to his friend William Richardson in 1737, "Although I were ill enough when I saw you [last], I am fourty times worse at present, and am no more able to be your guest this Summer, than to travel to America."[42] And to Richardson's niece the next winter, he admitted, "My traveling days are over." The Richardsons lived just over a hundred Irish miles from Dublin.[43]

At last Swift would not risk even a day's journey from St. Patrick's. "I long excessively to be in England," he wrote to Barber in 1735, "but am afraid of being surprised by my old Disorder in my head, far from help . . . and I dare not so much as travel here, without being near enough to come back in the Evening to lye in my own Bed."[44] The same year, he told Alexander Pope about the "cruel" attack of giddiness that had "seised" him during a ride outside of Dublin: "I have my own little regular Oeconomy with my very few Servants about me; and dare not venture to be a days Journey from this Town, for fear of taking a fit of giddyness that sincks me for a month, & by which I lose ground that I never quite recover. I was caught so some months ago in a Village six miles from hence, & with the utmost difficulty got home."[45] His sphere of action and mobility shrinking as his disorders got the better of him, the lost ground is both literal distance that he can no longer travel and metaphor of military retreat.

David Turner has written of disabled men in the eighteenth century that their disorders "made them excessively reliant on servants, or transformed them from a position of masterly command to infantile dependence." The prospect of dependency was especially difficult for a man of power and influence because "it might make [him] reliant on his social inferiors, or unable to exercise his ability to command them."[46] Swift could grumble, with delighted irritation, about friends from the upper orders who stopped by the deanery to wish him well in his illnesses, "I am vexed whenever I hear a knocking at the door, especially the Raps of quality, and I see none but those who come on foot."[47] Yet he complained more often that his illnesses confined him to the company and ministrations of domestics. He wrote to Pope in February 1728–29, "I see no creature but my servants and my old Presbyterian house-keeper, denying myself to every body till I shall recover my ears."[48] In "denying" himself to those solicitous well-to-do friends, Swift tried, at least narratively, to exert authority and influence. As we shall find, he found singular opportunities in the "sick role" to reimagine himself socially, as a man of power and influence. Here, however, bewailing his confinement to the deanery in his fits of giddiness and deafness, the prickly champion of liberties who always hated "Tyran[n]y and oppression" had to cede authority over his own body to agonizing physical "oppressions" and to cede social influence and power to his domestics.[49] Especially in his final years, we hear of Swift's pitiable dependence upon protective friends and servants.[50]

Swift's immobility and dependence undercut his own claims to masculine vigor. The Dean often scolded his sick friends for their sedentary habits, characteristically holding up his own exercise as example. For Swift, physical vigor was not only healthful humoral measure; it was also masculine identity. In boasting of his own athletic prowess to sickly male friends such as Pope and John Gay, Swift dug subtly at their diminished masculinity. To Pope he wrote, "The misfortune I most lament is your not being able by exercise to battle with your disorders, as I do by riding and walking."[51] Pope protested, "Infirmities have not quite unmann'ed me."[52] Swift countered, "You and I are valetudinarians of a direct contrary kind. I am almost every second day on horseback for about a dozen Miles."[53] If Pope "hath always loved a domestick life from his youth," their friend Gay was prone to corpulence and subject to "a rooted Lazyness." Swift wrote to him, "A coach and six horses is the utmost exercise you can bear, and this onely when you can fill it with such company as is best suited to your tast, and how glad would you be if it could waft you in the air to avoyd jolting; while I who am so much later in life can or at least could ride 500 miles on a trotting horse."[54] In 1733, Swift knitted his brow at Lord Harley's "Lazyness" and said of his own chronic giddiness, "I oppose it by constant riding and walking, wherein I wish you would follow my example."[55] Only a few years earlier in the *Essay of Health and Long Life*, George Cheyne had made a sort of hierarchy of exercise scaled according to levels of rigor: "*Walking* is the most Natural and effectual *Exercise*, did it not spend the *Spirits* of the tender too much," he wrote. "*Riding* a Horseback is less laborious, and more effectual for such. Riding in a *Coach* is only for the *Infirm*, and *Young* Children."[56] Couched in Swift's own recommendations that his friends exercise for health is a display of Swift's own masculine vigor and movement—and a feminizing of his friends, confined to their lazy, sedentary domestic lives. But confined to the deanery by his chronic illnesses, Swift must certainly have realized the irony of his own condition. So his ambivalent self-representations suggest.

Turner writes that because the domestic space was considered "feminine," men who were immobilized and confined to their bedchambers by disability often felt emasculated.[57] On more than one occasion, Swift represented himself feminized in his episodes of sickness. "I am forced to entertain you like an old Woman with my Aylments," he wrote to Ford in 1719.[58] Elsewhere, he represented himself both emasculated and socially diminished when he likened himself to a maidservant who might cry out for attention, "Oh, I'm very sick, if any body car'd for it!"[59] And perhaps most explicitly, Swift showed himself feminized in illness in poems to Stella. In the longish "To Stella, Visiting Me in My Sickness," he bewails his sufferings "in unmanly Strains." Stella in turn assumes masculine virtues, "a manly Soul ... molded ... with Female Clay." While the man of great motion and power languishes helplessly on his "sickly Couch," she takes heroic initiative, even tasting "each nauseous Draught" of medicine first on his behalf.⁶⁰ He also saw manly resolve in Stella's stoicism. During the shingles episode, Swift had represented himself in letters to his superior Archbishop King in the masculine, heroic discourse of uncomplaining suffering; with only a passing nod in one of several letters to the "cruel Disorder" that had laid him low, he was otherwise an able, important man, busy with London affairs.⁶¹ In poems to Stella, however, it is she who suffers without complaint while he lets loose his passions:

> And, when indecently I rave,
> When out my brutish passions break,
> With gall in ev'ry word I speak,
> She, with soft speech, my anguish chears,
> Or melts my passions down with tears:
> Although 'tis easy to descry
> She wants assistance more than I;
> She seems to feel my pains alone,
> And is a Stoic in her own.⁶²

In the same poem, Swift apologizes for the very ingratitude that he despised so much in others. "Ungrateful," he deems himself, "since to her I owe / That I these pains can undergo."⁶³ If this is a poem of contrition, it is also ironic self-representation. An ailing body, Swift is emasculate in his passivity and impotence.

Elsewhere Swift represented himself desexualized entirely. Ever self-observant, he had vowed even as a younger man that he would never "boast of [his] former beauty, or strength, or favour with Ladyes, &c." when he came to be old.⁶⁴ All the same, in ways that have provoked much biographical and critical debate, he courted the attentions of admiring younger women—Stella, Vanessa, Anne Acheson, and Lætitia Pilkington. In his age and illness, he grieved the loss of these attentions. "I have observed among my own Sex, and particularly in my self, that those of us who grow most insignificant expect most civility," he wrote to Mary Pendarves in his sixty-eighth year. "I am grown sickly, weak, lean, forgetfull, peevish, spiritless, and for those very reasons expect that you who have nothing to do but be happy, should be entertaining me with your Letters and Civilityes."⁶⁵ In 1735–36 he repined to Pope, "My state of health is not to boast of; my giddiness is more or less too constant.... What vexes me most is, that my female friends . . . have now forsaken me."⁶⁶ On the prospect of visiting England ten years earlier, he had promised that he would "venture all" and risk the trip if Pope could get him "two or three Harridan Ladys that will be content to nurse and talk loud" to him in his deafness.⁶⁷ Desexualized in illness, he had resigned the flatteries of the younger ladies to the ministrations of women whom he portrayed as old, shrill, and bossy. The ambitious man who prided himself on his masculine vigor and would be seen as a person of influence and power is sexless, neglected, and inconsequential.

We might think that correspondence and imaginative writing would become surrogates for the visits and conversation of friends that he could not enjoy in the confinement and isolation of his illness. Writing is social performance, too. For Swift it was a conversational mode. Having made a naughty remark to the ladies in the *Journal to Stella*, he caught himself, "Pshaw, what's all this I'm saying? methinks I am talking to MD [my dears] face to face."⁶⁸ In another letter, he wrote that he was gesturing as he talked to them on his way to bed: "All the while I was undressing my self, there was I speaking monkey things in air, just as if MD had been by."⁶⁹ As it disrupted his talk, then, his inability to write during fits of deafness and giddiness was also social withdrawal. He often ended a letter abruptly: "My head is too ill to write or think"; "This is a long Letter for an ill Head: So adieu."⁷⁰ Having just apologized to his friend Ford for prattling on in his "old Woman's Talk" about his illnesses, Swift signed off summarily, "—I can write no more for my Head, and so much the better for you—[.]"⁷¹ And so, his illnesses having forced him to withdraw from even the conversation of correspondence, he became further isolated.

Swift's recent biographer John Stubbs says that "writing had become for Swift not only a retreat but also a means of holding a still point amid his fits of dizziness, and staving off an existential vertigo that oppressed him even more."⁷² This may have been true at times. More often, however, Swift complained that the cognitive confusions brought by his giddiness, deafness, and tinnitus stymied or made nonsense of his writing. In 1724, he wrote to Chetwode, "I am now relapsed into my old Diseaze of Deafness, which so confounds my Head, that I am ill qualifyed for writing or thinking." Later in that letter, Swift begged that his friend "allow for this confused Paper for I have the Noise of seven Watermills in my Ears and expect to continue so above a Month."[73] Pressed by his bookseller Benjamin Motte to send revisions of *Gulliver's Travels*, he pleaded, "My Head is so confused with the returns of my deafness to a very great degree . . . that I am in an ill way to answer a Letter which requires some thinking."[74] To his fellow "Valetudinarian" Pope, Swift groaned, "My giddiness is more or less too constant. . . . I can as easily write a poem in the Chinese-language as my own."[75] In one of his final letters, he sighed, "I hardly understand one word I write."[76] This from the agile conversationalist and wit who had performed brilliant high-wire linguistic capers and still today draws admiration as the greatest prose satirist of the English language.

Earlier we situated Swift's complaints about his decaying intellect and memory and his fears of madness in the humoral narrative about fouled or impeded transmission of sense data to the understanding. The story about his declining cognitive abilities is also *social* narrative. Swift feared that as his giddiness, deafness, and tinnitus increasingly confined and isolated him, his disordered mind would at last cut him off irrevocably from the society by which he defined himself. In their social constructions of madness, early biographers like Samuel Johnson attributed what they saw as Swift's final madness to this very withdrawal from the world. Those who are isolated from society, deprived of the regulatory checks of conversation and company, may go mad. Johnson exhorted his own "disordered" friends to heed Robert Burton's injunction against madness, "Be not solitary."[77] Swift, he claimed, went mad because in his disorders and confinement, he had neither company nor conversation nor reading to "renovate" his mind.[78]

Some early biographers isolated him even further socially by committing him, as it were, to the "Hospital for Incurables" that he himself had funded in his will. "He died mad," said one, "among fellow-creatures similarly visited, but sheltered by his munificence," a claim made the more absurd by the fact that "St. Patrick's Hospital for Imbeciles" did not open until 1757, twelve years after Swift's death.[79] More routinely, his biographers show him as the pitiable, speechless old man roaming aimlessly for hours through the halls of the deanery. They make his complete social isolation all the more poignant by describing the busy comings and goings of servants, officious friends, and younger clergymen all around him.

While the facts of his late-life decline are certainly important, more significant here are the ways that Swift represented the disorders of mind. In writing about these, he attempted to objectify and contain them. As we have seen here, faced with the difficulties of expressing the subjectivities of illness, what it *felt* like physically and mentally to be a chronically sick person, he told instead the story of his social experiences. His body and mind disordered, the man of great political and social ambitions was forced to withdraw from the world of public affairs. He could not trust that his giddy body would perform in character as he would have it perform. Baffled by baffled hearing, "confined to [his] chamber" in the deanery, befuddled by his failing memory and cognitive confusions, Swift found himself increasingly isolated and emasculated, as well as dependent and obsolescent.[80] Personal identity, the way that he saw himself, and social identity, the way that he saw himself in relation to the world in which he lived, were muddled by humoral disorders. Because Swift's health mediated this identity, the disordering of his fluid body made that identity all the more indeterminate. The elusiveness of a fixed sense of himself may go far in explaining why Swift could never write a sustained and coherent autobiography.

Lætitia Pilkington mourned of Swift, "It is a very great Loss to the World, that this admirable Gentleman never could be prevail'd on to give us the Particulars of his own Life."[81] The truth, of course, is that autobiography is everywhere in Swift, in his comic apologias such as *Verses on the Death*, in those poems in which he casts himself as character and imagines how he must appear to others, and in grimmer verses such as "In Sickness" and "On His Own Deafness." As Brean Hammond remarks, "Swift's first important biographer was himself."[82] Claude Rawson rightly but more bluntly calls Swift, "for better or worse, one of the most egocentric writers in the language, but one who always took care to avoid seeming so," working instead by refractive self-irony and "defensive indirection."[83] Even so, too often the indirections and comic deflections in his self-representations frustrate any attempt to construct "the Particulars of his own Life." Notoriously, when Swift did tell stories about himself, he often gave different versions in different company. One such example is the story of his wet nurse's "abduction" of him when he was a year old. He told at least four different versions of the tale, some of them dramatically different.[84] This tendency to tell the same story differently, biographers have suggested, may have been elaborate mythmaking about his past. As Leo Damrosch remarks, Swift "liked to be mysterious toward everyone."[85] The different versions of his own story may also have simply been playful teasings and vexings of his audiences, which left his friends and earliest biographers both amused and bemused. Lord Orrery called him "my hieroglyphic friend."[86] Deane

Swift said of his cousin, "THE character of SWIFT is upon the whole so exceedingly strange, various, and perplexed, that I am afraid it can never be drawn up with any degree of accuracy."[87]

Because of Swift's scattered and often contradictory self-representations, in both correspondence and imaginative writings, this question of his identity—political, religious, national—has been much contested by biographers and critics. Was he Englishman or Irishman? Tory or Whig? Pious? Irreligious? Staunch maintainer of political orthodoxy and hegemony or ardent champion of individual conscience and civil disobedience? To some, he was "Anglo-Irish," the self-contradictions explained by the "existential dilemma" that came with displacement.[88] He was, say others, "a Whig in politics and Tory in religion."[89] One dubbed him a "skeptical fideist."[90] George Orwell called him famously a "Tory anarchist, despising authority while disbelieving in liberty."[91] And Orrery, for all of his complaints about his misspent genius, declared simply that Swift was sui generis: "I am pursuing the Dean through the mazy turnings of his character. But, they will easily be reconciled, when you consider, that of all mankind, SWIFT perhaps had the greatest contrasts in his temper"; "He was neither Whig nor Tory, neither Jacobite nor Republican. He was DOCTOR SWIFT."[92] Orrery's slippery resolution of the puzzling "contrasts in his temper" is to declare the Dean a singular character.

Without dismissing any such explanations, we might argue that one of the problems with trying to fix Swift's identity is the attempt of too many modern historians and biographers to organize his world neatly by imposing binaries upon it: Whig/Tory, Anglican / Roman Catholic, English/Irish. Frustrated when they cannot categorically fix Swift himself in those binaries, they speak of his "divided self" or "divided consciousness." Even Orrery frames his attempt to account for Swift's singular character in the very binaries that he would dissolve. But if the "divided self" that frustrates establishing his social and personal identities is "intolerable," as Patrick Reilly judges, it is so in part because the categories were never fixed in Swift's own day.[93] The nominal boundaries of partisan politics, religious doctrine and practice, and nationhood were always permeable and fluid. Swift cannot be situated firmly in categories that were themselves never firmly established.

Of course, the same could be said of many a writer of Swift's day. Behn, Defoe, Pope, Fielding, Sterne—all of them defy neat political, religious, and social categorization. What, then, makes Swift so peculiarly elusive? Why can we not pin the man down easily? Perhaps, as Michael McKeon and Seamus Deane argue, we must finally attribute the perplexing contraries in Swift and his works to his "omnivorous skepticism."[94] At the same time that he worried that order in the world was crumbling, he could not allow any ideology, myth, social position, or intellectual attitude to stand unchallenged, even his own. This skepticism made of him an unforgiving, hyper-aware self-observer, always checking and filtering his self-representations, imagining himself as others would see him. This would explain the ironic self-depictions and use of shifty "personae" that Rawson sees as self-concealment and deflection. The instinct of his skepticism was self-subversion; the *expression* of his skepticism was confusing and indeterminate self-representation. In another context, George Berkeley wrote of "a ridiculous, Sceptical Humor" that makes "every thing Nonsense and Unintelligible."[95] Swift's own "Sceptical Humor" would not allow him to tell the story of himself straight.

In this debate about Swift's indefinite selves, I suggest that we also see them as expressions of his disordered body. Like all humoral bodies, permeable and coextensive with the world outside of them, Swift's was ever fluid in the processes of unmaking and remaking. The unpredictable, disorienting, and sometimes terrifying fits of giddiness, deafness, and tinnitus made his sense of self all the more unstable. Swift might try to understand and express his uncertain body with humoral narrative, control it with medical interventions and regimen, and represent it ironically in scattered correspondence and imaginative writings. But he could never determine and fix it definitively. He was always "in a middling Way, between Healthy and Sick," he wrote to Sheridan in 1728.[96] Caught between the already tenuous binaries of health and sickness, balance and imbalance, order and disorder, Swift's personal and social identities were liminal. At times he was the entertaining conversationalist and social performer; at times, he was friendless and alone, isolated and immobilized socially by what became "almost a perpetuall Deafness and Giddyness."[97] He was the Drapier, the champion of Irish liberties whose birthday was celebrated by the citizens of Dublin with bonfires; he was the man forgotten, "left alone," languishing "obscurely" in Ireland.[98] And the "settlement of [his] health" never realized, so, too, his identity was unfixed and uncertain.[99] This humoral indeterminacy explains in part Swift's inability to write a sustained, coherent autobiography.

His single surviving attempt to write the story of his own life, found in manuscript after his death, is the disjointed fragment titled "Family of

Swift." Most biographers agree that he composed this piece sometime between 1727 and 1729, when he was about sixty.[100] An "Exile" in Ireland, beset by his chronic illnesses, most of his brilliant imaginative work behind him, his beloved Stella recently dead or dying (without a firmer date we cannot know), Swift found his world entropic. At this climacteric, he designed, it seems, to establish a personal identity by writing the story of his life. In fact, he spends most of the narrative reconstructing a family history in which to situate himself. Not until the thirteenth of barely twenty autograph pages does Swift finally announce his own birth in Dublin, posthumously to his father. In the same sentence, he tells the tale of having been abducted by his wet nurse, who spirited him away to England, where, according to his story, she raised him for three years before returning him to his mother and uncle in Dublin. Coming as it does after he has worked hard to establish his identity through an account of his family, this abduction tale disrupts and makes uncertain the very identity that Swift seems intent upon establishing in the fragment. A scant few pages, he abruptly and bitterly ends the narrative in his thirtieth year, when he was passed over for the Deanery of Derry because another candidate had bribed his way into the position.

Despite his attempt to establish an identity, the fragment shows the blurs and holes of that identity. Swift talks of family stories passed down from son to son, some of which are remembered, others forgotten. Although he would objectify himself by telling the story of his own birth and progress "in the character of a third person," he slips occasionally into the first person as archival researcher processing his materials.[101] Of one great family member Swift says, "I am ignorant whether he left heirs or no"; of a document that would be useful to his account he says, "I never could get a Copy, and I suppose it would now be of little use."[102] The manuscript itself is littered with erasures, smudgings-out, strike-throughs, and marginal corrections. All of these shifts and ruptures and second-guessings and gaps throw into question the reliability of the document. As Denis Johnston warned, we should not count upon the fragment for biographical facts.[103]

The autobiographical fragment seems at first troubling. Its incoherence, confusions, and abrupt ending suggest that Swift could no more determine his identity than he could impose order upon the anarchic humoral body that is writing that identity. How does one fix in place a "self" that is ever fluid, shifting, indeterminate? Identity is made, unmade, and remade, not in a tidy dialectical process but in the giddy chaos of constituent humors and desperate attempts to maintain some sort of equilibrium. Yet reading the fragment as the expression of Swift's humoral identity helps us appreciate better his gifts of impersonation and the instabilities of his narratives, which often shift in point of view or work by rhetorical indirection and doublespeak. While we should never reduce Swift to a mere material body, the man who could "never be sick like oth^r People, but always something out of th common way" was able to understand in ways that other writers could not that identity is performative, at times improvisational and, like his humoral body, fluid.[104]

7

Swift in the Sick Role

In our own day, by general acknowledgment, the clinical medicine whose authority is inscribed in social institutions, legal statutes, and professional language is the province of experts qualified by years of specialized education and practice. It claims the imprimatur of positivist science. Given the cultural ascendancy of the clinic, we trust that our doctors, in their greater knowledge, will tell us what is wrong with our bodies, even when we ourselves cannot, and then repair them. Certainly, there are challenges to both the practical and intellectual authority and the privileging of the clinic. We have only to witness the number of internet medical blogs; claims of natural and homeopathic remedies; and political-philosophical defiance of those such as Ivan Illich, who attacked the medicalization of Western society.[1] When we get sick, however, we generally submit to the authority of medical science and our trained physicians.

Having submitted thus to the authority of "medicine," said sociologist Talcott Parsons, sick persons accept the doctors' diagnoses and the expectations that come along with those diagnoses. That is, they perform in the "sick role." They behave *as* patients, following the doctors' orders and taking measures to get better. At the same time, in this sick role they have certain rights and exemptions—"sanctioned deviance"—because they are unable to perform expected daily duties or contribute meaningfully during their illnesses. Sick persons might get a "free pass" from work or school or social obligations; they might be forgiven for snapping impatiently at family and friends.[2] Of course, not everyone follows the doctor's orders or even consults a physician in times of sickness. But for those who do, there are implicit social contracts established and mediated by the authority of the doctor and the clinic.

The sick of Swift's own day also performed in various sick roles determined by social structures and relationships. As we saw in our discussion of the different medical resources and epistemologies competing with one another in early modern Britain, physicians and a medical "establishment" had only hit-or-miss authority. So, the sick person might not submit as readily to the doctor as the sick person of Talcott's modern clinical encounter does. Swift himself looked for relief from his chronic disorders wherever he could find it. But, despite his own skepticism about the doctors' authority and abilities, he sometimes invoked their orders to claim exemptions from social obligations when he found them serviceable. "I would have waited on Your Grace," he wrote to the Duke of Dorset in 1735, "if I had not been prevented by the return of an old disorder in my Head, for which I have been forced to confine my self to the Precepts of my Physicians."[3] Yet even without the doctors, he routinely played the sick role to avoid social obligations and entrapments, and he sometimes reacted testily when others did not honor his claims to sick exemptions pro forma.

In this context, we might consider a dramatic incident in Swift's life in which the pursuit of health framed his willful defiance of what he saw as capricious authority. Riding on the strand from Howth to Dublin in the winter of 1715–16, only a year or so after he had assumed the duties of Dean of St. Patrick's, Swift was harassed and driven off the road by an Irish peer, Lord Blayney, and his entourage. When he protested, Swift claims, Blayney threatened him with a loaded pistol. "Pray S^r do not shoot, for my horse is apt to start, by which I shall endanger my life," the Dean entreated. Having forced his will, Blayney rode on. Swift, outraged at both the insult and the peer's brutal haughtiness, drafted a petition to the Irish House of Lords, in which he claimed a right to the road and a right to exercise for his own health. This "humble Petition" begins with the plea that "your Pet^r is advised by his Physicians on account of his health, to go often on horse-back." At the same time that Swift questioned the doctors' authority—the same Swift who later flouted their cautions that he was exercising too much—he invoked that very authority in his appeal for justice: He had been riding under doctors' orders, after all. He ended with the same appeal to health: "Your Pet^r therefore doth humbly implore Your L^{d}shps in Your great Prudence and justice, to provide that he may be permitted to ride with safety on the s^d Strand, or any other of the King's high-ways, for the recovery of his health (so long as he shall demean himself in a peaceable manner)—." But he vowed also that he would not yield: "And Y^r Pet^{rs} health still requiring that he should often ride and being confined in winter to go on the same Strand, he is forced to enquire from every one he meets whether the s^d Lord be upon the same Strand; and to order his servants to carry arms to defend himself against the like or worse insult from the s^d Lord, for the consequences of which, Y^r Pet^r cannot answer." As "humble" as Swift claimed that his petition to the "Lords Spirituall and Temporal" was, we find here the temperament that made him such a trenchant satirist: prickly individualism; a keen sense of injured pride; ready outrage at insult, real or imagined. Here, too, we find the persistent targets of the champion of Irish liberties. He hated injustice of any kind, the high-handedness and thoughtless brutality of men in power, and the arrogance of those who would impose their will upon others. In this case, Swift clearly found the physicians' order serviceable—and authoritative. He must certainly have thought that the claims to pursuing health would legitimately stand against or level the claims of entitlement of a Lord Blayney.[4]

As in this formal protest that he be allowed to pursue his health without interference, what we know about Swift's illnesses comes largely from accounts of himself. While Swift left behind no sustained autopathography, we know his various performances in the sick role through the representations of himself in his correspondence, imaginative writings, and sundry fugitive pieces. Although some friends learned of his disorders secondhand, most heard the news from Swift himself. "I am very much concerned at the account you give me of your health," fretted Lord Howth in 1735.[5] And having received a letter from Swift after a lapse in correspondence, Charles Ford wrote, "The pleasure I had in not being quite forgot, was soon abated by what you say of your ill health. . . . Your giddiness and deafness give me the utmost concern."[6] This self-reporting of his afflictions raises the question of how he defined *illness* and raises issues of self-representation. "I am very much concerned at the disorder you complain of," wrote Mary Pendarves. "I hope you submit to take proper care of yourself; and that the next account I have of your health will be more to my satisfaction."[7] While there is no suggestion that Pendarves doubts Swift's "account" of his illnesses, there is an important subtext here: The reality of his illnesses is indistinguishable from his representations of himself sick. This blurring of illness and self-representation creates possibilities for performing illness. Knowing what is expected socially of the sick person—and what the sick person can expect of others—one might play the sick role for advantage.

In pleading exemptions and excuses in his illnesses, Swift played the sick role like others of his day. However, his social identity fluid, like his humoral body, he found singular opportunities for imagining and reimagining himself socially in his disorders, sometimes transgressively. Confined and isolated in his illnesses, he found community with "fellow-sufferers" in "sick talk"; in sick talk with the well-to-*do*, he imagined social elevation. Dependent upon servants in his helplessness, he imagined the privilege and ascendancy that he did not have by birth and that had not, at least by his own reckoning, been awarded to him for his abilities and merit. Emasculated by his disabilities, he reimagined himself young, athletic, and sexual. These imaginings in the sick role were yet further ways for Swift to impose order upon disorder. They were also ways to write his identity, however tentative and fluid it was.

Swift knew well what sick persons could expect of others. When his friends and correspondents were ill, he worried solicitously about them. "Madam, I am extremely concerned at the account you give of your health," he wrote to Jane Waring in one of his earliest surviving letters.[8] While he was in London, he cried to Stella, "God Almighty bless poor dear Ppt, and her eyes and head: What shall we do to cure them, poor, dear life?" "Pray Gd mend pooppts Health."[9] Many years later, Swift beseeched Pope, "Pray put me out of fear as soon as you can, about that ugly report of your illness."[10] His worries about the health of these and other friends—Oxford, Bolingbroke, Arbuthnot, Gay—are among the most persistent themes in his letters. Swift not only enquired personally of them but also presented them sympathetically to others. "My poor Friend Arthbuthnot [sic] I heartily pity, and would purchase his Health with the half of my Kingdom," he wrote to Ford in the early 1720s.[11] A decade later, he told another correspondent that Mary Barber "hath been afflicted with so many repetitions of the gout, that her limbs are much weakened, and Spirits sunk," and, he remarked, "neither could she be in much disposition to increase her volume [of verse]; for health and good humor, are two ingredients absolutely necessary in the poetical trade."[12] While there is nothing to suggest insincerity in Swift's concerns about his friends' health, the concern itself was a social expectation that came with the acknowledgment that they were "sick."

Throughout the many years of letters, Swift's correspondents in turn worried about his health. "I heard you were ill, and am heartily concerned for it," wrote Archbishop King in 1712. "I can only give you the assistance of my prayers, which I assure you I do with constancy."[13] "I have been under an unspeakable concern at an account I lately saw from Ireland of a return of your old disorders of giddiness and deafness," wrote another acquaintance years later.[14] The language that his friends used in expressing these concerns and sympathies is the same, again and again. Typifying such expressions are Edward Harley's condolence of 1727, "I was very much concerned to hear that you were so much out of order. . . . I should be glad to hear that you are well, and have got rid of that troublesome distemper, your deafness," and Ford's of a few years later, "I am extreamly concerned to hear the bad state of your health."[15] In some few cases, the idiom of sensibility creeps in. "Your letter would have given me the greatest pleasure of any thing I have ever met with," wrote Katharine Richardson, "had it not been for the complaints you make of your health, which give me a most sensible concern, as they ought to do every body that has any regard for this kingdom."[16] Given even the anxiety of "feeling" like this, Swift knew too well that sick talk, too, was prescribed and mediated by social forms:

> When you are *Sick*, your *Friends*, you say,
> Will send their *Howd'ye's* ev'ry day:
> Alas! that gives you small relief——!
> They send for *Manners*——; not for *Grief*——[17]

The sick role enforced an implicit social contract. For Swift, performance in this role was yet another way of imposing order on disorder.

David Womersley says that "social entrapment [was] one of the forms of vulnerable immobility which preoccupied Swift in his later years."[18] We can understand this entrapment in two ways. For one, Swift chafed at the constraining, artificial social forms of his day—the prescriptive "manners" that he both upheld and upheaved, parodying them in works such as *Polite Conversation* and poking at social propriety with what many of his contemporaries and biographers saw as eccentric behaviors. All the same, the manners that he challenged were the very forms that enforced social order in the world and the respect that Swift thought was owed him. Social entrapment could also mean, more basically, that Swift was obligated to *do* certain things: appear on schedule in certain places, perform certain duties for others, even respond readily to friends' letters. Conveniently, the very giddiness and hearing impairments that entrapped Swift, confining him to the deanery, also allowed him to wriggle free from such expectations. His body disordered by illness, the sick role exempted him from physical performances; it also exempted him from social obligations and gave him excuse for escape from awkward situations or intractable problems. When his efforts in the summer of 1714 to mend the fatal breach between Oxford and Bolingbroke failed, for example, he fled to the English countryside, writing to Thomas Walls in Dublin, "I have been in the Country these 5 weeks, and probably shall return to Town no more.... I sett abundance of People at a Gaze by my going away; but I layd it all on my Health."[19] That an "abundance of People" might wonder at his sudden departure during this crisis certainly gratified his sense of celebrity; at the same time, sickness allowed him an excuse for having failed to reconcile his two Tory friends. Swift's deafness and giddiness were mutually cause and explanation, or excuse, for his withdrawal from society.

In like fashion, Swift routinely used sickness to excuse himself from visits and other obligations. He asked that Thomas Wallis, vicar of Athboy, serve as proxy for a diocesan visitation from John Evans, the Bishop of Meath, because his "health will not suffer it."[20] Swift and Evans disliked each other. But Swift also used sickness to excuse himself from visiting those he got along with. "If I had not still continued (as I have been for three months) confined by deafness and giddiness," he wrote to Eaton Stannard, a lawyer friend, "I would have waited on you with my acknowledgements for your favour and goodness."[21] And to John Hoadly, William King's successor as Archbishop of Dublin, he apologized, "I have been a long time, and still continue so perpetually tormented with Deafness and Giddyness, that I am not fit for any Company or Conversation, and this disorder hath made it impossible for me to wait upon your Grace."[22] Swift wrote to Knightley Chetwode that during his final visit to England in 1727, he did not "go to Court, except when [he] was sent for and not always then." Knowing by this time that he was largely irrelevant in court affairs anyway, he added, "Besides my illness gave me too good an excuse the last two months."[23] Perhaps in part self-consolation, using sickness as excuse also could spur comic interchange.[24] Arbuthnot advised that Swift keep his sickness at the ready to escape social demands: "Your deafness is so necessary a thing, that I allmost beginn to think it is an affectation."[25] He joked that he could cure Swift's deafness, Pope wrote, "but he would not advise you, if you were cur'd, to quit the pretence of it; because you may by that means hear as much as you will, and answer as little as you please."[26] The Dean and his circle were well aware of how serviceable sickness could be.

The sick role scripted the rules of social performance for both the patient and those around him. It was understood. So Swift bristled when others did not grant him exemptions in his illnesses. He opened a letter of 1724 to Ford, "I wonder how You expect I can write Letters, when I am deaf and have been so these 2 Months and am afraid I shall never recover."[27] If this is good-natured scolding of his dear friend, Swift could also respond angrily when his claims of illness were not accepted as a matter of form. He wrote in outrage to Bishop Evans, who had refused to acknowledge his sickness as a valid excuse for his absence from the annual visitation: "I have received an account of your Lordship's refusing to admit my proxy at your visitation, with several circumstances of personal reflexions on myself, although my proxy attested my want of health; to confirm which, and to lay before you the justice and Christianity of your proceeding, above a hundred persons of quality and distinction can witness, that since Friday the 26th of May, I have been tormented with an ague, in as violent a manner as possible, which still continues, and forces me to use another hand in writing to you."[28] Swift was unquestionably a sick man. Usually we can tell from a pattern of reports over a certain time when he was being truthful in using illness as an excuse from social and professional commitments. But to doubt his word or challenge his claims, as Evans had, was to impugn his integrity. The embattled Swift would not abide this, even if he did sometimes find sickness useful for dodging obligations.

Swift might even claim humoral disorder as excuse for the viciousness of his satires. In more than one poem, he imagined that some persons will "complain / There's too much satire in [his] vein."[29] The line, which Swift used most famously in *Verses on the Death*, makes peccant humor of his intolerance of a wicked, foolish world. The satiric temperament was itself a sickness. "Drown the World," he wrote to Pope in 1725, as he was revising *Gulliver's Travels*: "I am not content with despising it, but I would anger it if I could with safety. I wish there were an Hospital built for it's despisers, where one might act with safety and it need not be a large Building, only

I would have it well endowed."³⁰ Bearing in mind Swift's claims elsewhere that he wrote from the body, it is difficult to know if he is speaking literally or figuratively in calling the "too much Satyr in his Vein" humoral disorder.³¹ The line appears in apologia poems, in which he defends the severity and offensiveness of his attacks on folly and wickedness. If satiric temper is foul humor, in the sick role Swift might be acquitted by Samuel Johnson, Walter Scott, William Makepeace Thackeray, and those others who complained that his immoderate anger became lunatic rage and mad misanthropy. Certainly, he must be allowed to bleed off the superfluous humor in restoring humoral balance.

When Swift began to plead sickness not only to excuse himself from social and professional obligations but also to explain cognitive failures—his decaying memory and inability to put thoughts into order—there were noteworthy implications for his imaginative writing. For Swift, this decay of memory and inability to organize his thoughts for writing were functions of his chronic illnesses. Even in his mid-forties, Swift had complained of memory loss. In his later years, he used it again and again as excuse. "My memory is so bad, that I cannot tell whether I answered a Letter from you, and another from Ld Bolin—that I received in Jan. last," he sighed to Pope.³² Later in life, he apologized to John Barber, "To shew my Memory gone, I wrote this Letter a week ago and thought it was sent till I found it this Morning."³³ The sick role gave Swift excuse for both his lapsing memory and the cognitive failures that addled his world. "About a Month ago I received your last Letter, wherein you complain of my long Silence," he wrote to Thomas Sheridan in 1737: "I have one Excuse which will serve for all my Friends. I am quite worn out with Disorders of Mind and Body; a long Fit of Deafness, which still continues, hath unqualified me for conversing, or thinking, or reading, or hearing; to all this is added an Apprehension of Giddiness, whereof I have frequently some frightful Touches."³⁴ Conversing, thinking, reading, hearing—through these, Swift understood and imposed order upon the chaos of human experience. When they faltered, the sick role consoled and excused his inability to enforce that order.

As evidence that Swift's contemporaries saw his disordered writing as sign of humoral disorder, we have a letter that Bolingbroke wrote him from exile in France: "I pity you the more. in reading y^r letters I feel y^r pulse, and I judg of y^r distemper as surely by the figures into wch you cast your ink, as the learned Doctor att the hand & urinal could do, if he por'd over y^r water. you are really in a very bad way."³⁵ Words are humoral excrements and Bolingbroke is physician, diagnosing Swift's illnesses from what he has written. As we have seen, Swift himself attributed any confusions and nonsense in his letters to the related disorders of body and mind. Yet even as the sick role gave him some excuse for this disordered writing, it allowed, and likely inspired, imaginative verbal play. In a letter to Henrietta Howard of 1727, he argued sickness as apology for the transpositions and substitutions of letters in his words: "I make nothing of mistaking untoward for Howard, well pull for Walpole, Slily for Ilay, Knights of a Share for Knights of a Shire, Monster for Minister; in writing *Speaker* I put an n for a p. and a hundred such blunders, which cannot be helped while I have a hundred oceans roaring in my ears, into which no sense hath been poured this fortnight, and therefore if I write nonsense, I can assure You it is genuin and not borrowed."³⁶ The apology reminds us that we cannot reduce Swift's writings to mere mechanical productions of his disordered body and mind, despite his own claims. His artful "mistaking one thing for another" ingeniously hits at his Whig enemies, the Prime "Monster" Walpole and his sneaky, share-grabbing political cronies: Archibald Campbell, Earl of Islay, who acted "Slily" as Walpole's informant, and Sir Spencer Compton, the "Sneaker" of the House of Commons, who had betrayed his Tory friends by going over to the Whigs.³⁷ This is hardly the nonsense of someone whose mind and writing were irrevocably discomposed by his chronic illnesses.³⁸

In humoral pathology, in fact, Swift found new imaginative opportunities. Among them, there are the brilliant Latino-Anglicus that he exchanged with Sheridan, his ingenious puns, and the coinages of *Gulliver's Travels* (Lilliputian, Brobdingnag, Yahoo, Houyhnhnm, and many others). All of them embody new linguistic order made from linguistic disorder. In the *Travels*, Swift also played games with size and perspective, shrinking bodies down and blowing them up. In the next chapters, we consider such ways in which he represented the physical and social experiences of illness in his imaginative writing. It is enough to know here that the sick role did more than excuse what Swift claimed were the disorders of his writing. It also licensed his wild imaginative play.

Olivia Weisser contends that sickness was "an important site of self-production in early modern England, a stage for constructing a sense of self."[39] We saw earlier how Swift himself invoked both biblical typology (the story of the fall) and family typology (the story of his grandfather the orchard thief) to give his personal sufferings meaning beyond themselves. His imagined figurations of himself, as ravenous Adam and as the heroic but unrewarded Royalist clergyman Thomas, helped Swift make sense of his illnesses. Simultaneously, they were important self-constructions, narratives that gave shape to an identity disordered by his humoral body.

In his ailments, Swift also found singular opportunities for constructing social identities. He forged a sympathetic community with other sick persons. He imaginatively conferred upon himself the social rank that he did not have by birth and had not been able to earn by merit and service. He even reimagined himself sexually, forming intimate relations with women who, like him, were chronically ill. Such were the opportunities that the fluid humoral body allowed. For Swift, then, the sick role was not only the performance of social forms, the expectations for how he should be perceived and for how he should act in his illnesses. It was, more profoundly, the reimagining of his social identity.

At the same time that he complained of increasing isolation in his progressive disorders, Swift formed an epistolary community with others who were sick. There were, to begin, those of his own social station, with whom he found some comfort in shared illnesses. He often exchanged enquiries about health with his friends—Stella, Pope, Gay, and others—and he had advice for them about diet, exercise, and management of the other nonnaturals. He expressly identified with sick acquaintances. Of his fellow Scriblerian and clergyman, the poet Thomas Parnell, Swift wrote in the *Journal to Stella*, "His Head is out of order like mine, but more constant, poor boy."[40] And after Matthew Prior's death in 1721, he complained, "I have been for some Weeks confined by a Deafness and Noise in my Ears (which disorder my Excellent Friend [Prior] was subject to)."[41] Many years later, he wrote to Barber and his wife, the poet Mary, "I wish we three valetudinarians were together we should make excellent company."[42] Swift shut the gates of this little de facto sick community to any but his "fellow-sufferers."[43] "You healthy People cannot judge of the Sickly," he sniffed at Charles Ford in 1720. He enforced the exclusion in a letter to the same four years later: "You are a Stranger to sickness and not a judge pour nous autres maladifs."[44] As we shall see later, Swift formed an even greater intimacy with Stella through shared illness, while pointedly excluding the third-party Dingley, whom he cast as crudely healthier and, as such, socially inferior.

Swift's fond hope that he spend time with his fellow valetudinarians was one thing in imagination, something different in reality. We have seen the unpretty portrait of himself sick being treated by Stella, who tended him "like an humble slave" while suffering silently in her own illness. In the verses, he is raving and "brutish"; Stella is "Stoic in her own."[45] To be sure, this representation is apologetically self-ironic. Be that as it may, it cynically undercuts any congenial ideal of "fellow-feeling" in shared illness. However much the sick role idealized the sympathy that one might expect or extend to others in illness, catering to sick persons could be difficult and often thankless. We see this strain especially in time that Swift spent with his fellow in illness Pope in the spring and summer of 1727.

Swift often commiserated with Pope about sickness and felt genuine concern about his health. "Pray let me have three lines under any hand or pothook that will give me a better account of your health; which concerns me more than others," he implored.[46] And he routinely exchanged medical notes with his younger friend. For his own part, Pope claimed brotherhood through shared infirmity. He wrote to Swift, "The natural imbecillity of my body, join'd now to this acquir'd old age of the mind, makes me at least as old as you, and we are the fitter to crawl down the hill together; I only desire I may be able to keep pace with you."[47] The two might find such kinship in illness. All the same, Swift seems to have resented the sad reminders of his own mortality and of the grief that must follow. "I am unhappy in sickly friends," he wrote to Pope in January 1730–31: "There are my L^d and Lady Bolin[gbroke] the Doct^r [Arbuthnot] you, and Mr Gay, are not able to contribute amongst you to make up one sturdy healthy person. If I were to begin the World, I would never make an acquaintance with a poor or sickly Man, with whom there might be any danger of contracting a friendship. For I do not yet find that years have begun to harden me."[48] Whereas shared sickness might bring some comfort to Swift, it also brought suffering and loss.

By the summer of 1725, it had been eleven years since Swift had seen his friends in England. He wrote to Pope that he would have visited long before if he had not been disabled by recurring deafness. But if Pope can get him the "two or three Harridan Ladys" who can nurse him and bellow at him in his deafness—and if he is still alive—he "will venture all" and brave the journey.[49] Upon this hint, Pope promised that there were women in his household who could accommodate his friend in his ailments: "If you come to us I'll find you elderly Ladies enough that can hallow, and two that can nurse, and they are too old and feeble to make too much noise; as you will guess when I tell you they are my own mother, and my own nurse."[50] In his studied self-representations, Pope often wrote letters (even to his intimate friends) with an eye toward publication. His concern for Swift's health here seems neither artful nor self-conscious, though. The offer of making accommodation for Swift's particular disorders is both sympathetic and specific.

After the almost immediate success of *Gulliver's Travels* in late 1726, Swift made a final visit to England the following April, no doubt eager to enjoy his newfound celebrity and perhaps to position himself one last time for a preferment in the English Church. During this time, he stayed with Pope in his villa at Twickenham. Despite the generous hospitality and accommodations, Swift soon tired of his time with the sickly Pope, whose tubercular condition made every movement painful. He himself was suffering from severe fits of both deafness and giddiness and claimed social embarrassment: "I am very uneasy here, because so many of our Acquaintance come to see us, and I cannot be seen."[51] Irvin Ehrenpreis writes, charitably, that "Pope's hospitality and good nature grew more impressive as the illnesses of the poet, his [own aged and infirm] mother, and their guest kept calling for attention."[52] But Swift confided to Sheridan that he found his friend's disabilities confining, his willingness to make himself agreeable indebting: "Mr. Pope is too sickly and complaisant; therefore I resolve to go somewhere else."[53] Despite his own disorders, Swift was still a man of great energies; in contrast, Pope was a frail invalid who had to be laced into a corset for support when he stood up.[54] He left Pope after four months, apparently with little warning, and went to his cousin Patty Rolt (Lancelot): "I will leave this Place, and remove to Greenwich, or somewhere near London, and take my Cousin Lancelot to be my Nurse."[55] Having given Pope "Pretence of some very unavoidable Occasions," Swift left for London on the last day of August.[56] By the end of September he was on his way back to Ireland.

Pope was hurt. He wrote to Swift, "Would to God I could ease any of them ['your complaints'], or had been able even to have alleviated any! I found I was not, and truly it grieved me. I was sorry to find you could think your self easier in any house than in mine." He hoped, if he lived long enough, "to visit [Swift] in Ireland": "[I would] act there as much in my own way as you did here in yours. [But] I will not leave your roof, if I am ill."⁵⁷ Swift responded shortly thereafter from Dublin, "I find it more convenient to be sick here, without the vexation of making my friends uneasy." He added that Pope's own illnesses made it difficult for him to care for a guest's as well: "It hath pleased God that you are not in a state of health, to be mortified with the care and sickness of a friend: Two sick friends never did well together; such an office is fitter for servants and humble companions, to whom it is wholly indifferent whether we give them trouble or no."⁵⁸ Sympathetic connections with fellow valetudinarians were comforting in the abstract. They were tiresome and demoralizing in reality. Nevertheless, in a world increasingly narrowed by his disabilities, such connections with other sick persons gave Swift some sense of community.

In his relations with well-to-do persons who were sick like him, he found more than this communal feeling. The socially aspirant Swift found new opportunities in linking himself to sick people of high status. In community with *these* people, he imaginatively conferred upon himself the rank and recognition for which he had always hungered.

As historians such as Roy Porter have shown, the traditional "three-class model" of a rigid social hierarchy—upper, middle, and lower orders—does not hold up against the facts on the ground.⁵⁹ There was much social mobility, at least among individuals, especially at the class margins. Younger sons of peers went into business, while the daughters of wealthy merchants married into titles. Even the enterprising sons of drapers, farmers, and coal miners might, in extraordinary cases, rise to rank in the Church or military or accumulate princely fortunes in business. Such, thought Swift himself, were the rewards for exceptional merit and industry. He acknowledged, perhaps with wincing self-irony, his own aspirations to social elevation, writing to Bolingbroke and Pope in 1729, "All my endeavours from a boy to distinguish my self, were only for want of a great Title and Fortune, that I might be used like a Lord by those who have an opinion of my parts." Characteristically, he undercuts his own desired ascendancy by reducing social rank to image and performance. Then, unconvincingly, he consoles himself that "the reputation of wit or great learning does the office of a blue riband, or of a coach and six horses."⁶⁰ That is, to be recognized as a man of wit and learning is itself enough. But here is sad comfort. We hear the voice of a man whose social identity and even parentage were never quite certain, a man hurt by neglect and the feeling that his services and talents have gone unrewarded.

For Swift, wit and learning and industry were themselves the currency by which he hoped to purchase social ascendancy. He wrote tellingly to Bolingbroke, "My Birth although from a Family not undistinguished in its time is many degrees inferior to Yours, all my pretensions from Persons and parts infinitely so; I a Younger Son of younger Sons, You born to a great Fortune.... [B]ecause I cannot be a great Lord, I would acquire what is a kind of Subsidium, I would endeavour that my betters shall seek me by the merit of something distinguishable instead of my seeking them."[61] He always hoped that he would rise by his own merits and agency, yet his experience taught him that his fortunes depended upon the recognition and rewards of those in power. He was ever disappointed in them. The positions of those grateful friends like Oxford and Bolingbroke were themselves too precarious to do him lasting good. Other men of influence, even Temple, were too often neglectful, forgetful, or capricious. In a later-life letter to Pope, Swift sighed of his celebrity as Irish patriot, "My popularity that you mention is wholly confined to the common people, who are more constant than those we miscal their betters. I walk the streets, and so do my lower friends, from whom and from whom alone, I have a thousand hats and blessings upon old scores, which those we call the gentry have forgot. But I have not the love, or hardly the civility of any one man in power or station."[62] Here are both the drawing of class lines and the rankling of a disappointed man, who always kept score of those "grateful" and "ungrateful."[63]

Even though his deafness and giddiness encumbered his clerical duties, social interactions, and writing, Swift himself never imputed the failure of his ambitions directly to his chronic disorders. We never hear nor does he suggest that he was passed over for a preferment in England because he would have been a bad health risk. Still, Swift often represents his confinement and isolation during illness as correlatives to the neglect and obscurity of his life in Ireland. Ruing his banishment to "this enslaved Country to which [he was] condemned during Existence, (for [he could not] call it Life)," he wrote in the same epistolary breath that deafness "hath confined" him to his "Deanry-House and Garden" and made him a "Speculative Monk."[64] Confinement to the deanery during episodes of giddiness and deafness was the spatial counterpart to his "Exile and Oblivion" in Ireland.[65] "I am now good for nothing," he wrote to Oxford's son Harley, "very deaf, very old and very much out of favour with those in Power. My dear Lord; I have a thousand things to say, but I can remember none of Them."[66]

The neglect and forgetfulness of his friends in his illnesses were sadly emblematic of the abandonment and ingratitude of powerful men.

Even as illness disabled and confined Swift, it gave him opportunities to imagine his own social ascendancy. In the sick role, he could claim not only sympathy and exemptions but also privilege and rank. In the permeability of social boundaries that came with illness, Swift made explicit connections between himself and the well-to-do. "I met Sir George Beaumont in the Pall-mall," he reported to Stella and Dingley. "I was telling him of my head; he said he had been ill of the same disorder, and by all means forbid me bohea tea; which he said always gave it him."[67] He clucked at titled friends like Bolingbroke and Sir Andrew Fountaine for their immoderate habits. And he scolded Lord Orrery, "You are neither fitted in body or Mind . . . for such a way of living."[68] In sick talk, his betters were his familiars, and illness was a mode of imaginative ascendancy. He wrote to Stella and Dingley, "Lady Kerry is just as I am, only a great deal worse . . . and we conn ailments, which makes us very fond of each other."[69] He imagined that Stella had her own sick talk with her own circle of friends: "Han't I seen you conning ailments with Joe's wife, and some others, sirrah?"[70] "Joe's wife" was the spouse of Joseph Beaumont, an Irish linen-draper. Stella might have held sick court with tradespeople and "some others," presumably from the lower orders. But in *his* illnesses, Swift stood with the most important people in England. After writing to the ladies in October 1712 that he was "deep in Pills with Assa fetida, and a Steel bitter drink," he accounted his "Head much better than it was": "The Qu, Ld Treas^r [Oxford], Ldy Masham and I were all ill togethr; but are now all better."[71] The queen; her favorite, Abigail Masham (who herself had begun in common circumstances); Oxford; and Swift, as he imagined himself through illness, were the power brokers of the nation.

Swift was particularly aware of the kinship he had in illness with Oxford, the political figure he admired most. "Did I ever tell you that lord treasurer hears ill with the left ear, just as I do?" he asked the ladies. "He always turns the right; and his servants whisper him at that only."[72] Not long after Oxford's death in 1724, Swift wrote to his son, "I have the Honor to be afflicted with the same Disease with Your Lordships Father, frequent Fits of Deafness."[73] Swift found a form of intimacy with Oxford in their shared disorder. This repositioning through illness, though, was not merely imagined social ascendancy. Swift knew well that sickness could serve his interests. In reporting to Stella and Dingley about the impaired hearing that he shared with Oxford, he added, "I dare not tell him, that I am so too, for fear he should think I counterfeited, to make my court."[74] Likewise, as we shall see, at the same time that he was commiserating with Henrietta Howard on their shared giddiness and deafness, he was also courting her influence in final hopes for an appointment in the English Church.

Because of "a continuance of giddyness," Swift complained, "a domestick Life is necessary."[75] Away from the world of public affairs, he was powerless, yet the sick role empowered him with a kind of social command. Likening himself to Oxford in the deafness they had in common, Swift wrote to his son Harley of his chronic illnesses, "While I am thus incommoded I must be content to live among those whom I can govern, and make them comply with my Infirmityes."[76] In 1727, he tried to entice the invalid Pope to visit him in Ireland with the promise of inferiors who would cater to their needs in sickness: "I have a race of orderly elderly people of both sexes at command, who are of no consequence, and have gifts proper for attending us; who can bawl when I am deaf, and tread softly when I am only giddy and would sleep."[77] He made the same appeal six years later: "There are at least six or eight gentleman of sence, Learning good humour & tast, able & desireous to please you, & orderly females, some of the bett[e]r sort, to take care of you."[78] These solicitous servants and family, "orderly" in the face of his disorders, were certainly of *much* consequence to Swift. His description of their comic deference is an ironic picture of himself in the sick role.

Because this role did in fact allow him to lord it over others, Swift could assume the airs of superior rank. Confined by illness, he complained to the Duchess of Queensberry, "I now hate all people whom I cannot comm[a]nd," adding in jest that "consequently a Dutchess is at this time the hatefullest Lady in the World" to him.[79] People of the lower ranks would certainly comply with his sick needs—and sick whims. Swift wrote to Pope in 1728, "I reckon that a man subject like us to bodily infirmities, should only occasionally converse with great people, notwithstanding all their good qualities, easinesses, and kindnesses. There is another race which I prefer before them, as Beef and Mutton for constant dyet before Partridges," he explained: "I mean a middle kind both for understanding and fortune, who are perfectly easy, never impertinent, complying in every thing, ready to do a hundred little offices that you and I may often want, who dine and sit with me five times for once that I go to them, and whom I can tell without offence, that I am otherwise engaged at present." The well-to-do of their acquaintance, said Swift, "are only fit for our healthy seasons."[80] Three years later, he wrote that "when a Man is Sick, or Sickly, great Lords and Ladies . . . are not half so commodious as middling folks, whom one may govern as one pleases, and who will think it an honor and happiness to attend us, to talk or be silent, to laugh or look grave just as they are directed."[81] Whatever wry comment Swift might be making about literary celebrity, these remarks convey his using the sick role to place himself socially higher than those in the "middle." That Lord Sunderland and Lord Somers had such compliant factotums was recommendation enough for Swift, he wrote to Pope: "I often thought you wanted two or three of either Sex in such an employment, when you were weary, or Sick, or Solitary, and you have my probatum est."[82] Privileges of rank could be reinforced in the sick role.

For Swift, social ascendancy in the sick role went even further. If he lorded over those "of no consequence" in his illnesses, Swift also commanded those of great consequence. On the prospect of visiting the Duchess of Queensberry in 1731, he wrote with mock imperiousness of the accommodations that she must make for him at her Amesbury estate:

> Valitudinarians must live where they can command, and scold; I must have horses to ride, I must go to bed, and rise when I please, and live where all mortals are subservient to me. I must talk nonsense when I please; and all who are present must commend it. I must ride thrice a week, and walk three or 4 miles besides every day. . . . If I wait on you, I declare that one of your women, which ever it is that had designs upon a Chaplain, must be my nurse[,] if I happen to be sick or pevish at your house: and in that case you must suspend your domineering Claim till I recover. . . . I promise you shall have your will six minutes in every hour at Aimsbury, and seven in London, while I am in health. But if I happen to be sick, I must govern to a Second.[83]

To indulge Swift in his illnesses, the Duchess must surrender her command; such are the privileges of the sick role. She responded that while she, too, "can scold & command," she also "can be Silent, & obey" but added feebly, "if she pleases."[84] Swift insisted that other well-to-do make similar accommodations. In one of his final letters, he pledged that he would visit Lady Orrery, "in spight of [his] two Grievances," deafness and giddiness. He added, "I will give my self the Honor and Happyness of Waiting on

Your Ladyship . . . upon a Promise that You will extend your voice untill you make me hear You."[85] To these friends of quality, the commands are jesting and good-humored. Nevertheless, Swift has imaginatively inverted the reliance and dependency of well-to-do disabled men upon their social inferiors. He is ordering around his social betters and commandeering *their* households in his illnesses.

As Swift reimagined himself socially, so he reimagined himself sexually in his illnesses, establishing curious, sometimes intimate relations with women who, like him, were chronically ill. Some of them, such as Lady Kerry and Henrietta Howard (later the Countess of Suffolk), were his social superiors; as we find, at least in his relations with Howard, his kinship in illness becomes at once socially and sexually transgressive. But it is his relationship with Stella in sickness, which has been given little attention by biographers and literary critics, that compels particular interest first. Because Stella's correspondence to Swift during his London years does not survive, we can only infer what she sent to him about her own health and her solicitudes about his. In *his* talk of illness and health specifically to Stella, often to the exclusion of the third-party Dingley, we see a distinctive intimacy formed in sickness.

In the *Journal*, we hear Swift at his tenderest when he asks over and over about Stella's health: "I am sure 'tis the grief of my soul to think you are out of order"; "Pray God, Ppt's illnesses may not return!"[86] "Sure you don't deceive me, Ppt, when you say you are in better health than you were these three weeks," he scolded, "for Dr. Raymond told me yesterday, that Smyth of the Blind-Quay had been telling Mr. Leigh, that he left you extreamly ill; and in short, spoke so, that he almost put poor Leigh into tears, and would have made me run distracted."[87] Beneath what seems comic representation of Stella's health as town gossip and the image of Swift's running mad through London, likely in his cassock, there is genuine worry and affection. We hear this even when he guards himself against sentimentality with his "little language": "Gd be thank^d that Tp^t im bettr of her disoddles [disorders]; pray God keep her so."[88] The health of the woman he loved profoundly was one of Swift's persistent concerns, not only in the *Journal* but also in the often-anxious letters that he wrote to others when he and Stella were apart. Infantilizing her by enquiring about her "disoddles," Swift would fix her in time so that illness and decay and mortality can never reach her.

In his inquiries about Stella's well-being, we see a particular pattern emerging as Swift connects his own health with hers, often conjoining the two syntactically in a *maladie à deux:* "My health continues pretty well; pray God Ppt may give me a good account of hers."[89] Making a symmetry of sickness, he writes, "I . . . hope to hear that Ppt has been much better in her head and eyes; my head continues as it was, no fits, but a little disorder every day."[90] He and Stella are bound sympathetically in their chronic disorders. "I hoped ppt would have done with her illness," he wrote in 1712. "But I think that we both have tht Faculty never to part with a Disorder for ever; we are very constant."[91] Constancy here takes on new meaning if we consider that shared illness is in its own way shared affections.

So focused is Swift in his concerns about Stella's health that we forget that Rebecca Dingley was also party to the letters. But she is excluded from this sick talk. While fostering sympathetic kinship with the chronically ill girl, Swift peremptorily dismisses Dingley—because she is healthy. "How does poor Ppt?" he asks. "Dd [dear Dingley] is well enough. Go, get you gone, naughty girl, you are well enough."[92] In a letter of March 1710–11, after wishes that the palsy water he sent "may do my dearest little Ppt good" and then a long turn to literary news, inquiries about mutual friends, even a report on his servant Patrick's pet bird, he remarks, "And I suppose Dd is so fair and so fresh as a lass in May, and has her health, and no spleen."[93] In the tête-à-tête between the sick persons, Dingley is eavesdropper or afterthought. Worse, Swift would have the healthy woman serve the ill, reading and writing for Stella, whose eyes were delicate: "Poor dear Ppt, don't write in the dark, nor in the light neither, but dictate to Dd; she is a naughty healthy girl, and may drudge for both."[94] Stella, like Swift exceptional and privileged in the sick role, commands the ministrations of the sturdy, dull, and hale Dingley.[95]

Swift often advised both ladies to walk for health, but while the chronically ill Stella, like him, had to watch her diet, he presumed that the healthy Dingley need not worry about such restraint. Enviously watching the Lord Keeper Simon Harcourt "champing and champing" on "delicious peaches" while he himself "durst not eat one," he wrote, "I wished Dd had some of them, for poor Ppt can no more eat fruit than pdfr [that is, himself]."[96] On the prospect of the ladies' going to Wexford in the summer of 1711 so that Stella could drink the mineral waters for her health, Swift enjoined them to "love one another, and be good girls; and drink pdfr's health in water, madam Ppt; and in good ale, madam Dd."[97] He was bewildered later to find that Dingley had taken the waters, too: "But why Dd drinks them I cannot imagine; but truly she'll drink waters as well as Ppt: why not?"[98]

Even years later, while he and the ladies were staying in rural Quilca with the Sheridans, Swift represented Dingley as the outsider, self-preoccupied and unconcerned with her sick companions, while he and Stella were both ill: "Mrs. *Dingley* full of Cares for herself, and Blunders and Negligence for her Friends. Mrs. *Johnson* sick and helpless: The Dean deaf and fretting."[99] While we cannot put too much stock in punctuation, which Swift used irregularly, the conjunctive colon marries Stella and Swift in their illness. Dingley is set off alone with a period.

In sick talk with his beloved Stella, Swift could imagine "constant" and exclusive romantic relations; in sick talk with women "of quality," he could imagine both intimacy and social ascendancy. Of "poor Lady Kerry, who is much worse in her head than I," Swift wrote to Stella, "We are so fond of one another, because our ailments are the same; don't you know that, Madam Ppt?"[100] There is comic teasing to jealousy here, with Kerry cast as the other woman in sick relations. There is also social reimagining. In sick talk with a Lady Kerry, Masham, Orkney, or Germain, a Duchess of Ormonde or Queensberry, Swift could establish connections with high-ranking women in shared physicality.

The most sexually suggestive of such relations in shared illness was that with Henrietta Howard.[101] Alexander Pope had introduced Swift to Howard. In trying to entice the Dean to visit him in England, he had promised supplying the "elderly Ladies . . . that can hallow" to him in his deafness. He added, "I can also help you to a Lady who is as deaf, tho' not so old as your self."[102] Howard, the lady in question, was then about thirty-six, Swift almost fifty-eight. Swift responded, "I have almost done with Harridans and shall soon become old enough to fall in love with Girls of Fourteen." And then of Howard, he added, "I am glad she visits you but my voice is so weak that I doubt she will never hear me."[103] When he did visit England in 1726, he quickly established an acquaintanceship with her, no doubt in part because he still cherished lingering ambitions for a clerical appointment in England. Although Howard was "no Party-woman," said Pope, Swift must certainly have known that she was mistress to the Prince of Wales, even though she maintained discretion and propriety.[104] Perhaps she could work her influence with George for Swift's benefit.[105]

In his first surviving correspondence with Howard, written after his return to Dublin in 1726, Swift established a mutual sick-relation: "Dr Arbuthnot lately mortified me with an Account of a great Pain in your Head[.] I believe no Head that is good for any thing is long without some

Disorder, at least that is the best Argument I have for any thing that is good in my own."[106] Although Swift was never one to sentimentalize illness or to see sickliness as a sign of refined sensibility, as did the "nervous" of the later eighteenth century, he does suggest here that the disorder he shares with Howard betokens superior intellectual endowments.[107]

In the summer of 1727, when Swift was staying with Pope at Twickenham, he and Mrs. Howard exchanged a quick series of letters over six days, during which he forced a kind of intimacy through their shared disorders. On August 12, he had written to Sheridan that he was miserably ill and was planning to leave England soon. Two days later, in the first of his letters to Howard, who was only a couple of miles away at Richmond, Swift was surprisingly jaunty. With only the most perfunctory opening civility, he began, "Madam. I wish I were a young Lord, and you were unmarryd. I should make you the best husband in the world, for I am ten times deafer than ever you were in your life, and instead of a few pain[s] in the face, I have a good substantial giddyness and Head-ake; the best of it is, that although we might lay our heads together, You could tell me no secrets, that might not be heard five rooms distant."[108] He imagined, that is, that they would be heard throughout the house as they screamed at each other in their shared deafness.

There are comic raillery and playful performance here. There is also blunt physicality. Sharing Swift's chronic disorders, Howard is an "understanding Body."[109] In his sixtieth year, Swift casts himself as young, rakish, noisy, and titled, in a marital relation with a social superior twenty-two years his junior. Sick bed is sex bed. And Swift makes Howard's attentions exclusive. He effaces any rival male so that he enjoys her sole attentions, replacing not only her husband but also her lover, the newly crowned monarch (and this on the very day that George was visiting Richmond). This sick talk, then, is both sexually and socially transgressive. Because Swift says that the secrets that he and Howard bawl at each other will "be heard five rooms distant," illness is also public performance, however comic. It is important to Swift that his social ascendancy and his sexuality be recognized.

At the end of this first letter, as if to acknowledge that he has taken liberties, Swift says that the newly elevated Queen Caroline herself remarked that he "was an odd sort of man" who would "speak freely to Princes."[110] Responding two days later, Howard pointedly, even if playfully, checked this overstepping: "I did desire you to write me a Love letter but I never did desire You to talk of marrying me. I had rather you and I were dumb as well as deaf for ever then that shou'd happen; I wou'd take your giddyness, your head-ake or any other complaint you have, to resemble you in one circumstance of life. so that I insist upon your thinking your self a very happy man, at least when ever you make a comparasion [sic] between you and I."[111] Despite her gentle reprimand, Howard, in the indeterminacy of her own disorders, can also remake herself. Unhappily married to a husband whom Lord Hervey described as "wrong-headed, ill-tempered, obstinate, drunken, extravagant, brutal," she would gladly take on Swift's greater ailments to be unmarried, like him.[112] As Swift could reimagine himself socially and sexually in the sick role, so Howard would buy her freedom with the currency of illness and reimagine her own identity.

Howard having tamped down his flirtatiousness, Swift reasserts rhetorical control with protective self-irony in his next letter. No longer the rakish husband but no less high-ranking, he is now "like a great Minister in a tottering condition."[113] He then retreats further by putting his disorders into a medical context, however ironically: "I chiefly valued my self upon my bad head and deaf ears. if these be no charms for you, I must give over. . . . [S]ince my best qualityes will not move you, I am so desperate that I resolve to get rid of them as soon as possible and accordingly am putting my self into the apothecary's books, and swallowing the poisons he sends me by the Doctors orders."[114] Here the appeal to the doctors' authority and his role as dutiful patient are rhetorically serviceable. He can play the sick role to draw back protectively from the very intimacy that he had imagined in their shared illnesses.

Responding to a second gently scolding note from Howard in a final letter of their exchange, Swift famously diagnoses his own ailments, attributing them to his reckless youthful gluttony at Richmond, as we saw earlier. At the end of his explanation for the disorders that once brought him into Howard's metaphorical bed, he closes, "So much for the calamityes wherein I have the honor to resemble you; and you see your sufferings are but children in comparison of mine."[115] In his illnesses, his body unstable and his identity fluid, he had cast himself as Howard's social equal and bedmate. Tracing back in this last letter what he calls elsewhere his "old Disorders," Swift now reasserts differences in both degree of illness and age and recasts himself and Howard in the father-daughter relationship that so often characterized his associations with younger women. In so doing, he desexualizes himself, protectively. But even here he reaffirms sexuality and masculine vigor. If his claim to having eaten the hundred golden pippins at one sitting is confession of humoral self-abuse, it is also grandiose boast. This would have been a prodigious feat, something worthy of Swift's favorite Gargantua or his own Gulliver in Lilliput. The story of his gorging upon apples is a reimagining of himself young and unrestrained. It is also his original sin, of course. And here, too, is shared sexuality. Like Adam, Swift is sexualized in his sin of appetite. The fact that Mrs. Howard, chronically disordered by her own "bad head, and deaf ears," was residing at Richmond when he wrote, implicitly bound her to him in that fall.[116] It was there that Swift had eaten all those apples so many years earlier.

At the end of this letter to Howard, as a final way of restoring distance and decorum, Swift resorted to characteristic self-protective comic and ironic representation of himself in his illnesses. In response to his promise to swallow the apothecary's "poisons," Howard, who had been urging him to visit, asked him to write her "if *poison* or other Methods" prevent him from coming in person.[117] Swift seized upon the opportunity for wordplay: "I wish the *poison* were in my Stomack (which may be very probable considering the many Drugs I take) if I remember to have mentioned that word in my Letter. But, Ladyes who have poison in their eyes, may be apt to mistake in reading—Oh, I have found it out; the Word *Person* I suppose was written like *Poison*. ask all the friends I write to, and they will attest this mistake to be but a trifle in my way of writing, and could easily prove it if they had any of my letters to shew."[118] The artful transpositions and substitutions of letters discussed earlier and his apology for writing nonsense follow. Swift is able to lay the blame for any indiscretions upon his disorders and to protect himself through refractive irony. One of his favorite refuges.

The letters to Howard plot the imaginative possibilities that Swift found in illness. A would-be rake playing on shared physicality, Swift, in his age and sickness, insinuated himself into the epistolary bed of a woman more than twenty years his junior. As "husband" in illness to a noblewoman (and one he hoped would use her influence to promote his ambitions), he also imagined social rank. But gently rebuffed, he restored the decorum of social boundaries by playing the role of doctors' patient, telling the story of his humoral disorders, reaffirming the difference in age, and resorting to comic and ironic self-representation. Over a correspondence of only five days, Swift navigated chronic illness, ambition, and sexuality—all through sick-talk in the sick role.

8

Gulliver's Travels and Swift's Travails

As Swift's modern biographers have uniformly accepted the retrospective diagnosis of Ménière's disease and then written his life and experiences through the lens of the modern clinic, so literary critics have made a critical lens of that diagnosis and found in his works imaginative representations of his Ménière's symptoms. One brief but representative article finds direct correspondences between Gulliver's hearing impairments and the "informational isolation" that comes with Ménière's disease.[1] Another, more recent essay on Swift's sicknesses claims that "every symptom of this mystery sickness [Ménière's disease]—down to the anxiousness and the way it forced his friends to shout—appears in *Gulliver's Travels*."[2] Even Clive Probyn, in an otherwise valuable article on Swift and the medical profession of his day, makes the unusual statement that one of Swift's poems "indicates the Galenic reading Swift had done in order to understand for himself the debilitating bouts of labyrinthine vertigo (Ménière's syndrome) which afflicted him."[3] Galen would obviously have had little to say about a disorder that was not created until the mid-nineteenth century, and he would have been baffled by the clinic's conception of the body.

Within the logic of retrospective diagnosis, such readings of Swift's works are useful. For one, they make the case that Swift was writing *from* the body, that is, that his bodily experiences somehow affected what he wrote and how he wrote it. Seeing events in a work like *Gulliver's Travels* as imaginative representations of Ménière's symptoms is serviceable as analogy: If we understand the physical and mental sufferings of Ménière's patients, we can appreciate better how Swift represents his own disabilities and anxieties. But reading his works through the lens of the clinical diagnosis misdirects and limits our understanding of Swift's imaginative representations of his experiences as a sick person. As I hope that my study has made clear throughout, this interpretation uses the wrong body as referent. Swift wrote not from the clinical body of Ménière and John Bucknill but from the fluid, ever-shifting humoral body that he knew; he represented his disorders not as "entities" that fit neatly into a disease taxonomy but as messy imbalances lurching his entire system into chaos that had somehow to be contained. The clinical diagnosis makes symptomatology of lived experience. In turn, a clinical reading of Swift's imaginative writing becomes an exercise in drawing one-to-one correspondences between Gulliver's experiences and the discrete symptoms of the modern disease. Knowing, for example, that the Ménière's patient typically loses hearing in the left ear first, one reader focuses on Gulliver's turning his right ear to hear on several occasions.[4] Another sees his transformation from optimist to misanthrope as representation of Swift's own vertigo, an "otological symptom" of his Ménière's disease.[5] Using the retrospective diagnosis in this way as a critical lens constrains our reading of his imaginative works, as it does our reading of his life. Reducing "disorder" in all of its comprehensive meanings to a categorical disease entity and Gulliver's experiences to clinical symptoms, this reading cannot appreciate as fully how Swift imaginatively represents the lived experience of his illnesses, the chaos of body, confusions of senses and faculties, social disabilities and embarrassment, indeterminacies of identity, and fears of madness. Nor does it appreciate that a work like the *Travels* is yet another way for Swift to impose order on disorder, of a piece with the humoral explanation of his illnesses, his regimen, and his performances in the "sick role."

Before turning to the ways in which Swift imagined the experiences of illness in the *Travels*, we need to theorize briefly the much-debated issue of self-representation itself in his works. Formalists, especially those who read and teach works like "A Modest Proposal" and the *Travels*, would make an absolute separation between the author and his "personae": Swift is one person; the too-rational projector and gullible traveler are distinct, other persons. But those such as Irvin Ehrenpreis respond that we can never, finally, extract the historical Swift, his attitudes, and his experiences from his writings.[6] Claude Rawson has argued that, even in "A Modest Proposal," the attitudes of Swift's speaker are never entirely distinct from his own. Author and speaker "are neither the same nor separable," contends Rawson.[7] To insist that a modest proposer, Grub Street hack, freethinker, or Gulliver is a separate character—or even a "character" at all—is to insist upon textual unity that does not exist and to miss Swift's "unofficial energies" beneath the text.[8]

The argument that Swift is representing his disordered *body* is all the more problematic when we ask whether the "personae" or "voices" that Swift presents are themselves embodied or are mere abstractions floating free of physical connections. Certainly, there are bodies, of sorts. To choose from among the best-known, the Grub Street hack who tells the *Tale of a Tub* announces that his "whole Work was begun, continued, and ended, under a long Course of Physic."[9] The modest proposer, surrounded by bodies in a culture of consumption, likes his children seasoned with pepper and salt to his own tastes. The voyeurs of the "scatological" poems are preoccupied with the nauseating physicality of the women they spy on, even if they will not acknowledge their own. In all of these works, Swift is confronting and representing imaginatively the intractable materiality of his own body. Among all of his embodied "characters," however, Gulliver, who eats, breathes, reports on his daily bodily functions, and moves about in the various worlds that he inhabits, is most substantially a body living among bodies, even if he is not entirely coherent as character or consistent in his attitudes.

That Gulliver's physicality is prominent—and precarious—has much to do, I would say, with Swift's apparent need to represent imaginatively his own experiences as a sick man at the time that he wrote the *Travels*. The composition history of the work supports the argument that Swift found source material in his own disorders. The tale almost certainly originated in the Scriblerian project begun in 1714, when he and his "brothers" set out to parody "all the false tastes in learning" and Swift apparently took on the task of writing Scriblerus's travels.[10] But while Gulliver's adventures likely germinated in Scriblerian follies, Swift wrote the *Travels* itself between 1721 and 1725.[11] During these several years, he suffered fits of giddiness and deafness more frequently and for longer periods than he had at any previous time. In the first surviving mention of the work, he reported to Charles Ford in

April 1721, "I am now writing a History of my Travells . . . but they go on slowly for want of Health and Humor."[12] In almost every letter in which he updates his friends on the progress of the work until its publication in late October 1726, he complains of his giddiness, deafness, and tinnitus.

If Swift thought that his "ill head . . . dispose[d] [him] to blunders," however, he also found imaginative possibilities in sickness.[13] His disordered head, he had claimed to Henrietta Howard, was his "best Argument . . . for any thing that is good" in it.[14] By his own testimony, his illnesses thus served as creative catalyst. Gulliver's experiences often imaginatively represent Swift's own disabilities. Moreover, his particular disorders of body, senses, and mind confused and destabilized all of those categories by which he would make sense of the world. Linguistic, epistemological, and even ontological order uncertain, Swift could imagine fantastic bodies, new languages, monstrous identities. He might turn the indeterminacies of perception, language, and identity itself to satiric purposes. His own disordered humoral body was his imaginarium.

At the first level of representation in the *Travels*, we find imaginative depictions of Swift's recurring physical ailments—giddiness, deafness, and tinnitus. Twelve times larger than the inhabitants of Lilliput, Gulliver looks down dizzily from his great height; shrunken to one-twelfth the size of the Brobdingnagians, he is always in fear of falling. The "treble and Countertenor Voices" of the Lilliputians are those of the few friends that Swift would "suffer" to see him in his deafness, like the diminutive Pilkingtons.[15] Those whom he would not are like Gulliver's Brobdingnagian farmer host. Gulliver says, "He spoke often to me, but the Sound of his Voice pierced my Ears like that of a Water-Mill."[16] In 1724, as he was completing the *Travels*, Swift himself apologized to Knightley Chetwode that "the Noise of seven Watermills in [his] Ears" "confused" his thinking and writing.[17] The chronic physical disorders, born of humoral imbalances, were source materials for Swift's imaginative writing.

In Lilliput, Swift establishes his protagonist as the humoral body writ large. Gulliver consumes vast amounts of food and drink. Having agreed to the articles of liberty, he is granted a daily "Quantity of Meat and Drink, sufficient to the Support of 1724 *Lilliputians*."[18] His evacuations are awesome. Gulliver recounts of his time tethered to the beach, "I was able to turn upon my Right [side], and to ease my self with making Water; which I very plentifully did, to the great Astonishment of the People, who conjecturing by my

Motions what I was going to do, immediately opened to the right and left on that Side, to avoid the Torrent which fell with such Noise and Violence from me."[19] Subsequently chained in the abandoned Lilliputian temple, Gulliver explains apologetically to his "candid Reader" how he managed "the Necessities of Nature": "I was under great Difficulties between Urgency and Shame. The best Expedient I could think on, was to creep into my House, which I accordingly did; and shutting the Gate after me, I went as far as the Length of my Chain would suffer; and discharged my Body of that uneasy Load. . . . From this Time my constant Practice was, as soon as I rose, to perform that Business in open Air, at the full Extent of my Chain." This business of the humoral body, *performed* as it is, becomes a communal project: "Due Care was taken every Morning before Company came, that the offensive Matter should be carried off in Wheel-barrows, by two Servants appointed for that Purpose."[20] Such prodigious defecating and urinating, sweating, eating, drinking—all strike awe in the tiny Lilliputians: Feeding him "as fast as they [can]," they show "a thousand Marks of Wonder and Astonishment at [his] Bulk and Appetite."[21] In the magnitude of Gulliver's consumptions and evacuations, Swift writes the humoral body as something gigantic and monstrous.

In book 2, it is the Brobdingnagians who are the humoral bodies gigantized: porous, sweating, urinating. The inescapable realities of the humoral body disgust Gulliver. Even with her "weak Stomach," the queen of Brobdingnag swallows "at one Mouthful, as much as a dozen *English* Farmers could eat at a Meal" and drinks "above a Hogshead at a Draught." Her consumptions, says Gulliver, are "for some time a very nauseous Sight."[22] He is sickened, too, by the appalling evacuations of the Brobdingnagian maids of honor, who unabashedly perform their natural humoral functions in front of him: "Neither did they at all scruple while I was by, to discharge what they had drunk, to the Quantity of at least two Hogsheads, in a Vessel that held above three Tuns."[23] What's more, Gulliver is "much disgusted" by "a very offensive Smell" that comes "from their Skins." In a rare moment of self-recognition, however, he remembers, "An intimate Friend of mine in *Lilliput* took the Freedom in a warm Day, when I had used a good deal of Exercise, to complain of a strong Smell about me."[24] This moment of dawning reflection upon the offensiveness of his own humoral body foreshadows what he will discover in the final book of the *Travels*, the adamant reality that humans are "filthy *Yahoos*."[25]

Having imaginatively represented his own humoral body in Gulliver himself and the Brobdingnagians, Swift then imagines that body disordered by giddiness, deafness, and noise in the ears. In the opening chapter of book 2, the Brobdingnagian farmhand who discovers Gulliver in the field holds him "in the Air above sixty Foot from the Ground"; the tiny, giddy hero "resolve[s] not to struggle in the least . . . for fear [he] should slip through [the giant's] Fingers."[26] That same day, the farmer places him on the dinner table, "which was thirty Foot high from the Floor." Gulliver recalls his terror: "I was in a terrible Fright, and kept as far as I could from the Edge, for fear of falling."[27] Later, in the most dramatic and suggestive representation of Swift's own giddiness, Gulliver is snatched up by a Brobdingnagian monkey, who carries him to a rooftop. There it crams nauseating victuals into his mouth while a crowd gathers to watch the spectacle. At last the monkey drops Gulliver on a ridge of the roof and escapes. "Here I sat for some time five Hundred Yards from the Ground," he says, "expecting every Moment to be blown down by the Wind, or to fall by my own Giddiness, and come tumbling over and over from the Ridge to the Eves."[28] After he is rescued and his "dear little Nurse" Glumdalclitch has picked out "the filthy Stuff the Monkey had crammed down [his] Throat," says Gulliver, "I fell a vomiting, which gave me great relief."[29] We recollect the waves of nausea that came with Swift's own fits of giddiness and his frequent recourse to vomits for restoring balance to that giddy body.

Throughout the *Travels*, Swift also imagined his deafness and tinnitus. Lilliputian voices are tiny but shrill enough to pierce muffled hearing. Immobilized on the beach in Lilliput, the bewildered Gulliver wakes to hear the "confused Noise about [him]," then "a shrill, but distinct Voice" crying out, "*Hekinah Degul.*"[30] The voice of the Lilliputian emperor, he says later, "was shrill, but very clear and articulate, and I could distinctly hear it when I stood up."[31] Brobdingnagian voices are thunderous, booming "many Degrees louder than a speaking Trumpet" (a megaphonic device being proposed in Swift's day as a method for communicating with the deaf).[32] In Brobdingnag, Gulliver becomes so used to bawling at the top of his lungs to be heard by the giants that the English ship's captain who brings him home at the end of book 2 wonders "to hear [him] speak so loud; asking [him] whether the King or Queen of that Country were thick of hearing."[33] In book 3 of the *Travels*, Swift represents his own "thickness of . . . hearing" in Gulliver's encounters with the ludicrous "flappers."[34] So "wrapped up in Cogitation" are the Laputans that anyone who is "able to afford it" employs a menial to rouse him from his abstraction when he needs to hear or speak. Armed with rattles made of "blown Bladder[s]" filled with pebbles or dried peas, this "flapper" gently "strike[s] with his Bladder the Mouth of him who is to speak, and the Right Ear of him or them to whom the Speaker addresseth himself."[35] Here is a comic image of the deafness that stymied Swift's own hearing and understanding.

In the *Travels*, Swift also imagined his own tinnitus, confusing and frightening. Perched high on the dinner table with the Brobdingnagian farmer's family, Gulliver would show his gallantry and respects by drinking the health of his host's wife. In his loudest voice, he bawls out a toast to "her Ladyship." This makes "the Company laugh so heartily" that, in a pointed parallel to Swift's own tinnitus, Gulliver is "almost deafened with the Noise." The next moment, a cat purrs with a "Noise ... like that of a Dozen Stocking Weavers at work." Then an infant screams in "a Squall that you might have heard from *London-Bridge* to *Chelsea*."[36] In the din and confusion of these noises, collapsed into a single episode, Swift imaginatively represented the "noise in [his] head, which deafen[ed] [him]."[37]

A clinical reading of *Gulliver's Travels* finds in episodes like these the classic triad of symptoms that indicate Ménière's disease: vertigo, deafness, and tinnitus. In humoralism, however, there is no abstracting of discrete symptoms from the lived experience of sickness, as there is in the retrospective diagnosis. A reading of the work through the critical lens of this clinical diagnosis cannot evince as fully how Swift represents in Gulliver's experiences the physical sufferings, confounding of senses and understanding, embarrassed bodily performances, and indeterminacies of personal and social identity that he suffered in his disorders. Like all sick persons, Swift lacked a ready vocabulary for expressing the lived experience of his chronic illnesses. Representing them imaginatively as Gulliver's experiences was one means of doing so.

In the *Travels*, shifts of scale and perspective disorient. Bodies are shrunk down and blown up. Gulliver's senses are too weak or too acute. Noises are almost inaudible, or they deafen him. From the opening scene in Lilliput, Swift represents the ineffable disordering of his own senses as they converged in his giddiness, deafness, and tinnitus. Pinned by ligatures to the beach in Lilliput, Gulliver awakens to find himself on his back, "not able to stir" or to move arms, legs, or head: "I could only look upwards;

the Sun began to grow hot, and the Light offended mine Eyes." Unable to see anything but the sky, he hears "a confused Noise" about him. Then he feels "something alive" moving across his body. When he is finally able to wrench one arm free and to loosen his bindings on one side "with a violent Pull, which gave [him] excessive Pain," the Lilliputians launch a volley of "above an Hundred Arrows," which cause Gulliver to groan "with Grief and Pain." Resolving at last to remain still, he hears "the Noise [of their voices] increasing," and then in his right Ear he hears "a Knocking for above an Hour"; the Lilliputians, it happens, are building a huge platform on which to wheel their submissive, disabled captive to the capital.[38] In Gulliver's jumbled perceptions, Swift imagined the anarchy of his own disordered senses and sensations—sights, sounds, feelings—that he could not sort out.

In Brobdingnag, the chaos of body and senses becomes more frightening because Gulliver is yet more helpless and vulnerable. We see this especially in the scene in which the eagle who has absconded with his "Traveling-Box" drops it from a great height into the sea. Its giddy passenger, Gulliver spins in a disorienting nightmare fall, made all the more terrifying by the fact that he cannot make sense of what is happening to him in the moment: "In a little time I observed the Noise and flutter of Wings to encrease very fast; and my Box was tossed up and down like a Sign-post in a windy Day. I heard several Bangs or Buffets . . . and then all on a sudden felt my self falling perpendicularly down for above a Minute; but with such incredible Swiftness that I almost lost my Breath. My Fall was stopped by a terrible Squash [splash], that sounded louder to mine Ears than the Cataract of *Niagara;* after which I was quite in the Dark for another Minute."[39] In his free fall, Gulliver experiences the chaos of giddiness, thunderous noise in the ears, and convergence of the senses that characterized Swift's own disorders. Given Swift's penchant for wordplay, the fact that the protagonist falls with "Swiftness" connects Gulliver all the more with the Dean himself. Puns disorder language by collapsing more than one denotation into a single homograph or homophone. Even in Swift's wordplay there are possibilities for representing the physical and cognitive confusions associated with his humoral disorders.

In these experiences of Gulliver, Swift represented the subjectivities of illness, what it felt like to be a man disordered by giddiness, deafness, and auditory clamor. But as was the Dean himself, Gulliver is also a social body, observed and defined by those around him. In Gulliver's experiences, Swift represented himself as, he imagined, others saw him in his disorders: comic spectacle, helpless invalid, and unmanned object of pity. This ironizing of his experiences exemplifies the peculiar "double consciousness" about which we have already spoken, the conflated expression of his own lived experience and his imagining of how others saw him. It was yet another method for imposing order on his disorders.

Gulliver is, from the outset, a celebrity body, something gawked at, scrutinized, puzzled over. "As the News of my Arrival spread through the Kingdom" of Lilliput, he recalls, "it brought prodigious Numbers of rich, idle, and curious People to see me"; as the monstrous "*Man-Mountain*" takes gigantic strides through the metropolis, the "Garret Windows and Tops of Houses [are] so crowded with Spectators, that I thought in all my Travels I had not seen a more populous Place."[40] In Brobdingnag, Gulliver is first a "little Creature" gaped at by the bewildered farmer and his hinds.[41] Then his "Master" begins displaying him for money: "All the neighbouring Gentlemen from an Hundred Miles round, hearing of my Fame, came to see me at my Master's own House. There could not be fewer than thirty Persons with their Wives and Children; (for the Country is very populous;) and my Master demanded the Rate of a full Room whenever he shewed me at Home, although it were only to a single Family." "Finding how profitable" Gulliver is, the farmer then designs to show him in "the most considerable Cities of the Kingdom" and "all the Towns by the Way."[42] Not long after, he becomes the object of scientific scrutiny when the Brobdingnagian King's "three great Scholars" "examined [his] Shape with much Nicety."[43] In Houyhnhnmland, too, Gulliver is a body observed. He recounts of the first Houyhnhnm he meets, "The Horse started a little when he came near me, but soon recovering himself, looked full in my Face with manifest Tokens of Wonder."[44] Having led Gulliver to his own house, the same creature, now his "Master," puts him side by side with a Yahoo for comparative observation and is fascinated in particular with his clothing. As Gulliver later undresses, his "Master observed the whole Performance with great Signs of Curiosity and Admiration."[45] Even the Yahoos gawk at Gulliver and mimic his actions. His body is at once strange and familiar to them. In fact, only in Laputa does Gulliver's body not excite much observation. Upon his arrival on the floating island, itself a symbol of abstracted senses, he is "surrounded by a Crowd of People" who behold him "with all the Marks and Circumstances of Wonder."[46] But then the wacky intellectuals, seemingly unaware of their own materiality, treat his body with complete indifference.

Swift himself, ever aware of how others perceived him, feared that his giddiness and hearing impairments would embarrass his public performance. "I very seldom go to Church for fear of being seised with a Fit of Giddyness in the midst of the Service," he wrote to John Barber in 1735.[47] In Gulliver's pratfalls and failed athletic performances, Swift imagines the fool he must look in his own giddy fits. Indeed, Gulliver looks quite silly when, "with much difficulty," he raises his thimble-sized "Dram-cup" of "small Cyder" to toast the health of the Brobdingnagian farmer's wife. He speaks in an English wholly unintelligible to the family. When the company laugh at the ridiculousness of his puny performance, Gulliver is so disoriented by the "great surprize" of finding himself in a body so out of its nature (and tipsy from drink), he trips embarrassingly: "I happened to stumble against a Crust, and fell flat on my Face."[48] Here is the tottering Swift himself in fear of tumbling, walking "like a drunken Man," made ridiculous in company.[49]

Like his giddiness, Swift's hearing disorders embarrassed him socially. In his deafness, he fussed that he could "bear no Company but Trebles and counterteners" and complained that he was confined to "a scurvey home" where he could "command people to speak as loud as [he] please[d], before the vexation of making a silly figure and tearing the Lungs of [his] friends."[50] In the *Travels*, Swift comically represents his own deafness and tinnitus as not only physical but also social impairments. They impede conversation and understanding. Disoriented upon waking in Lilliput, Gulliver listens to a tiny-voiced official's long harangue, "whereof [he] understood not one Syllable."[51] Dangled in the air by the huge farmworker who stumbles across him in Brobdingnag, he desperately calls out for mercy in his strange tongue; the fieldhand is amazed "to hear [Gulliver] pronounce articulate Words, although he could not understand them."[52] Later in the same book, when Gulliver is put on the stage for money, his "Master's" daughter Glumdalclitch asks him "Questions as far as she knew [his] Understanding of the Language reached": "I answered them as loud as I could."[53] In this scene and others, sense disorders are inseparable from cognitive disorders.

Swift's making the problems of understanding ever more difficult (and absurd), Gulliver has to manage his hearing and speaking through gibberish. In each of the fantastic lands that he visits, he is struck first not by words but by inarticulate sounds: Pinned down on the Lilliputian beach, he hears great shouts in "a very shrill Accent."[54] The "Noise" of the Brobdingnagians' voices is "so High in the Air, that at first [he] certainly thought it was Thunder."[55] The Houyhnhnm he initially meets "neigh[s] three or four times, but in so different a Cadence" that Gulliver almost starts to believe that the horse is "speaking to himself in some Language of his own."[56] Only the Laputans, abstracted from their senses, do not make "conversation" with Gulliver. Seeing their island floating overhead, a crowd of people looking down at him, he "call[s] and shout[s] with the utmost Strength of [his] Voice." Although they plainly see him, they make "no Return to [his] Shouting." When Gulliver appeals to them "in the humblest Accent," he "receive[s] no Answer." At last, one distinguished-looking Laputan calls "out in a clear, polite, smooth Dialect, not unlike in Sound to the *Italian*": "Therefore I returned an Answer in that Language, hoping at least that the Cadence might be more agreeable to his Ears. Although neither of us understood the other, yet my Meaning was easily known, for the People saw the Distress I was in."[57] Even when he imagines with these Laputans and the Houyhnhnms that they are "speaking some language of [their] own," it is at first all nonsense: *Borach Mivola, Splacnuck, Hlunnh*, and the most impressive *Fluft drin Yalerick Dwuldum prastrad mirplush.*[58] These are the playful sounds of infant babble, the idiot's tongue, and the ludic nonsense-sense of Swift's own extravagant word games and "little language" ("ourrichar Gangridge") of the *Journal to Stella.*[59] Yet we can imagine these uttered noises, too, as the hardly intelligible, shrilled and squeaked sounds that Swift himself half-heard and misheard through his baffled ears and "stufft" head, jumbled and distorted by fouled humors. Disordered by deafness and tinnitus, he had to make sense of these unintelligible sounds; in a similar way, Gulliver imposes grammatical and syntactic sense upon the nonsense of the gibberish that he hears—and then speaks. Significantly, when he returns to England at the end of his travels, he finds only two nominal differences between Yahoos and people: Humans hide their filthy humoral bodies behind clothes and "use a Sort of *Jabber.*"[60] His own English is only more "horrible Howlings of the *Yahoos*," somehow to be sorted out and made sense of.[61]

Public performances of the body conversant are social activities. In Gulliver's pratfalls, confused hearing, and addlement, Swift imagined his own body tottering in the pulpit and his own vexed colloquies. In the *Travels*, he also represents the helplessness that he felt in his invalidism, the diminishment of masculine vigor by which he defined himself, and the uncertainties of his identity, personal and social. Especially in Brobdingnag, Swift represents himself reduced to childlike helplessness in his disorders. Like Swift, Gulliver is confined to the domestic sphere, his little box, "close[d] on every Side, with a little Door for [him] to go in and out, and a few Gimlet-holes to let in Air."[62] Like Swift, tended to in his illnesses by Stella and kind domestics, Gulliver must rely upon the attention and protection of the farmer's nine-year-old daughter: "I called her my *Glumdalclitch*, or little Nurse."[63] Already infantilized, he suffers further humiliation as a simian baby. After spiriting Gulliver up to the rooftop, the monkey first cradles him "as a Nurse doth a Child she is going to suckle." He relates the vile outcome: "The Monkey was . . . holding me like a Baby in one of his Fore-Paws, and feeding me with the other, by cramming into my Mouth some Victuals he had squeezed out of the Bag on one Side of his Chaps, and patting me when I would not eat."[64] After his rescue, the solicitous Glumdalclitch nurses Gulliver back to health. Confined and helpless, Gulliver has no choice but to cede authority to his "dear little Nurse." He is, as the name Grildrig would have it, "girl thing."[65]

In the previous chapter, we saw how Swift reimagined himself socially and sexually in the sick role. Even reduced in his illnesses to his rooms in the St. Patrick's deanery, he would "command and scold," insisting that others make accommodations for him. In the *Travels*, Swift parodies his own attempts to assert authority in his disorders. In Lilliput, his huge body in order, Gulliver nominally governs a vast household of compliant underlings: "An Establishment was also made of Six Hundred Persons to be my Domesticks."[66] Nevertheless, he submits to the "Commands" of the Lilliputian emperor, as he submits to the orders of other "masters" in every place he visits. Swift himself had always a "perfect Hatred of Tyran[n]y and Oppression"; Gulliver's submissions to the commands of his many "masters" throughout the work are ironic representations of his own failures to assert autonomy.[67] Ill and broken, confined to the walls of the deanery, Swift could exercise power only over his small domestic corner of Ireland. And it is with this little hope that the Portuguese ship's captain convinces Gulliver to "return to [his] native Country, and live at home with [his] Wife and Children." There, says Gulliver, "I might command in my own House, and pass my time in a Manner as recluse as I pleased."[68] Swift himself might command in his own home during episodes of giddiness and deafness. In Brobdingnag, puny, helpless Gulliver makes commands, too. He "orders" servants to accommodate his needs. Glumdalclitch takes him out for air "at [his] own Desire."[69] And he insists on more than one occasion that the "Queen's Dwarf," who plays malicious tricks upon him, be "pardoned at [his] Desire."[70] Such magnanimity from such a tiny speck of a creature.

In the *Travels,* Swift reflects also upon the unsteady manliness that was both cause and effect of his diminished authority in the world. Again and again, Gulliver would display his masculinity—physical vigor, athleticism, and heroic exploits—and assert himself as a sexual being. Again and again, he fails. Sometimes he makes a ridiculous spectacle of himself in these performances. In his male sexuality, he is not just absurd; worse, he is exploited and attacked and narratively neutered. Through Gulliver's pitiful, albeit comic displays of masculinity, Swift ironically represented his feelings that in his chronic disorders, he, too, was emasculated.

Like Swift, Gulliver prides himself on his athletic abilities. He swims, walks, rows, and uses "a good Deal of Exercise."[71] In Lilliput he gobbles up ground in walking, "ten Yards at every Stride."[72] Challenged by Lilliputians "to shew them some Proofs of [his] prodigious Strength . . . [he] readily oblige[s] them."[73] In Brobdingnag, too, Gulliver would display his manly athleticism. The queen asks him "whether a little Exercise of Rowing might not be convenient for [his] Health"; she has "her own Joyner," "an ingenious Workman," outfit a little "Pleasure-Boat with all its Tackling" for him. The joiner then builds a giant trough, "of three Hundred Foot long, fifty broad, and eight deep."[74] Here Gulliver rows for both diversion and exercise. Such athletic activities imaginatively represent Swift himself in his regimen. But they are also performances of manhood. Gulliver rows his little boat vigorously, proud to impress "the Queen and her Ladies" with his "Skill and Agility."[75]

Gulliver might try to exhibit his own masculinity with feats of physical vigor and abilities, but because his body is weirdly out of place in the various worlds in which he finds himself, he suffers frequent athletic failures and mishaps, often laughable, sometimes pathetic. He thinks that he has impressed the Brobdingnagian queen and her ladies with displays of masculine athleticism; they, however, "thought themselves [merely] agreeably entertained." Sometimes, his masculine energies fail him all together. When he tires of rowing in the little trough that the Brobdingnagians have built for him, he puts up the tiny sail on his boat; "then," he says, "my Business was only to steer, while the Ladies gave me a Gale with their Fans; and when they were weary, some of the Pages would blow my Sail forward with their Breath."[76] Here is Swift himself, at the mercy of his nurses and domestics. In another instance, Gulliver has his athletic abilities tested when the Queen's dwarf, in mischievous envy, drops him into a large bowl of cream. He tumbles "over Head and Ears." He reminds his readers and himself, "If I had not been a good Swimmer, it might have gone very hard with me." (This self-reassurance falters in view of his "swallow[ing] above a Quart of Cream" before his "little Nurse" Glumdalclitch rescues him.)[77] In such attempts to insist upon his masculinity through athletic prowess, Gulliver goes to absurd lengths, as when he challenges the dwarf to a wrestling match—thumping his little chest imprudently, for in such an encounter he would have been quickly flattened and embarrassed by his thirty-foot opponent. But he feistily continues in his attempts to prove himself; these attempts always end in comic failure. In the most humiliating and memorable failed physical performance, he tries to impress the Brobdingnagians with his leaping abilities. Walking with Glumdalclitch and friends, he sees a "Cow-dung in the Path" and "must needs try [his] Activity by attempting to leap over it": "I took a Run, but unfortunately jumped short, and found my self just in the Middle up to my Knees." The story of Gulliver's short-jumping quickly makes the rounds in court, "so that all the Mirth, for some Days, was at [his] Expence."[78] Such failed physical performances are Swift's own, and the laughter of the Brobdingnagians at his expense is the laughter that he imagines from others who see him as comic spectacle and his own laughter as he observes himself tottering, tripping, failing. During a country stay in 1721, he wrote, "I row or ride every day, in spite of the rain, in spite of a broken shin, and falling into the lakes, and several other trifling accidents."[79] To the degree that Swift could laugh at his own athletic mishaps, Gulliver's physical misadventures are self-ridiculing parody. In all of the activities in which Gulliver would perform his athletic "Skill and Agility"— leaping, rowing, swimming, wrestling—he is made ridiculous, his failures representations of Swift's own.

Throughout the *Travels*, there are also parodic enactments of the riding that Swift prized above all other exercises for restoring humoral balance and for exercising his manliness. "In an ugly State of Health by the disorder in my Head," he wrote once to Ford, he wished for nothing more than "the medicine of an unfoundred trotting Horse."[80] Even into his age, he routinely rode a dozen miles three times a week. In Lilliput, of course, Gulliver cannot ride for exercise. In fact, in a comic reversal of Swift's own riding, one article of Gulliver's liberty decrees that, in an emergency, he must carry a *horse*: "If an Express require extraordinary Dispatch; the *Man-Mountain* shall be obliged to carry in his Pocket [both] Messenger and Horse."[81] In later books, however, Swift comically imagines his own riding. In Brobdingnag, Gulliver is several times on horseback, once traveling from one market town to another, a distance of about twenty miles: "I was terribly shaken and discomposed in this Journey, although it were but of half an Hour. For the Horse went about forty Foot at every Step; and trotted so high, that the Agitation was equal to the rising and falling of a Ship in a great Storm, but much more frequent."[82] Swift himself rode to cure his giddiness; Gulliver's ride in Brobdingnag is itself vertiginous. In Houyhnhnmland, riding is out of the question. The horses are outraged that Gulliver would even imagine such a thing. His "Master, after some Expressions of great Indignation, wondered how we dared to venture upon a *Houyhnhnm*'s Back." The weakest among the Houyhnhnms, he says, "would be able to shake off the strongest *Yahoo*; or by lying down, and rouling upon his Back, squeeze the Brute to Death."[83] Swift himself as rider is Yahoo here. This imaginative parodying of his own riding and his other exercises is comic self-portraiture, a way of ironizing his own experience. But Swift may also have been expressing doubt about the efficacy of his regimen. "I ride often every week, & walk much; but am not better," he despaired to John Gay in 1730.[84] And to Pope a few years later, he wrote, "I continue to ride & walk, both of which, although they be no cures, are at least Amusements."[85] If Gulliver's amusing athletic failures parody his own "immoderate" exercising for health, Swift may have been pausing here to reflect on the futility—or fatuity—of his lifelong regimen.

Gulliver is made to look a "silly figure" in still other performances of masculine endeavors. For a crowd of Brobdingnagian spectators, he shows his expertise with sword and pike: "I drew out my Hanger, and flourished with it after the Manner of Fencers in *England*. My Nurse gave me Part of a Straw, which I exercised as a Pike, having learned the Art in my Youth." In his antic gestures, Gulliver is a tiny, silly spectacle. He himself calls these displays "Fopperies."[86] Sometimes, however, his very animal survival forces him into heroic battle with other "little Creature[s]": rats, flies, and birds.[87] As Gulliver is rowing one day in Brobdingnag, a loathsome frog climbs up on his boat, making "it lean so much on one Side, that [he is] forced to balance it with all [his] Weight on the other, to prevent overturning." As proof of masculine heroism, he insists that he "deal with it alone": "I banged it a good while with one of my Sculls, and at last forced it to leap out of the Boat."[88] In such encounters, he imagines himself as epic hero, his bravery and "Dexterity . . . much admired."[89]

On the one hand, in Gulliver's heroic performances, Swift, like his many contemporaries who traded in mock genres, is subverting the various classical forms that he admired and, at the same time, highlighting the sad shortcomings of his own decidedly unheroic age. In doing so, because heroic narratives are also masculine discourses, Swift's mock-heroic portrayal of Gulliver's would-be heroism subverts cultural stories about manly bravery, physical strength, and virile resourcefulness. On the other hand, this subversion also registers the vicissitudes of Swift's own performative body. Indeed, the masculine heroic narrative is undercut by the unavoidable actualities of the humoral body itself. Just before the rats threaten him on his huge Brobdingnagian bed, Gulliver finds himself in precarious urgency: "Some natural Necessities required me to get down." Having heroically dispatched one of the rats with his sturdy hanger and driven the other off, he must still attend to the urgent "natural Necessities": "I was pressed to do more than one Thing, which another could not do for me."[90] Neither bravery nor martial manliness can stay or slay excretory functions. One may kill a big rat, but one cannot vanquish the need to urinate and defecate. If such comic and ironic juxtapositions of heroic exploits and base excretory functions upend larger cultural narratives about masculinity, they represent as well the diminishment of Swift's own masculinity, which was subject to humoral realities.

It is also through the increasingly serious challenges to Gulliver's sexualized masculinity—that is, manhood enacted through erotic presence—that Swift represents his lived experiences as a man whose humoral disorders affected how, and how much, he might lose and recuperate sexual masculinity. Ironic representations of Gulliver's sexuality register Swift's ambivalent sense of his own humorally disrupted sexuality. In Lilliput, Gulliver's sexual organ is laughable. To indulge "a fancy of diverting himself," the Lilliputian emperor has Gulliver stand like the Colossus of Rhodes while a contingent of foot soldiers and cavalry march between his legs. Although the soldiers are commanded to "observe the strictest Decency, with regard to [his] Person," some cannot help looking up as they pass beneath. "And, to confess the Truth," says Gulliver, "my Breeches were at that Time in so ill a Condition, that they afforded some Opportunities for Laughter and

Admiration."⁹¹ At once ridiculous and awesome in a body so out of place, Gulliver is freakishly well-endowed; the more sexually masculine he is, the more his sexual masculinity cannot be taken seriously. In Gulliver's paradoxical emasculation, Swift represents what it feels like to experience the unmanning brought by illness.

In Brobdingnag, Gulliver's sexual identity is completely crushed in his encounters with the maids of honor in their private closet. These girls strip him "naked from Top to Toe" and lay him "at full Length in their Bosoms" for their entertainment and "Pleasure," treating him "without any Manner of Ceremony, like a Creature who had no Sort of Consequence."⁹² Used thus by the Brobdingnagian maids of honor, Gulliver feels insulted. Most abashedly to the belittled man in his encounters with the girls, the "handsomest among these Maids of Honour, a pleasant frolicksome Girl of sixteen, would sometimes set [him] astride upon one of her Nipples; with many other Tricks." He hopes that the "the Reader will excuse [him] for not being over particular" in describing such tricks further.⁹³ This image of Gulliver's riding astride the girl's huge nipple deflates both his masculine sexuality and his athletic pretensions. Riding for Swift was almost exclusively a masculine pursuit; he boasted about his abilities, recommended it to his male friends for their health, and gibed them good-naturedly for their inabilities.⁹⁴ In Gulliver's adventures with the Brobdingnagian maidens, however, riding turns to comic representation of the emasculation that came with Swift's ailments.

His sexual pride insulted by the Brobdingnagian maids of honor who treat him as a "Creature" of no "Consequence," Gulliver resorts to his only means of rescuing his sexual identity, the narrative itself. He is quick to insist that the girls' "naked Bodies" are "very far from being a tempting Sight, or from giving [him] any other Motions than those of Horror and Disgust."⁹⁵ While the word "Motions" means emotions, it is sexually suggestive as well; in claiming that *he* is not aroused by the girls, Gulliver is trying to salvage some vestige of sexual pride. Gulliver's puny declaration could be Swift's own. His "female friends" having "forsaken" him in his age and illness, Swift parodies his own feeble attempts to reaffirm himself as a sexual being, a man of "Consequence."⁹⁶

The most devastating injury to Gulliver's sexual being is yet to come. From his being sexually exploited in book 2 (one wonders for what "many other Tricks" the sixteen-year-old female uses him), he goes in book 4 to being sexually attacked by a Yahoo maiden.[97] As he bathes naked in a river one day, "a young female *Yahoo*," "inflamed by Desire," as he later conjectures, leaps into the water and, says Gulliver, "She embraced me after a most fulsome Manner." Only when Gulliver's protector gallops over to rescue him does she quit "her Grasp, with the utmost Reluctancy." She stands "gazing and howling all the time" as he is donning his clothes. "I was never in my Life so terribly frighted," Gulliver writes. What terrifies him most in this encounter is the undeniable realization that he, too, is Yahoo: "I could no longer deny," he says in self-horror, "that I was a real *Yahoo*, in every Limb and Feature, since the Females had a natural Propensity to me as one of their own Species."[98] Worse, sex is procreative, producing more gross humoral bodies and thus more putrid matter. When Gulliver returns to England at last, in a parallel to the river scene in Houyhnhnmland, his own Mary Gulliver takes him in her arms and kisses him. Gulliver falls "in a Swoon for almost an Hour."[99] He reflects in disgust that he has created more bestial bodies by mating with "that odious Animal": "And when I began to consider, that by copulating with one of the *Yahoo*-species, I had become a Parent of more; it struck me with the utmost Shame, Confusion and Horror."[100] Little wonder that it is Gulliver himself who suggests that the Houyhnhnms castrate the Yahoos to "put an End to the whole Species."[101] Sex—and sexuality—are dead to him.

9

Gulliver's Ordeals as Swift's Order

Through Gulliver's experiences, then, Swift expresses the physical, psychological, and social experiences of living in his own giddy body, isolated from company and conversation by deafness and befuddled by auditory din. Concurrently, he could imagine himself as others might look upon him in his disorders, as a "silly figure," unmanned and unable. How are we to explain this ambivalent representation of himself disordered—expressing and ironizing his experiences at the same time? We might start by considering early eighteenth-century attitudes toward disability and deformity, which attitudes Swift himself shared. Cartoons, "jest books," broadsides, and other popular forms of print culture typically made unpitying fun of deaf, blind, limbless, and crooked persons. The deaf man who responded inappropriately, sometimes with unwitting bawdry, to something he had misheard or not heard at all was a stock caricature in such jests. So, too, were dwarves and persons with crooked spines, often depicted as "apes" or "monkeys."[1] (Swift would certainly have seen cartoons of his friend Alexander Pope, often depicted by his enemies as "bow-backed AP^e.") Along with such representations, there were also *performances* of disability and deformity. In public diversions, crowds gawked at misshapen and monstrous persons: giants, dwarves, "Prodigies and Strange-births."[2] And disabled and deformed beggars appealed for charity in the streets of Dublin and London.[3] Increasingly a new culture of sentimentality and "fellow-feeling" would see these unfortunate persons as "piteous objects." The charitable—but decidedly unsentimental—Swift did not. Patrick Delany reported that the Dean kept a "Seraglio" of female beggars in the neighborhood of St. Patrick's, all of them disabled or deformed: "One of these mistresses wanted an eye: another, a nose: a third, an arm: a fourth, a foot: a fifth, had all the attractions of AGNA's *Pollipus:* and a sixth, more than all those of AESOP's hump." "For distinction's sake, and partly for humour," Swift named them "Cancerina, Stumpa-Nympha, Pullagowna, Fritterilla, Flora, Stumpantha." Although he "saluted them with all becoming kindness," the affectionate mock-pastoral names suggest that he also saw deformity and disability as laughable.[4] His apologist in *Verses on the Death* says of Swift, "He spar'd a Hump or crooked Nose, / Whose Owners set not up for Beaux."[5] Perhaps he spared them in his print satires. But not so in his affectionate ridicule of the disabled street beggars.

Simon Dickie states that the spectacle of a deformed or disabled person in the early eighteenth century evoked "an automatic and apparently unreflective urge to laugh at weakness simply because it is weak."[6] Swift understood this urge to laugh. In *Verses on the Death*, he imagines how others must see and talk about him, as dizzied, deaf, and addled old fool. In a remarkable moment of self-reflection in Brobdingnag, Gulliver similarly imagines himself as ridiculous spectacle. Perched hundreds of yards above the ground after the monkey absconds with him, the tiny man clutches the roof tiles in giddy terror. Aware of how ridiculous he appears to the crowd of Brobdingnagians who are gaping at the spectacle, he notes that "many of the Rabble below could not forbear laughing." "Neither do I think they justly ought to be blamed" for their laughter, says Gulliver of the gawkers, "for without Question, the Sight was ridiculous enough to every Body but my self."[7] In Gulliver's absurdity, Swift imagined his own. Forsaken in "a nation of slaves," confined to the deanery for weeks in his illnesses, he sees himself as weak and "silly figure."[8] Observing another like himself, he would laugh, too.[9]

Swift's ironizing of his own experiences as a sick person is a function of his "double vision," the ability to express his own experiences at the same time that, as an observer, he stands outside of his experiences. Certainly, this duality relates to the profound skepticism that Michael McKeon, Seamus Deane, and others have discussed. But as I have suggested throughout this study, this skepticism has its corollary in—is a function of, if we are to accept Swift and his contemporaries on their own terms—his disordered body. As Swift ravels and unravels his and others' every behavior and motive, so his body is caught ever in a shuttle of humoral order and disorders.

Ironizing his own experiences as a sick person in *Gulliver's Travels* distances Swift from himself; this creates an imaginative space in which he may construe and control his experiences.

Gulliver's Travels was an opportunity for Swift to imagine the physical, psychological, and social experiences of humoral disorder. It is also an essay on identity. Because the humoral body and the world outside existed on the same continuum, his social identity was not merely correlative to his body; it resided in that body, unstable and out of order. Here we needn't resort to a postmodern notion of identity as ever-provisional and indeterminate: The indeterminacies of Swift's identity inhered in his fluid, uncertain humoral *constitution,* disordered by "crasie" confusions of senses and faculties. In the *Travels,* Swift imagines and represents these indeterminacies of his own identity by embodying them in Gulliver. In each of the fantastic kingdoms, Gulliver is a body out of place, something inchoate, which can never quite be fixed. Here is Swift's own protean body, liquid and shifting, never quite fixed. The "slippage" of Gulliver's identity is Swift's own.

That Gulliver's being exists in print does not set certainly or contain his essenceless self. He represents what eludes representation: He is a monstrosity. In a brilliant study of the eighteenth century's imagining of monsters, Dennis Todd writes that "in the monstrous, the boundaries which articulate form and identity begin to dissolve toward an unnameable amorphousness."[10] In naming something, one imposes order. But because there is nothing else like it in nature and no taxonomy by which to classify it, a monster defies even a name that would define it, that would draw distinctive boundaries around it. Gulliver himself is a celebrity body in the various fantastic worlds, a spectacle that evokes admiration, awe, terror, and wonder. But he also defies definition. In Brobdingnag, he suffers "the Ignominy of being carried about for a Monster."[11] He is advertised first as "a strange Creature . . . in every Part of the Body resembling an human Creature; [who] could speak several Words, and perform an Hundred diverting Tricks."[12] Then he is turned over to the Brobdingnagian scientists, who try to determine what he is:

> These Gentlemen, after they had a little while examined my Shape with much Nicety, were of different Opinions concerning me. . . . One of them seemed to think that I might be an Embrio, or abortive Birth. But this Opinion was rejected by the other two, who observed my

Limbs to be perfect and finished; and that I had lived several Years, as it was manifested from my Beard; the Stumps whereof they plainly discovered through a Magnifying-Glass. They would not allow me to be a Dwarf, because my Littleness was beyond all Degrees of Comparison; for the Queen's favourite Dwarf, the smallest ever known in that Kingdom, was near thirty Foot high. After much Debate, they concluded unanimously that I was only *Relplum Scalcath,* which is interpreted literally *Lusus Naturæ* [a sport or "freak" of nature].[13]

The gigantic scholars make their determination of Gulliver's identity exclusively as an observed body, a physical object. And in naming him, they place him, finally, in that category of creatures whose identity cannot be defined. As Orrery declared "DOCTOR SWIFT" a singular character, so Gulliver is sui generis, a one-off who can "not be produced according to the regular Laws of Nature."[14] While Gulliver would have us think that the various fantastic beings that he encounters are monsters in their littleness or bigness or grotesqueries, it is he who is monster, an indefinable body out of order.

There are other confusions that arise from the indeterminacy of his body, some comic, some terrifying. In Lilliput Gulliver, who is ambiguously "Man Mountain," is accused of having a sexual affair with the Treasurer Flimnap's wife, who, "the Court-Scandal ran," "had taken a violent Affection for [his] Person" (that is, his body). He goes to inordinate lengths to defend himself and the "excellent Lady" against this charge. Both Lilliputians and Gulliver himself have collapsed his physical identity. Never once does Gulliver invoke, or even apparently imagine, the obvious defense, the physical impossibility (or certainly inadvisability) of having a sexual affair with a woman one-twelfth his size.[15] The size ratio reversed in Brobdingnag, there are similar confusions of body-identity. Gulliver reflects upon the terrifying episode with the monkey, "I have good Reason to believe that he took me for a young one of his own Species." More monstrously, the monkey who seems to want to "suckle" Gulliver is male.[16] Species, sex, maternity, all are confused here, a dissolving of discrete identities in a repugnant physical encounter.

In book 4, for all of their reason, that faculty of mind by which one makes sense of things perceived, the Houyhnhnms can never quite place Gulliver. His Houyhnhnm "Master" finds that in his "Head, Hands and Face,"

Gulliver "exactly resemble[s]" the Yahoos.[17] But the horses are perplexed by his features, behavior, and tractability. Gulliver, they decide, is "a wonderful *Yahoo*, that could speak like a *Houyhnhnm*, and seemed in his Words and Actions to discover some Glimmerings of Reason."[18] Here, too, he is lusus naturae. If Houyhnhnm reason cannot finally fix Gulliver's identity, however, Yahoo nature does not fail. Of the Yahoos, says Gulliver, "I have Reason to believe, they had some Imagination that I was of their own Species, which I often assisted myself, by stripping up my Sleeves, and shewing my naked Arms and Breast in their Sight, when my Protector was with me: At which times they would approach as near as they durst, and imitate my Actions after the Manner of Monkeys, but ever with great Signs of Hatred; as a tame *Jack Daw* with Cap and Stockings, is always persecuted by the wild ones, when he happens to be got among them."[19] In Swift's day, "jackdaw" was byword for any silly, prattling, or conceited fellow. The pet jackdaw here, dressed sportively by its owner in cap and stockings, is something unnatural and ludicrous. It is an emblem of human vanity.[20] In its ridiculous affectation, it is also a creature whose identity is indeterminate, pretending to be something beyond its base nature.

In his discussion of monsters, Todd speaks of the particular attention that gawkers at popular diversions gave to those "creatures that blurred the distinction between men and beasts": dwarves and giants; boys covered with fish scales or hedgehog quills; animals trained and dressed to mimic humans; clever horses, elephants, spaniels.[21] Monsters compel the horrified fascination of those who look upon them, says Todd, because they "blur the boundaries between the bestial and the human."[22] They trouble us because they put our own identity into question. This uncertain identity explains Gulliver's ambivalence in his initial encounter with the monstrous Yahoos. At first, his detached scientific gaze enforces the distinction between himself and the creatures so seemingly unlike him. His opening description of the Yahoos sounds like something from the pages of the Royal Society's *Philosophical Transactions*. Then he recoils in disgust: "I never beheld in all my Travels so disagreeable an Animal, or one against which I naturally conceived so strong an Antipathy."[23] Something so different and so disgustingly like ourselves.

Ultimately, Gulliver cannot gainsay what he determines is his own Yahoo identity. Though the Houyhnhnms laugh at his being mauled by the "young female *Yahoo*," Gulliver cannot. For him the event does nothing less than shatter his sense of who and what he is. He becomes a human manqué. Human on the Great Chain of Being, Gulliver would be Houyhnhnm but finds himself Yahoo. Swift has figured this slippage of identity into the creature names themselves, *Yahoo* and *Houyhnhnm*, each near-punning on the word *human*. The convergent words disorder Gulliver's identity: Is he human? Yahoo? Houyhnhnm? But Gulliver's body, like Swift's own, is also *humoral*, a term resonant in the syllabic sliding of those words *Yahoo*, *Houyhnhnm*, and *human*. The confusion of identities, like all the others, is a confusion of fluid bodies. If we see this welter of bodies and identity in the context of humoralism, we understand better how Swift wrote from his own physical experiences. The Yahoos that Gulliver wants so desperately to distinguish himself from are humoral bodies ungoverned. They gluttonize on "every thing that [comes] in their Way, whether Herbs, Roots, Berries, corrupted Flesh of Animals, or all mingled together" until they are "ready to burst."[24] They "suck... with great Delight" on an intoxicating root, which "would make them sometimes hug, and sometimes tear one another; they would howl and grin, and chatter, and roul, and tumble, and then fall asleep in the Mud."[25] They let loose their passions, screaming, scratching one another, groaning in melancholy. They are unrestrained in their sexual appetites. They void their excrements indiscriminately. In other words, there is no attempt to regulate the non-naturals. The Yahoos are Swift's unblinking representation of the humoral body uncontained, reduced to exchanges of foul matter with the world around them in their ungoverned consumption and evacuations. The runny, tumultuous Yahoo body is Gulliver's, too. If throughout the *Travels*, he has been a body in search of an identity—or an identity in search of a body—he has, it seems, found both. That this body is humoral is reinforced by the liquid reflection that Gulliver sees of himself after he can "no longer deny" that he is Yahoo: "When I happened to behold the Reflection of my own Form in a Lake or Fountain, I turned away my Face in Horror and detestation of my self; and could better endure the Sight of a common *Yahoo*, than of my own Person."[26] "Person" is body; the humoral body is ever-fluid, like the image in water.

If Gulliver is repulsed and engrossed in his first encounter with the Yahoos, it is with much less ambivalence that he rejects his own humoral body. Having promised the "dear Reader" that he "would *strictly adhere to Truth*," and protesting his bookseller's omissions and insertions, he nevertheless shies at giving them details about his bodily functions.[27] After discharging his "Body of [its] uneasy Load" in Lilliput, he vows that "this was the only Time [he] was ever guilty of so uncleanly an Action" and hopes that his "candid Reader will give some Allowance, after he hath maturely and impartially considered [Gulliver's] Case, and the Distress [he] was in."[28] Enforcing the denial of his own natural functions, he registers his disgust with the oozing, excreting bodies of the Brobdingnagian maids-of-honor. And recounting the incident in which a Yahoo "Cub" "voided its filthy Excrements of a yellow liquid Substance, all over [his] Cloaths," Gulliver adds that "perhaps [he] might have the Reader's Pardon, if it were wholly omitted."[29] He demurs at the messy functions of the humoral body. Narrative concealment of these functions has its counterpart in Gulliver's concealment of his physical self. In a prefatory letter to his "Cousin SYMPSON," Gulliver says that humans "only differ from their Brother Brutes in *Houyhnhnmland*, because they use a Sort of *Jabber*, and do not go naked."[30] In Houyhnhnmland, he tries desperately to hide his naked Yahoo body with clothes: "I had hitherto concealed the Secret of my Dress, in order to distinguish myself as much as possible, from that cursed Race of *Yahoos*."[31] Gulliver says of his Houyhnhnm "Master," "He was most perplexed about my Cloaths, reasoning sometimes with himself, whether they were a Part of my Body; for I never pulled them off till the Family were asleep, and got them on before they waked in the Morning."[32] When his clothes begin to wear out and Gulliver finds "it in vain to [hide his body] any longer," he strips down in front of his "Master," who "observe[s] the whole Performance with great Signs of Curiosity and Admiration."[33] Gulliver begs "that the Secret of [his] having a false Covering to [his] Body might be known to none" but his "Master."[34] He does not want to acknowledge his own humorally messy Yahoo body.

Gulliver's denial of this Yahoo body—consuming, excreting, chattering unintelligibly—is not Swift's own. Swift himself was forced to confront his disordered body every day in trying to contain it, with humoral narrative, medical interventions, regimen, and imaginative representation. Gulliver is, rather, like those voyeurs of the "scatological" poems, repelled and horrified to face, yet unable to look away from, the actual bodies that society would have us conceal. Gulliver also registers the outrage of those readers who have found Swift's "excremental vision" objectionable. Edward Young, for example, apostrophized, "O *Gulliver!*. . . . In what ordure hast thou dipt thy pencil? What a monster has thou made of the—*Human face divine?*"[35]

Countering objections of this tenor, his friend and early commentator Patrick Delany argued that Swift was, sanatively, forcing us to confront the realities of our own Yahoo bodies. Putting this into the terms of medical humoralism itself, he said that Swift was "an able physician, who had, in truth, the health of his patients at heart, but laboured to attain that end, not only by strong emeticks, but also, by all the most nauseous, and offensive drugs, and potions, that could be administered."[36] Acknowledge the humoral body, insists Swift, as a first measure of acknowledging the material realities of the human condition. It takes Gulliver the entirety of his travels to accept this materiality and its excremental facts. In the very opening scene, in which he would try to enforce the distinction between himself and the filthy Yahoos, "at least forty" of them come "flocking about [him] ... howling and making odious Faces." Then they "discharge their Excrements on [his] Head." Gulliver is "almost stifled with the Filth, which [falls] about [him] on every Side."[37] He might try to conceal his own humoral functions with polite apologies to the "gentle Reader" and dainty circumlocutions. To little effect: The Yahoos confront him (and the reader) with the undeniable excremental nature of us all.

As function of its humoral disorderliness, the Yahoo body ails. Gulliver observes that Yahoos are "the only Animals in [Houyhnhnmland] subject to any Diseases." When these "sordid Brute[s]" get sick, there are natural cures for righting the humoral imbalance. To remedy their gluttonies, "Nature had pointed out to them a certain *Root* that gave them a general Evacuation." And when, by their "Nastiness and Greediness," they contract the "*Hnea Yahoo,* or the *Yahoo's-Evil,*" the Houyhnhnms intervene with their rational medicine. An emetic, "the Cure prescribed is a Mixture of *their own Dung* and *Urine,* forcibly put down the *Yahoo*'s Throat."[38] This use of a vomit follows exactly from the principles of humoral medicine that Gulliver himself has described to the Houyhnhnm "Master." The purgative forces the dyscrasial Yahoo body back into balance by vacuating it of foul or harmful excrements. Gulliver, extensively trained in medicine himself, endorses the cure: "This I have since often known to have been taken with Success: And do here freely recommend it to my Countrymen, for the publick Good, as an admirable Specifick against all Diseases produced by Repletion."[39] If the cure seems gratuitously foul to us and Gulliver's enthusiasm for it yet more evidence of his blind reverence for Houyhnhnm reason, we should remember that not only disreputable "empiricks" but also celebrated physicians of

Swift's own day (such as Sir Hans Sloane and Thomas Willis) touted the curative and prophylactic powers of animal dung—from dogs, pigs, horses, peacocks, and geese—and even human urine and feces.[40] There were also the revulsive vomits and clysters, asafoetida, "devilish" hiera picra, and "nasty" steel drops and "dyet" drinks that Swift himself took to remedy his disorders. The "receipt" for curing the "Yahoo's-Evil" is written from his own humoral experiences.

If the Yahoos represent the humoral body uncontained, the Houyhnhnms are humoral bodies in perfect balance (eucrasia). They maintain that natural balance by observing the best virtues of Hippocratic-Galenic rational medicine. Regulating their food and drink, "each Horse and Mare eat their own Hay, and their own Mash of Oats and Milk, with much Decency and Regularity."[41] Controlling their passions, the Houyhnhnms feel neither "Jealousy, Fondness, Quarreling, [nor] Discontent."[42] Exerting their equine bodies, they "train up their Youth to Strength, Speed, and Hardiness, by exercising them in running Races up and down steep Hills . . . and when they are all in a Sweat, they are ordered to leap over Head and Ears into a Pond or a River."[43] In short, the Houyhnhnms maintain humoral balance by regulating the non-naturals in a disciplined regimen. As *"the Perfection of Nature,"* they themselves are never sick.[44] They are well because their lives are well-regimented. And because "they are subject to no Diseases," they "can have no Need of Physicians."[45]

Management of the non-naturals in regimen was a way for Swift himself to govern the unruly body by keeping the fluid humors in check. It was one measure, however tenuous, of maintaining an identity separate from anarchic matter. That Gulliver, like Swift, follows a careful Houyhnhnm regimen is Swift's representation of his own attempts to distinguish himself from repulsive Yahoo humoral nature, even if he had to acknowledge and face it unblinkingly every day. Disgusted by the foul meat that the Yahoos eat, Gulliver instead dines upon oat cakes, milk, and "wholesome Herbs, which [he] boiled, or eat as Salades with [his] Bread."[46] Like the Houyhnhnms, he disciplines his body with exercise: "I fell to imitate their Gait . . . which is now grown into a Habit; and my Friends often tell me in a blunt Way, that *I trot like a Horse.*"[47] His body tempered by his regimen, Gulliver maintains humoral balance. "I cannot but observe," he says of his time in Houyhnhnmland, "that I never had one Hour's Sickness, while I staid in this Island."[48] His regulated humoral body proof against the *"Hnea Yahoo,"* Gulliver does not need the medical interventions of vomits and purges. Swift cannot resist taking yet another hit at the doctors of his day: In Houyhnhnmland, says Gulliver, there is no "Physician to destroy my Body."[49]

We recall Swift's resignation to his being always "in a middling Way, between Healthy and Sick, hardly ever without a little Giddiness or Deafness, and sometimes both."[50] In *Gulliver's Travels*, he imaginatively represents this oscillation between humoral order and disorder as the opposition between Houyhnhnm discipline and Yahoo chaos. Like Swift, Gulliver would "fence against" humoral imbalance with a strict regimen. In the end, though, he can no longer ignore the ineluctable fact of his own humoral body: He—and all other humans—are Yahoo. While Gulliver would finally repudiate the humoral body, however, Swift himself would confront and try to reform it. Through all of his efforts—explaining his illnesses in an intelligible diagnostic narrative, trying to correct imbalances with medical interventions and regimen, casting himself in various sick roles, and representing his disorders imaginatively in works such as *Gulliver's Travels*—Swift tried to impose order on his body. But the governance of the disordered body is no less governance of the disordered world: "I desire that my Prescription of living may be published... for the benefit of Mankind," he had written tongue-in-speak to William Pulteney.[51] Gulliver has a similar plan, but he is entirely serious. He insists upon Houyhnhnm governance of our foul Yahoo bodies.

10

Voyages Out and Voyages Back

Navigating Madness

Whether, when, and in what sense Swift did become "mad"—these are questions addressed in chapters 2 and 3. As these issues pertain to *Gulliver's Travels*, however, further complexities arise. Reading Gulliver as humoral body helps us engage these questions, and the two stories of Swift's madness that have guided some who have read the *Travels* as psychoautobiography. One is that in his final years, Swift lapsed into a "state of ideotism," deprived at last of memory and understanding and voice. Readers who knew him in life, such as Lord Orrery and Lætitia Pilkington, saw the "mortifying Sight" of the Struldbruggs of book 3 as Swift's nightmare imagining of what he might—and did—become.[1] The other version is that Swift was "lunatic," gnashing his teeth with savage indignation against the world. Prosecuting this version of his madness, readers such as Johnson, Scott, Thackeray, and Gosse saw Gulliver not as representation but as symptom: His misanthropic ravings and final repudiation of Yahoo humankind are Swift's own. Both versions of how Swift's own purported madness subtends *Gulliver's Travels* may be countered with, or at least qualified by, envisioning Gulliver's mental disorders as a function of Swift's humoralism. Gulliver's mad misanthropy is no more symptom of Swift's own lunacy than the images of excremental females are symptoms of Freudian coprophilia. Rather, like the Struldbruggs, mad, misanthropic Gulliver is ironic self-*imagining*, a representation of how it might end for Swift. As such, it is yet another means of controlling disorders of body and mind. In the work, Swift imaginatively represents "lunacy" in the fantastic voyages and final raving misanthropy of Gulliver himself; he represents "idiotism" in the vacant, pitiable Struldbruggs.

In a letter to Pope of 1734, Swift lamented of his "two inveterate Disorders, Giddyness & deafness," "I have lost by those deseases much of my memory, which makes [me] commit many blunders, in my common Actions at home, by mistaking one thing for another."[2] By this time, he felt profound horror at the prospect of dying of the cephalic disorders that distressed him. And so, said his early readers, he had represented this terror imaginatively in the nightmare spectacle of decayed memory, the Struldbruggs. These "Immortals," whom Gulliver encounters in the kingdom of Luggnagg, are cursed that they "should never dye."[3] At first "struck with inexpressible Delight" at the prospect of immortality, the projector Gulliver imagines that if he were a Struldbrugg, he would reform humankind with examples of "the Usefulness of Virtue" from his "own Remembrance, Experience and Observation."[4] He then learns the horrifying facts: Although the Struldbruggs live forever, they grow increasingly disordered in body and mind. They lose teeth and hair and taste. They become more and more grotesque in their passions. Here is the humoral body dissolving, without the mercy of final dissolution.

More frightening to Gulliver—and to Swift himself—is the decay of the Struldbruggs' memories: "They have no Remembrance of any thing but what they learned and observed in their Youth and middle Age, and even that is very imperfect."[5] For example, "in talking they forget the common Appellation of Things, and the Names of Persons, even of those who are their nearest Friends and Relations."[6] In his final years, Swift himself mourned the "utter Loss of [his] Memory": "I cannot recollect the Names of those friends who come to see me twice or oftner every Week."[7] In *Verses on the Death*, he represented himself benignly as addled old fool who forgets his friends and tells the same stories again and again:

> Besides, his Memory decays,
> He recollects not what he says;
> He cannot call his Friends to Mind;
> Forgets the Place where last he din'd:
> Plyes you with Stories o'er and o'er,
> He told them fifty Times before.[8]

The Struldbruggs are a dreadful version of this same forgetful fool.

After Swift's death, his earliest readers saw the Struldbruggs as horrified prolepsis. Pilkington wrote that although she revered the Dean's "sacred Memory," his lapsing into the very idiocy that he had imagined in the Struldbruggs was fitting punishment for his indiscriminate savaging of mankind. He might justly satirize "the Vices of human Kind," conceded Pilkington. But in ridiculing "Infirmities"—a word that she does not explain—Swift "seem'd to have done a displeasing Act to Heaven, inasmuch as he was [himself] punished with them all in a remarkable manner": "He lived to be a *Struldbrugg*, helpless as a Child, and unable to assist himself."[9] Orrery, too, found irony in Swift's becoming at last the creature that he had imagined. But more interested in understanding Swift's psychology than in casting moral judgments, he saw the Struldbruggs as expressions of the Dean's greatest fears of what he would become in his dotage. "He probably felt in himself the effects of approaching age, and tacitly dreaded that period of life, in which he might become a representative of those *miserable immortals*," speculated Orrery. "His apprehensions were unfortunately fulfilled. He lived to be the most melancholy sight that was ever beheld."[10] Orrery, who knew Swift in his final years, said that he often lamented "the state of childhood, and idiotism, to which some of the greatest men of this nation were reduced before their death." He always sighed heavily and gestured uneasily when he thought of these sad spectacles, "as if he felt an impulse of what was to happen to him before he died." Swift "certainly foresaw his fate" not merely in the sad examples of the Duke of Marlborough and Lord Somers but also in the humoral disorders of his own body and mind. "His frequent attacks of giddiness, and his manifest defect of memory, gave room for such apprehensions," said Orrery.[11] Deane Swift protested that the comparison of Swift with Struldbrugg "insult[ed] the ashes of so bright a genius with infirmities of his latter days."[12] Still, Orrery's explanation of Swift's decaying memory and final imbecility conformed with humoral theory: The "giddiness in his head" that Swift himself ascribed to that youthful gluttonizing on fruit confounded his senses, addled his understanding, and at last "compleat[ed] its conquest, by rendering him the exact image of one of his *Struldbruggs*."[13]

Orrery could see the Struldbruggs as imaginings of the "utter deprivation of the senses" that Swift feared. With his comments on Yahoos and Gulliver's mad misanthropy, however, there is a signal shift in his reading of the *Travels* as psychoautobiography. The Yahoos are evidence of Swift's own lunacy; Gulliver's mad misanthropy is Swift's own. "In painting [the] Yahoos he becomes one himself," wrote Orrery.[14] He who could imagine such creatures is himself depraved. Samuel Johnson, too, saw the Yahoos as evidence of lunacy. "The greatest difficulty that occurs, in analysing [Swift's] character," he wrote, "is to discover by what depravity of intellect he took delight in revolving ideas, from which almost every other mind shrinks with disgust." He asks why Swift would dwell upon "disease, deformity and filth." While he leaves the question unanswered, the Yahoos are clearly a symptom of this "depravity."[15] How else, ask Orrery, Johnson, and the others, are we to explain the representation of ourselves as revulsive Yahoos than by ascribing it to a depraved imagination, ungoverned by reason? How else, too, are we to explain Gulliver's mad repudiation of Yahoo-mankind than by seeing it as Swift's own? In the "last part of his imaginary travels," frowned Orrery, "SWIFT has indulged a misanthropy that is intolerable."[16] Edmund Gosse, who had explicitly linked Swift's misanthropy with his chronic giddiness, saw "the awful satire of the Yahoos" as "the first literary expression" of his "rage and despair."[17] Thackeray famously cast Swift as depraved "monster gibbering shrieks, and gnashing imprecations against mankind,—tearing down all shreds of modesty, past all sense of manliness and shame; filthy in word, filthy in thought, furious, raging, obscene."[18] Surely anyone who would savage our godly sensibilities by forcing us to confront the Yahoo nature that we would like most to deny in ourselves must be lunatic.

Having insisted that we see Gulliver as character, not as Swift himself, Edward Stone argued years ago that he goes insane at the end of the *Travels*.[19] Michael Seidel suggests that Gulliver is insane all along; perhaps, in fact, the whole mad tale is a "stay-at-home invention, the fancy of a homebound lunatic."[20] Historically sensitive readers such as Michael DePorte and Christopher Fox have reached the same conclusions by placing Gulliver within Locke's psychology of "consciousness" and definitions of madness contemporary to Swift himself.[21] Such studies are valuable in establishing Gulliver's lunacy, independently. It is Gulliver, not Swift himself, who is Bedlamite.

Here, however, I want to reconnect mad Gulliver with Swift himself, not by reading the character's misanthropic rantings as Swift's own, as did Orrery, Johnson, Thackeray, and all those others, but by reading them as imaginative renderings of himself disordered—and then recovered. Sending Gulliver off into "remote nations of the world," Swift would have us stand back and see our human foibles and follies, vicious behaviors, and corrupt institutions at a safe remove. But without being too paradigmatic, I suggest that we can also read each of Gulliver's journeys out as representation of Swift himself, "lunatic" in body and mind, each journey back as recovery. With each voyage out, Gulliver, like Swift himself, is a "crasie" body at sea, senses confused, understanding confounded, boundaries between self and others and body and world indeterminate and provisional. Like Swift in his fits of giddiness, deafness, and tinnitus, he is torn from the salubrious company and conversation of friends and family. Each voyage home, except the last, is an imaginative return to humoral order. Gulliver's body back in its proper place among like-bodied people, senses and understanding restored to order, social roles as husband, father, and friend reestablished, Swift has imagined recovery of his own body and mind.

Earlier we saw how Swift was able to express the subjectivities of illness in Gulliver's experiences: what it *felt* like to be living in a body that he could not trust, that would not function as he willed it, senses scrambled, understanding jumbled. Reframing the representations of disorder now in the discussion of his madness, we can see the disorienting shifts in perspective and scale, hallucinatory transformations of bodily forms, and unintelligible gibberish in each strange world as the stuff of insanity. Gulliver's narrative is a lunatic's tale. Fittingly, with his return from every fantastic kingdom, he must prove his sanity; that is, he must show that his disordered senses and understanding have been put back in order. When Gulliver tells the tale of his adventure in Lilliput, the ship's captain who brings him home to England thinks he is "raving, and that the Dangers" he has undergone have "disturbed [his] Head."[22] Likewise, he says, the captain who rescues him from Brobdingnag "concluded [he] was raving," "began again to think that [his] Brain was disturbed," and felt "sorry to have taken so ill a Man into his Ship." The captain imputes Gulliver's odd behavior "to some Disorder in [his] Brain."[23] When Gulliver returns to his own house, his wife, daughter, and servants decide that he has "lost [his] Wits."[24] But in returning home from Lilliput, Brobdingnag, and Laputa, Gulliver is restored to senses and sanity; so Swift could imagine the restoration of his own wits and understanding.

Gulliver's lunacy entails his separation from—and eventual repudiation of—mankind. This detachment from other humans is forecast from the beginning. One reason for his embarking on his sea life is that he has "few Friends" in London who can support him in his career as surgeon.[25] Absurdly, Gulliver tries to insinuate himself into friendships with

Lilliputians, Brobdingnagians, Laputans, and Houyhnhnms. These relations are provisional and dubious. The friendship between him and Reldresal, "principal Secretary for private affairs" in Lilliput, is "well known to the World"; it is this "intimate" Reldresal who suggests that, as a more merciful solution to the "Gulliver problem" than poisoning him, his eyes be put out and he be left to starve.[26] The Great King of Brobdingnag speaks of him with jocular condescension as "My little Friend *Grildrig*."[27] In book 3, a particular Luggnuggian friend of his—"(so he thought fit to express himself)"—chuckles behind his back as Gulliver holds forth on notions of immortality.[28] In Houyhnhnmland, Gulliver at last does "not feel the Treachery or Inconstancy of a Friend."[29] But he *has* no friends there. While the Houyhnhnms celebrate "universal" "*Friendship* and *Benevolence* [as] the two principal Virtues" among them, they do not extend their friendship to Gulliver himself.[30] "Friendship, we say," wrote Swift himself, "is created by a resemblance of humours."[31] If we literalize "humours" here as natural constitution, Gulliver's kinship is not with Lilliputians, Brobdingnagians, Laputans, or Houyhnhnms; to his own disgust, it is with Yahoos.

As Gulliver tries to establish relations with these strange others in strange lands, his familiars—family and friends—become themselves alien. Having "spent the greatest Part of [his] Life in travelling," he is, by virtue of circumstance, already separated from humankind, both physically and psychologically.[32] Book by book, this alienation grows. Home for only two months after his time in Lilliput, his "insatiable Desire of seeing foreign Countries would suffer [him] to continue no longer."[33] Returned to England from Brobdingnag, he looks "down upon the Servants, and one or two Friends who were in the House, as if they had been Pigmies, and [he] a Giant."[34] Only two months later, having been restored to "good Health" (mentally as well as physically, we presume), he ships out again.[35] After his return from Laputa, he is gone again after only five months spent at home. He would have remained "in a very happy Condition," he says, if he "could have learned the Lesson of knowing when [he] was well."[36] At the end of the first three books, then, Gulliver recovers his wits and his human identity. He recovers neither after his return from Houyhnhnmland.

When he returns to England from Lilliput, Brobdingnag, and Laputa, he returns also to rehabilitated senses and sanity. In the final book, there is no such recovery. Don Pedro de Mendez, the decent Portuguese captain who brings Gulliver home at last, listens to his story about Houyhnhnms and

Yahoos "as if it were a Dream or a Vision" but indulges him in kind forbearance.[37] His fellow Englishmen think Gulliver *mad*. He has "great Reason to complain, that some of them are so bold as to think [his] Book of Travels a meer Fiction out of [his] own Brain; and have gone so far as to drop Hints, that the *Houyhnhnms*, and *Yahoos* have no more Existence than the Inhabitants of *Utopia*."[38] Having encountered both Houyhnhnms and Yahoos, he rejects all humans and returns to England only when Don Pedro convinces him that "it was altogether impossible to find such a solitary Island as [he] had desired to live in."[39] Gulliver scorns the "poor Wife" whom he has left "big with Child" as a foul Yahoo with whom he has "copulated." Inverting the spirit of communion, he forbids wife and children from touching his bread or drinking "out of the same Cup."[40] Mad, misanthropic recluse in his house in Newark, Gulliver shuns the company and conversation of people but talks with his "two young Stone-Horses" "at least four Hours every Day. . . . [T]hey live in great Amity with [him], and Friendship to each other."[41] Toward the very end of his narrative, he has begun to permit his "Wife to sit at Dinner with [him], at the furthest End of a long Table." Nonetheless, "the Smell of a *Yahoo* continuing very offensive," he always keeps his "Nose well stopt with Rue, Lavender, or Tobacco-Leaves."[42] Fittingly, these three plants were "aromaticks" thought to prevent plague. They had more specific medical uses as well: Tobacco was advised in curing the acute fever of an ague; lavender and rue calmed the passions.[43] Nicholas Culpeper said that a "Decoction made with the Flowers of Lavender [and other herbs] is very probably used to help . . . the giddiness or turning of the Brain."[44] But there is no curing fever, calming lunatic passions, or restoring Gulliver to society: "My Reconcilement to the *Yahoo*-kind in general might not be so difficult, if they would be content with those Vices and Follies only which Nature hath entitled them to. . . . But, when I behold a Lump of Deformity, and Diseases both in Body and Mind, smitten with *Pride*, it immediately breaks all Measures of my Patience."[45] The ironic subtext smirks at the reader: Gulliver might claim that in writing his *Travels*, his "sole Intention was the PUBLICK GOOD," that is, making us confront our Yahoo nature. He himself repudiates that nature.[46]

In this final book, there is no narrative closure in a recovery of wits and human identity. Gulliver, who would be horse, will whinny madly in the stable with the stone horses. In Gulliver's increasing isolation from people, Swift could imagine his own. "Quite worn out with Disorders of Mind and

Body; a long Fit of Deafness . . . to [which] is added an Apprehension of Giddiness," he complained that his "Friends have all forsaken" or "utterly dropped" him.⁴⁷ Yet as Swift tells it, it is he who shut the door to *them*. In the early 1720s, confined to the deanery with his disorders, he figured himself "an unsociable Creature, hating to see others, or be seen by [his] best friends."⁴⁸ If he is "visited seldom" during his giddy fits, he himself "visit[s] much seldomer."⁴⁹ At home he denies himself to "every body," except those Lilliputians whose shrillness can pierce through his muffled hearing: "I . . . refuse all People who have not hearable Voices."⁵⁰ Even these he suffers "as seldom as possible."⁵¹ Patrick Delany groused in comic verse, "DEAR Sir, I think 'tis doubly hard / Your Ears and Doors shou'd both be barr'd." His body and faculties disordered, Swift, like his character, has shut himself away from company and conversation. Delany might plead, "Methinks, a Friend at Night shou'd cheer you, / A Friend that loves to see and hear you."⁵² But for friends now, Swift has only giddiness and deafness, the mad humors of his "crasie" body.⁵³ Like Gulliver, he has removed himself from society.

"Be not solitary," Johnson enjoined the melancholic Boswell. That, he said, is the "great direction which Burton has left to Men disordered like you."⁵⁴ He blamed Swift's own increasing isolation for his lunacy. As the "fits of giddiness and deafness grew more frequent, and his deafness made conversation difficult," wrote Johnson, his eventual withdrawal from all company and conversation "left his mind vacant to the vexations of the hour, till at last his anger was heightened into madness."⁵⁵ Only a year after publishing the *Travels*, Swift wrote morosely to Sheridan, "I am strongly visited with a Disease that will at last cut me off; if I should this Time escape; if not, I have but a poor Remainder, that is below any wise Man's valuing."⁵⁶ If he means (as is likely) that his disorders will finally kill him, he also fears that they will at last cut him off from society and that he will die "in a rage, like a poison'd rat in a hole."⁵⁷ As the Struldbruggs represent the idiotism into which Swift feared he would lapse, so Gulliver's final rejection of humans represents the lunacy that Swift feared his disorders of body and mind would come to at last. In Gulliver mad, he can see himself in the glass. But it is image, not himself. In showing Gulliver as irrevocably mad in his self-appointed "exile" and confinement, Swift was imposing order on his own disorders. Ironizing his own experiences in *Gulliver's Travels* was Swift's own imaginative act of recovery. Imagining this recovery was crucial to a man suffering from chronic disorders for which there was no narrative closure.

Frank Brady, Claude Rawson, and others have challenged claims that Gulliver is "ironic persona"; he is never entirely coherent, as we might expect of a novelistic character, nor is he entirely distinct from Swift himself.[58] There, however, is the very definition of the fluid humoral body and never-quite-determinate humoral identity. By returning Swift to his humoral body, we can make sense of Gulliver as character. Gulliver, like Swift, is at once subject and object, at once representing the experiences of his own disordered being and ironizing those experiences to put them at a distance. Through Gulliver Swift has imagined the battle between order and disorder playing out in his own humoral body.

Conclusion

Returning Swift to the humoral body in which he lived helps us appreciate more fully his own experiences as a chronically ill person and restores narrative and representational authority to the man himself. It frees us from the rigid teleology that sees his chronic disorders as symptoms that led inevitably to madness rather than as lived experiences. Returning Swift's disorders to his own understanding and representation of them frees us from the reductive biomedical model of disease and the interposing authority of the modern clinic, and it helps us comprehend better the fluid nature of both his body and his social identity. It helps us understand the sometimes desperate measures that Swift took to manage that body, his performances in the "sick role," and his varied representations of himself ill. Paradoxically, returning him to his early modern body also opens up new opportunities in reading imaginative works like *Gulliver's Travels*. It allows us to see the ways in which he represented both his experiences and his identity as a sick person. Finally, with Swift's own fluid and permeable humoral body as referent, we get a more profound understanding of his anxieties about social and cultural disorder than the studies of his politics, religion, and aesthetics, which abstract his ideas from his body, can give us by themselves.

The word *disorder* mediates Swift's physical sufferings and disabilities, the decline of his cognitive abilities, the disruptions to his social life, and the indeterminacies of his social identity. But in the humoral system, the body itself is coextensive with the world outside of it. As Swift's humoral body was the contested site in a battle between physical and psychological order and disorder, so it was also referent for political, religious, social, and aesthetic order and disorder. Understanding the microcosmic-macrocosmic relations of humoral body and world helps explain the smoldering tensions between order and disorder that we find in both the man and his work. Swift was preoccupied with upholding orthodox beliefs and institutions—at the same time that he challenged and subverted those very beliefs and institutions at every turn.

The lines between social, political, and humoral bodies of Swift's early modern world were permeable and uncertain. In *Absalom and Achitophel*, John Dryden memorably represents the blurring of boundaries among these bodies. Describing the Exclusion plot fomented by malcontents who threatened the "peaceful raign" of Charles II, he begins with the concept of humoral digestion as metaphor. The "Multitude" have been fed lies, which are "swallow'd in the Mass, unchew'd and Crude."[1] The social and political disorder that follows is *humoral* disorder:

> This Plot, which fail'd for want of common Sense,
> Had yet a deep and dangerous Consequence:
> For, as when raging Fevers boyl the Blood,
> The standing Lake soon floats into a Floud;
> And ev'ry hostile Humour, which before
> Slept quiet in its Channels, bubbles o're:
> So, several Factions from this first Ferment,
> Work up to Foam, and threat the Government.[2]

Although Dryden would metaphorize social disorder as humoral disorder—"as . . . so . . ."—the boundaries between natural body and body politic are indistinct. Social disorder is not separate from but continuous with humoral disorder; government of the political body is government of the humoral body. A few lines later, memorializing the Earl of Shaftesbury, leader of the "Petitioners" for Exclusion, as the villainous Achitophel, Dryden makes social disorder a *function* of bodily disorder. Shaftesbury is himself a frail, deformed body that can hardly contain its dangerous humors:

> Restless, unfixt in Principle and Place;
> In Pow'r unpleas'd, impatient of Disgrace.
> A fiery Soul, which working out its way,

Fretted the Pigmy Body to decay:
And o'r inform'd the Tenement of Clay.³

Here is not a solely figurative representation of a scheming politician; it is a literal description of a humoral body disordered and uncontained.⁴

Other writers, nonimaginative and imaginative alike, placed physical, social, and political bodies on the same continuum. The first volume of *Tristram Shandy* closes with the claim that "the bilious and more saturnine passions, by creating disorders in the blood and humours, have as bad an influence, I see, upon the body politic as body natural."⁵ In book 3 of *Gulliver's Travels,* Swift himself comically collapses any distinctions between body politic and natural body when he literalizes political disorder as humoral disorder. There a projector in the Academy of Lagado who insists upon "a strict universal Resemblance between the natural and the political Body" proposes an infallible scheme for curing political ills with the same prescriptions used to restore humoral balances: "Lenitives, Aperitives, Abstersives, Corrosives, Restringents, Palliatives, Laxatives, Cephalalgicks, Ictericks, Apophlegmaticks, Acousticks."⁶ Some of these numbered among the medicines that his friend and physician John Arbuthnot had prescribed for Swift; others, like the "cephalalgicks" and "acousticks," for treating cephalic disorders and deafness, respectively, would have served him well in his own disorders. The Dean is writing his satire on government from the experiences of his own disordered body. For Swift, the humorally disordered world was no mere abstraction or comic prop. Thrown into disarray by his confused and convergent senses, his world was topsy-turvy. With his own disordered body as referent, recreating his experiences as a chronically ill man helps us understand not only his concerns with maintaining order in the world but also his own notorious subversions of that very order, perpetrated, he said, "to vex the world."⁷

Fixated on political, religious, and social order, Swift was ever anxious about disorder in the larger world. The seismic disruptions of the English Civil War and the beheading of a king still resonated profoundly, especially for the man who traced the upheavals of his own family to the "great Rebellion and usurpation."⁸ Swift blamed the mad enthusiasms of the Commonwealth for the displacement of his family from their native England to Ireland. His grandfather Thomas had lost his livings in the Civil War because of his Royalist allegiances. Of Thomas's sons, "four were settled in

Ireld (driven thither by their sufferings, and by the death of their father)."[9] This displacement helps to explain Swift's own hopes for an appointment in the English Church, a return of the patrimony that he felt was rightfully his.

Already thirty-three years old at the turn of the eighteenth century, Swift had lived through most of Charles II's reign; the serious business of Exclusion, during which the Tories and Whigs had germinated as partisan groups; and the deposal of the Catholic James II and the installment of William and Mary in the Glorious Revolution of 1688. These disruptions had profound impact upon Swift's life and ambitions. When James turned to Ireland for help in restoring himself to the English throne, Irish Protestants worried about a Catholic Jacobite uprising. "The Troubles then breaking out," Swift himself went to England for safety in 1689. There he "was received by Sr Wm Temple," who employed him on and off as private secretary for some ten years.[10] Temple, a moderate Whig who supported the Glorious Revolution as a commonsense solution to the political disorder of the day, was the longtime acquaintance of William III; in fact, it was he who had negotiated the marriage of William and Mary. Swift adopted Temple's brand of Whiggism and was himself entrusted with communications between Temple and the king.[11] But when the Whigs began threatening the institutional political and religious order that Swift saw as a dike against chaos, his political sympathies shifted. The Whig attempts to remove the Test Act agitated him especially. This act (more properly, series of acts) enforced Anglican orthodoxy against Roman Catholic recusancy and Protestant dissent by requiring that all persons in civil, military, or church office take the Oath of Supremacy, which denied the doctrine of transubstantiation and recognized the monarch as head of the English Church. They also had to receive the Anglican form of communion. Deeply committed to maintaining these institutional forms and order, Swift turned his allegiances to the Tories, who vowed to preserve the Act. "The prejudice of the Tory is for establishment," Samuel Johnson was supposed to have said, "the prejudice of the Whig is for innovation."[12] Swift found order, however tenuous, in the preservation of establishment.

Fearing that political and religious worlds were always on the precipice of disorder, Swift also worried that language itself, that discursive form of order, was slipping into chaos. There were the venial trespasses against linguistic forms—misspellings of words by his beloved Stella and others of his acquaintance.[13] There was also the irritating modish slang of the fashionable set, which Swift satirized in *Polite Conversation*, one of his last publications.[14] But most worrisome to him, as to his admirer George Orwell so many years later, was the fast and loose use of language to exploit others: the cant of religious enthusiasts that had provoked the English Civil War; the meaningless windy drone of nonconformist preachers that he pilloried in *A Tale of a Tub*; the manipulations of the lawyers "bred up ... in the Art of proving by Words multiplied for the Purpose, that *White* is *Black*, and *Black* is *White*, according as they are paid."[15] So concerned was Swift with what he saw as the deteriorations and abuses of language that in 1712 he wrote a serious *Proposal for Correcting, Improving and Ascertaining the English Tongue*.[16] In this pamphlet, one of the few works to which he signed his name, he calls for the founding of an academy in England "for *Ascertaining* and *Fixing* our Language for ever."[17] The order of language, insisted Swift, had to be regulated against both decay and abuse.

In his position as dean of St. Patrick's, Swift also demanded rigorous observation of established forms. He kept a watchful eye on his subordinates and, Patrick Delany reported, he took notes on the performances of visiting preachers and corrected their missteps: "As soon as any one got up into the pulpit, he pulled out his pencil, and a piece of paper, and carefully noted every wrong pronunciation, or expression, that fell from him. Whether too hard, or scholastic (and of consequence, not sufficiently intelligible to a vulgar hearer) or such as he deemed, in any degree, improper, indecent, slovenly, or mean; and those, he never failed, to admonish the preacher of, as soon as he came into the chapter-house."[18] In his open *Letter to a Young Gentleman, Lately Enter'd into Holy Orders*, written by "a Person of Quality," Swift spends more time counseling the clergyman on matters of performance in the pulpit than he does in discussing doctrinal matters, laying out clerical duties, or warning against the snares of society. He has advice on choice of words and quotations, inflections of voice, appeals to passion, turns of wit, and even the way in which the clergyman should write his sermons out on paper for easier reading. In this letter, Swift also gives his famous "true Definition" of literary *style* as the "Proper Words in proper Places."[19]

Swift, who usually delighted in the company of others, had rules of order for conversation as well. He "talked a great deal in all companies, without engrossing the conversation to himself," said Deane Swift. "His rule of politeness in this case was, that every man had a right to speak for a minute;

and when that minute was out, if nobody else took up the discourse, after a short pause of two or three moments, the same person had an equal right with any of the rest of the company, to speak again, and again, and again, and so on during the whole evening."[20] Swift, we are told, was always consulting his watch. We can only imagine here the performance of conversation, at once carefully regulated and amusing, governed always by the Dean.

Swift insisted, too, on forms of respect. His cousin Deane recollects that on one occasion, Swift's "indignation took instant fire" when a correspondent addressed him chummily as "Dear Swift": "DEAR SWIFT, said he! What monstrous familiarity is here!" When the impertinent writer signed himself Swift's friend, the Dean "was out of all patience. My friend! my friend! . . . pish, psha; my friend!" But, said Swift, "He is a lord, and so let it pass."[21] On another occasion, a bishop sent his servant to ask a favor of Swift. Swift refused to grant the bishop's request because, he grumbled, "he ought to have come himself, and not sent his servant to me upon such a message."[22] Swift, said Deane, "knew to a point the respect that was due unto him; which he took care to exact without any sort of abatements."[23] This expectation that he be properly addressed was not mere arrogance; it was the nominal enforcement of social rank. Insisting upon "due" respect appropriate to his own "point," Swift was ever making a social—and thereby personal—identity.

In seeking to preserve social order, Swift expected practiced performance even of servants. Dining with Lord Orrery in Dublin, he kept notes of a servant's missteps: "I am thinking," Swift remarked to Orrery, "how often, if your servant had been mine, I should have chid him for faults which I have seen him commit; and I find the number of times amount to twenty-two." The servant's faults, said Orrery, were all failures of form: "not giving a plate with the right hand; not taking off a dish with both hands; putting the plates too near or too far from the fire; and such kind of trifles."[24] Tendering a retrospective psychological diagnosis, some recent commentators suggest that Swift's preoccupation with such "trifles" was a sign of an obsessive compulsive disorder and that, in the face of existential uncertainty, he tried to find protective security in trivial details and repetitive rituals.[25] But there is more to it. To Swift, forms were crucial to preserving order in the face of the modernity that Claude Rawson calls "the dissolution of orderly standards and categories."[26] The carefully circumscribed performances of servants at dinner were no less significant to enforcing this order than religious rituals, linguistic forms, and class boundaries—permeable and tenuous as Swift always knew they were.

For all of his anxiety about maintaining order in the world, few people of his day presented their own beliefs so ambiguously; few perpetrated greater disorders of social forms and language—greater cultural mischiefs—than Swift himself. At the same time that he would attack the superstitions and tyranny of the Papists and the mad enthusiasms of the Dissenters, his own (apparent) defense of reasonable Anglicanism in *A Tale of a Tub*—refracted as it is through the crackpot ramblings of the teller, the irreverent ribaldry, and the fits and halts of the allegory itself—is so disjointed and oblique that many readers, including Queen Anne, were convinced that its author was entirely irreligious. In his writings about Protestants in Ireland, he often subverts the "very conservatism he upheld in church affairs," says Joseph McMinn.[27] As a clergyman in the Church of Ireland, he nominally represented English interests in Ireland; at the same time, he was the "Hibernian patriot" and anonymous M. B. Drapier, with a bounty on his head for "promot[ing] Sedition among the people."[28]

Swift also subverted the very forms of respect and ritual performance that, he insisted, enforced social order and rank. "There are persons who complain," he wrote,

> There's too much satire in my vein,
> That I am often found exceeding
> The rules of raillery and breeding,
> With too much freedom treat my betters,
> Not sparing even men of letters.[29]

As evidence of his "Incivility," Pilkington told the story of Swift's once addressing the Lord Lieutenant of Ireland as "You, Fellow with the blue String."[30] Samuel Johnson took Swift to task for such liberties. Himself the poor petitioner who famously rebuked the Earl of Chesterfield for turning him away at his door, Johnson nonetheless "insisted on the duty of maintaining subordination of rank." In respecting rank, said Johnson, "I consider myself as acting a part in the great system of society, and . . . I would behave to a nobleman as I should expect he would behave to me."[31] In his *Life of Swift*, Johnson criticized Swift for his violations of social manners:

> It may be justly supposed that there was in his conversation, what appears so frequently in his Letters, an affectation of familiarity with the Great, an ambition of momentary equality sought and enjoyed by the neglect of those ceremonies which custom has established as the barriers between one order of society and another. This transgression of regularity was by himself and his admirers termed greatness of soul. But a great mind disdains to hold any thing by courtesy, and therefore never usurps what a lawful claimant may take away. He that encroaches on another's dignity, puts himself in his power; he is either repelled with helpless indignity, or endured by clemency and condescension.[32]

Johnson understood Swift's behavior perfectly but not his motives. Begrudging the ingratitude and neglect of those whom he had served faithfully (we saw earlier), Swift felt that he deserved social elevation for his merits and service. His "transgression[s] of regularity" challenged the very structure that he had come to see as failing him.

Furthermore, Swift violated the forms of language that he himself was so concerned about maintaining. Although he was ever "tormented by the dangerous plasticity of language," he indulged in exhaustive, sometimes exhausting wordplay.[33] There is in the *Journal to Stella* the "little language" that he shared with Stella and Dingley. There are also outrageous puns throughout his correspondence; elaborate word games, especially with his fellow language prankster Thomas Sheridan; and neologisms in his imaginative works. It is Swift, after all, who gave us words like *Lilliputian* and *Yahoo* and the name Vanessa.[34] In one of the most brilliant disorderings of language, he and Sheridan exchanged letters in hybrid "Latino-Anglicus" and "Anglo-Latinus," which ingeniously spliced together Latin and English words.[35] Such clever word games celebrated the imaginative possibilities for language, and they showed the permeability of linguistic forms and precariousness of linguistic order.

As Swift unstitched the norms of "correct" language, so he also broke social expectations by slipping in and out of character in company. His bookseller George Faulkner claimed that in his youth, Swift played the roles of a number of people—"a waggoner's boy, a boot-catcher, an ostler, a waiter at a tavern . . . a weaver, a shoemaker. . . . a footman to a lady"—in order to know "a variety of life, in all shape whatever, from the beggar to the prince."[36] "As he was an excellent mimick," said his biographer Sheridan, he once "personated the character of an aukward Country Parson to the life," a parody made all the more ironic by the fact that after taking orders in the Irish church, Swift himself was a poor country parson in Kilroot.[37] Lætitia Pilkington recounted that on another occasion, Swift suddenly lifted up "Part of his [clerical] Gown to fan himself with" and, "acting in Character of a prudish Lady," quipped, "I never could bear to touch any Man's Flesh—except my Husband's."[38] Subverting the dignity of his own social bearing and of sex roles, the grave clergyman teased the company's expectations—and got away with bawdy badinage. Swift, remarks Rawson, had an "almost magical inventiveness as a mimic."[39] This fluidity of character and the ability to ventriloquize people of all social levels served him well in his satiric works. But they also played with social forms, turning people's preconceptions on their heads and making his identity as they understood it slippery and elusive.

While Swift's mimicry and odd social performances are sometimes regarded as eccentricities, they are of a piece with his notion of the "bite," convincing people first of some serious idea and then pulling the rug out from beneath their convictions. In suggesting how his friend William Tisdall could get the better of Stella, Swift explained the game: "I'll teach you a way to outwit Mrs. Johnson: it is a new-fashioned way of being witty, and they call it a bite. You must ask a bantering question, or tell some damned lye in a serious manner, and then she will answer or speak as if you were in earnest: then cry you, Madam, there's a bite. I would not have you undervalue this, for it is the constant amusement in Court, and every where else among the great people."[40] The bite itself, which Swift exploited in elaborate practical jokes like the *Bickerstaff Papers* and satires like "A Modest Proposal" and "An Argument Against Abolishing Christianity," counts for its effect upon the disruption of order—what is expected—and what one then gets. It is an ironic teasing of social forms and perceptions.

Swift hated disorder. Swift delighted in disorder. He was highly entertained when his servants tore apart a wall new-made by roguish masons and when he saw a monkey wreak mayhem in a kitchen. "I built a wall five years ago," he wrote to Bolingbroke in 1729, "and when the masons play'd the knaves, nothing delighted me so much as to stand by while my servants threw down what was amiss: I have likewise seen a Monkey overthrow all the dishes and plates in a kitchen, merely for the pleasure of seeing them tumble and hearing the clatter they made in their fall."[41] Such zany entertainments had no meaning for Swift, of course, without an appreciation for the *order* thrown into chaos. So, too, the effects of his disruptive social performances rested in prescribed norms, the typology of "manners" and "polite conversation" that Swift turned on its head in his violations of social forms and his impersonations. Similarly, the effects of Swift's anarchic wordplay depend upon "correct" forms of language. The egregious puns, the brilliant Latino-Anglicus, the nonsense words—all are defined still by forms of syntax and grammar. Such play puts order and disorder into continual tension.

Certainly, we may attribute Swift's acute awareness of the confusions of order and disorder to the political conditions of post–Civil War Britain that forced him to seek safety in England; to the internecine religious conflicts in which he engaged; to the economic and social upheavals of the long eighteenth century; and to the exceptional conditions of his own life as an "Anglo-Irish" man insecure in his parentage and disappointed in his political and religious aspirations. We may also ascribe his anxieties about disorder in the world to the "omnivorous skepticism" that could never let forms and institutions and myths stand unchallenged, even when they enforced the order he so desperately sought.[42] But as I hope that this study has also made clear, the tensions between order and disorder were a reality of Swift's humoral body, coextensive with the world outside of it. His chronic "Giddyness," "Deafness," and "noise in [his] Ears" disoriented him, occluded his senses and understanding, and confounded his identity. His humoral explanation of his illnesses, medical interventions, and regimen; often ironic representations of himself ill, even mad; and performances in the "sick role"—all were attempts to impose order upon a humoral body ever on the precipice of disorder.

Swift and his imaginative works certainly warrant more discussion than the limits of a single study permit. Here I can only suggest some biographical and critical possibilities that come with our historicizing of Swift's body and his understanding of his illnesses. While I do give some attention in earlier sections to the ways in which Swift's disordered body confused his identity, there is more to be said about his curious "character" and often puzzling behavior, which have implications for his imaginative work. Swift loved pranks, April Fool's jokes, and "bites." If we are to accept the anecdotal testimony of Lætitia Pilkington and others, he was also given to sudden unpredictable and at times erratic shifts of mood and behavior. The unpredictable shifts of humoral balance will not by themselves explain or excuse his mischiefs and occasionally bizarre behavior. But seeing Swift as a humoral body helps us appreciate what modern clinical psychology does not, that as his "Vexatious Disorder[s]" threw that body into disarray, so he understood something about how to "vex the world" by subverting its forms of propriety and decorum.[43]

We need also to give more attention to the way that Swift's humoral disorders shaped his satiric methods. Returning Swift to his humoral body helps us appreciate the gifts for mimicry and physical caricature that served him well in his satires. The certainty of his own bodily performance undermined by humoral disorders, he understood the fluidity of identity. He often teased in and out of character in conversation and correspondence. And he wrote more often in "voice"—earnest social arithmetician, doughty English traveler, canting enthusiast, Grub Street hack—than in propria persona. These "characters," New Critics dogmatized, must always be taken as "ironic personae," who stand in antithesis to the "norm" or "correct view" that Swift himself would argue. The problem, says Rawson, is that, forced by New Critical dicta into the "mechanical routine" of separating authors and speakers, readers have been "terrorized . . . into believing that poets never said anything directly."[44] Swift could speak directly, even in the indirections of his personae. Understanding the confusions and indeterminacies of his humoral body encourages new ways to read Swift's "characters" as something both of himself and outside of himself.

We have seen the possibilities for reading Swift's representations of his humoral disorders in *Gulliver's Travels*. Beginning with the premise that Swift is imagining his humoral body gives us new ways to read both the content and form of other works as well. There are, of course, the handful of autobiographical poems in which Swift represents himself disordered: "In Sickness," *Verses on the Death,* and "On His Own Deafness." Reading these as imaginings of his humoral disorders helps us appreciate not only the experiences that Swift depicts but also his attempts to impose order on disorder with comic and ironic self-representation and with the formal features of verse.

Furthermore, a humoral reading suggests new interpretive possibilities for the so-called scatological poems and those that "anatomize" women. The pastoral "nymphs" Corinna, Chloe, and Cælia are presented as repulsive bodies disordered, consuming and defecating, their loathsome parts inventoried by horrified male voyeurs. Contextualized within the social forms "of delicacy and decorum," the apparent preoccupation with excretory functions in these poems, no less than in *Gulliver's Travels*, has shocked and offended some readers' polite sensibilities.[45] It has convinced others of Swift's aberrant psychosexuality, others of his misogyny.[46] In these disgusting, anatomized female bodies, says Carol Houlihan Flynn, Swift presents his own fears of cultural disorder: "Women threaten to scatter reason, waste energy, and destroy the possibility of civilization."[47] But if we think about the objectified "nymphs" not only as female bodies but also as *humoral* bodies, we might appreciate better Swift's representations of his own disorders. Corinna, Chloe, and Cælia are, like all persons, playing out Swift's own daily humoral experiences, consuming, excreting, spitting, sweating, trying to impose order on the unruly body.

Humoralism gives us a narrower and, I would argue, a more historically apt cultural context in which to place the apparent preoccupation with excretory matters that have offended so many of Swift's readers. All of the foul bodily functions to which they object—"frowzy Steams," "sweaty Streams, / Before, behind, above, below," "Dirt, and Sweat, and Ear-wax," "Snot," "Moisture of her Toes," "shits," and "Humours gross"—are humoral excrements. However offensive the male voyeurs (and fussy readers) find these bodily functions, here is Swift's exposition of humoral nature. All the more urgent perhaps because Swift himself was forced to confront it hour to hour, all the more brutal because he must destroy the fatuous romanticizing denial that the body is materially connected with the world outside of it in continual exchanges mediated by the six non-naturals.

What is it, then, that so horrifies the male voyeurs—Strephon, Cassinus, and the window-peeper of "A Beautiful Young Nymph Going to Bed"? Certainly the reality beneath the appearance and the blasting of their fatuous ideals. But it is also the stark and unavoidable confrontation with the naked Ya-humoral body that they, like Gulliver, have tried so hard to deny. If all bodies are humoral, however, why the particular disgust and horror at *women's* bodies? In short, because of the way that humoralism gendered persons. Menstruating and lactating, along with performing all of the other excretory functions, the female body was thought to be "moister," more porous, more dangerously fluid and unstable. Men's bodies were more fibrous and solid.[48] In the women, the voyeurs and anatomizers of Swift's poems must confront the humoral body writ large, as does Gulliver with the Brobdingnagian maids of honor. In the culture of denial, men insist that women conceal these anarchic bodies in their closets and privies and behind masquerade garb: "Lace, Brocades and Tissues."⁴⁹ They are further hidden in the social protocols of delicacy and decorum. Likewise, linguistic and literary forms conceal the women's chaotic bodies. The men would contain these foul bodies with their classical and pastoral tropes, their euphemisms, and what Helen Deutsch calls "a veritable encyclopedia of circumlocutions." So discreet is the nymph Chloe at the privy that, as the politest description of her defecating would have it, "None ever saw her pluck a Rose."⁵⁰

If we see the women of the "unspeakable" poems as humoral bodies, what terrifies the men is not the abstract scattering of reason and wasting of energy that Flynn speaks about. It is, rather, the embodied threat of oozing humoral mess. In the context of humoralism, then, Swift is not expressing his own fears of cultural disorder that women bode. Rather, he is going after those Strephons and Cassinuses who would disavow the realities of their own bodies. Swift himself will have none of this. Faced with the exigencies of his disordered humoral body, he would shock his readers into acknowledging their own humoral instability. His appalled voyeurs serve as stand-ins for all persons who would refuse to accept their own real bodies. The very structures of the poems force readers to face their own humoral anarchy. As Deutsch remarks, in the "scatological poems," Swift "delight[s] in exploding euphemisms by juxtaposing them with the bodily functions they conceal."⁵¹ Another of his favorite rhetorical tricks is apophasis, drawing attention to the "Things, which must not be exprest," by denying their existence.⁵² "No Humours gross, or frowzy Steams" issue from the nymph Chloe:

> No noisom Whiffs, or sweaty Streams,
> Before, behind, above, below,
> Could from her taintless Body flow
> . . . .
> Her dearest Comrades never caught her
> Squat on her Hams, to make Maid's Water.
> You'd swear, that so divine a Creature
> Felt no Necessities of Nature.⁵³

No person, Swift would say, is exempt from the "Necessities of Nature."

While the men of these poems do everything they can to avoid and repudiate the unruly humoral body, the women heroically do what they can to put theirs back in order again for public display. From the "Confusion" of Cælia's humoral body, order springs, and "Tulips [are] rais'd from Dung."[54] The anatomized Corinna collects her "scatter'd Parts" and with "Anguish, Toil, and Pain" gathers "up herself again."[55] Imposing order on the chaos of their humoral bodies, these women represent Swift's own lifelong efforts to put himself together again. If readers object that the women are presented as mere stage-forms—prosthetic parts held together with spirit gum and white lead and smeared with gaudy "Dawbs of White and Red"—Swift has made his point about containing the body all the more forcefully.[56] Bodily form and per*form*ance are the means by which Swift himself tried to impose order upon the disorder of his humoral body. Without form, says the speaker of "The Progress of Beauty," matter cannot subsist.[57] That women's bodies are more humorally fluid, porous, and excretory than men's makes their putting themselves back together again all the more extraordinary.

If we understand Swift's humoral disorders, we can also appreciate better what are often seen as the incoherent forms of his works. As his disordered body and intellectual faculties confused and frustrated his attempts to make sense of them—and of the world around himself—so the generic confusions of imaginative writings frustrate expectations for formal unity and attempts by readers to categorize them by genre.

Gregory Lynall argues that Swift would never say that "the faults in men's minds [can] simply be attributed to bad vapours or faulty hydraulics."[58] Nevertheless, while the Dean himself shuddered at the notion that a body could be reduced to a mere machine, he sometimes spoke of his own writing as a mechanical production of his own. In correspondence of early 1722–23 to John Gay during a fit of giddiness, he hoped that his friend was "good at reading ill hands."[59] That Swift wrote with "ill hands" suggests that his handwriting was hardly legible, perhaps because he could not control his physical performance. At the same time, in his letter, those hands expressed his illnesses. His illegible writing to Gay was the *autograph* of the disordered humoral body.

We should never reduce his imaginative writings to mere machine-like productions of his body, even if Swift himself did in such instances (with what sincerity it is hard to tell). Still, caught always between a body disordered and a body in order, he would have appreciated the precariousness and provisionality of anything "certain," including traditional literary forms. This understanding of the tentativeness of forms registers in works such as *A Tale of a Tub* and *Gulliver's Travels*. The *Tale* is ostensibly stitched together by the story of brothers Peter, Jack, and Martin, an allegory about the Reformation. But the Grub Street hack who tells the tale rambles into arcane allusions that are sometimes cued by tenuous associations and puns, and he digresses at great length about offhand topics, including critics, madness, and even digressions themselves. Although genre had been theorized as early as Aristotle, there is no fixing the *Tale* generically. The same is true of *Gulliver's Travels*. It has been variously called novel, fantastic travel narrative, parody of new science report, inverse spiritual autobiography, and, as a way to comprehend its generic mess, Menippean satire.[60] There are literary precedents in Cervantes, Robert Burton, and Swift's beloved Rabelais. Even so, the generic indeterminacies of the *Tale* and *Gulliver's Travels* are correlative to—and expressive of—the ever-precarious, wobbly order of Swift's own humoral body.

Understanding the disorders of this body also helps us appreciate Swift's other games with form. Subversions of traditional poetic genres such as the pastoral, elegy, and landscape poem are his stock-in-trade.[61] And as we have seen before, there is ingenious wordplay, which subverts the very linguistic—and cultural—order that Swift himself had insisted upon in his proposal for purifying the English language. Swift's unrelenting skepticism likely provoked him to undo forms and traditions and myths. But in a fluid and uncertain humoral body made all the more chaotic by the bewildering of his senses, few other writers could ever have *imagined* such disorders.

Finally, understanding that the humoral body is always in the process of being made and unmade and remade, we can appreciate better Swift's imaginative constructions and destructions and reconstructions. In his earliest surviving letter, Swift wrote to a friend from Sir William Temple's house at Moor Park, "You know, that there is somthing in me which must be employ'd, & when I am alone, turns all for want of practice into speculation & thought; insomuch that in these seven weeks I have been here, I have writt, & burnt and writt again upon almost all manner of subjects, more perhaps than any man in England."[62] More than forty years later, he wrote to Pope of his declining powers, "God be thanked I have done with every thing & of every kind that requires writing, except now & then a Letter, or, like a true old Man Scribbling trifles only fit for children or Schoolboys of the lowest Class at best, which three or four of us read & laugh at today, & burn to Morrow."[63] We might attribute the ephemeral making and unmaking and remaking of what he has "writt" to the thoroughgoing skepticism that would not let anything stand. We might say of Swift that he was a singularly restless man who could never sit still or be satisfied or that he was caught precariously between the classical world and modernity. But as I hope this study has made clear, we may say also that the processes of constructing and tearing down are the processes of his "crasie" humoral body, as it was caught always in heady rounds of balancing and unbalancing and rebalancing.

APPENDIX

Prescriptions for Swift from John Arbuthnot

Throughout Swift's correspondence, we hear occasionally of his taking certain medications for his chronic disorders: the Jesuit's bark, asafoetida, hiera picra, and various unspecified pills and tonics provided by doctors and friends. To my knowledge, however, only two formal prescriptions survive, both of them from his physician and intimate friend John Arbuthnot. The first of these, excerpted from a letter of December 1718, appears at the beginning of a long, gossipy excursion through news of mutual friends and public affairs: "I have done good lately to a patient & a freind [sic] in that Complaint of a Vertigo by Cinnabar of Antimony & Castor, made up into Bolus's with Confect of Alkermes. I had no great opinion of the Cinnabar but trying it amongst other things my freind found good of this prescription; I had tryd the Castor alone befor, not with so much success. small quantitys of Tinctur Sacr: now & then will do yow good."[1]

Here Arbuthnot explicitly prescribes for the giddiness from which Swift had suffered much in the months before. While he seems generally to have shied away from metal cures like mercury and antimony, cinnabar of antimony, "a Composition of Mercury, common Sulphur, and crude Antimony sublimed," was prescribed by some for vertigo and epilepsy.[2] It was used also as a diaphoretic and as a *"salivating Medicine"* to "dissolve, and evacuate the *Mucous* and *Coagulation* of the *Lympha*, by Dividing and Cutting the Parts asunder."[3] Even if Arbuthnot was an iatromechanist who focused on strengthening the fibrous solids of the body rather than balancing out fluid components, both of these interventions accorded with the humoral logic of dislodging and expelling the superfluous or peccant humors that might have caused Swift's giddiness. Castor, a reddish-brown "odoriferous animal-substance" taken from the beaver, was "looked upon as one of the capital nervine and antihysteric medicines."[4] And the tinctura sacra

("Tinctur Sacr") was a name applied to a variety of cordials and electuaries, most used as purgatives but also regarded as a "sovereign Preservative" against seasonal "Distempers that affect the Head."[5] Arbuthnot directs that Swift combine the cinnabar of antimony and castor into a bolus with "Confect of Alkermes," a confection that included the "juice" of the kermes, a red scale insect; presumably this would be more palatable. All of the suggestions here are for cephalic disorders such as Swift's own, noxious or superfluous fluids that had accumulated in the head.

Arbuthnot's second letter, of November 1730, is devoted almost exclusively to prescriptions for Swift's disorders. It begins,

> The passage in Mr popes Letter about your health dos not Alarum me both of us have had this distemper these 30 years. I have found that Steel the warm Gumms & the Bark all do good in it. therefor first take the Vomit A then every day the Quantity of a Nutmeg in a Morning of the Electury markd B with five spoonfulls of the Tinctur Mark'd D. take the Tinctur; but not the Elect in the afternoon yow may take one of the pills marked C at any time when yow are troubld with it or 30 of the drops markd E in any vehicle evn water. I had a servant of my owin that was cur'd merely with vomiting. Ther is another med[icine] not mentiond which yow may trye the pull Rad [Val] sylvestris about a scruple of it twice a day.[6]

Following a postscript in which he reports that he has "recommended Dr Helsham to be physician to the Lord Liewtenant," Arbuthnot encloses prescriptions for the five compounds labeled A–E; this is followed by a receipt for bitters:

A

℞ pulv. Rad. ipecacuanhæ ℈s.

B

℞ Conserv: Flavedin. Aurant., Absynth. Rom. an ʒvj. Rubrqui. Martis in pollem Redact. ʒiiij. syrup C succo Kermes, q.s.

C

℞ As. Fœtid. zij. Tinctur. Castor q. s. M. fiant pilulæ xxiv

D

℞ Cortic. peruvian elect: rubrqui. Martis an ʒj. digere tepide in vini Alb. Gallic. ℔ij per 24 horas postea fiat colatura.

E

℞ sp. cc. cerv., sp. Lavandul., Tinctur. Castor. an ʒij. Misce.

[*Enclosure*, f. 8ᵛ]

Take of Zedoary Root one drachm Galangal
Roman wormwood of each two drachms orange peel a drachm
Lesser Cardamon seeds two scruples
Infuse all in a Quart of Boyling Spring water for six hours. Strain it off and add to it four ounces of Greater Compound wormwood water[7]

While Arbuthnot never discusses a specific diagnosis here, his own iatromechanical approach to restoring health focuses not on the heat of the stomach, as Galen's humoralism had, but on the strength and elasticity of the fibers that circulated the fluids through the body. The goals of Arbuthnot's iatrophysics and the old humoralism were nevertheless the same, to attenuate the fluids through proper digestion so that the solids can drive them efficiently through the body, preventing the pathological accumulation of any one humor in any one part. His prescription maps a standard course of treatment for purging the body of foul humors, strengthening the stomach for proper digestion, and preventing the buildup of fluids that would clog the system. Swift is, first, to purge with ipecac ("Rad. ipecacuanhæ" of "Vomit A"), to cleanse the stomach of foul excess. Then he is to take medicines to encourage proper digestive functions. Roman wormwood ("Absynth. Rom." in the "Electuary markd B"), one of the "warm Gumms," was "a strong bitter" used to strengthen the stomach; the authoritative *Edinburgh New Dispensatory*, published forty years after Swift's death, says that it "was formerly much used . . . against weakness of the stomach."[8] An early eighteenth-century English pharmacopoeia claimed that "there is not a chronic distemper in which it is not serviceable."[9] Like Roman wormwood, the Jesuit's or Peruvian bark ("Cortic. peruvian" in "the Tinctur markd D"), best known as a cinchonic antimalarial medicine, was also an astringent "corroborant [that is, strengthener] and stomachic" used to encourage appetite.[10] "Succo kermes" in electuary "B," the juice of kermes that we saw in Arbuthnot's letter of 1718, was also considered a "corroborant."[11] While Arbuthnot speaks of steel remedies in his explanation, "Rubrqui. Martis" in the same compound was specifically iron rust, considered to have an "aperient [gentle laxative] virtue."[12] But like wormwood and the bark, it could also be "an astringent to others"; that is, it would constrict mucous membranes, thereby reducing the secretions that might otherwise accumulate in the head, and would tone the fibrous parts of the body.[13] Swift complains of taking chalybeates—a word denoting iron salts, taken from the Greek word for steel—especially during the fall and winter of 1712–13, when he was "extremely out of Order with a Giddiness in [his] Head."[14] But he seems to have been convinced that the steel compounds worked, no matter how repugnant he found them: "I . . . take some nasty steel drops, & [my] head has been bett^r this week past."[15] And weeks later: "I take some steel drops; & my Head is pretty well."[16]

Many of the medicines in Arbuthnot's armamentarium, then, were used to stimulate proper digestion and assimilation of the humors by strengthening the stomach and preventing excessive secretion of the phlegm that would impede healthy physiological processes. Included among the medicaments are also those used specifically in nervous and cephalic disorders. Asafoetida ("As. Fœtid." in "the pills marked C"), "the strongest of the fetid gums," was used routinely "in hysteric and different kinds of nervous complaints."[17] As we saw in Arbuthnot's letter of 1718, castor ("Tinctur. Castor" in the same medicine) was prescribed for nervous disorders and hysteria. The pills in "C" were considered "antispasmodics"; that is, they would prevent muscle spasms and epilepsy. We recall here the concern by both Arbuthnot and Peter Shaw that vertigo might eventuate in epilepsy or an apoplexy. The solution of lavender in "the drops markd E" was "a warm stimulating aromatic . . . principally recommended in vertigoes, palsies, tremors, suppression of the menstrual evacuations; and in general in all disorders of the head, nerves, and uterus."[18] The wild valerian that Arbuthnot suggests in his instructions ("pull Rad [Val] sylvestris") was a medicinal herb long thought to have a "warming" effect and used to calm nerves and to cure insomnia. The addendum following item E in the prescriptions is a recipe for a bitter tonic, used, like the other bitter medicines (wormwood and the Jesuit's bark), as a digestive aid.

NOTES

ABBREVIATIONS

Accounts	The Account Books of Jonathan Swift
Correspondence	The Correspondence of Jonathan Swift, D.D.
GT	Gulliver's Travels
JS	Journal to Stella: Letters to Esther Johnson and Rebecca Dingley, 1710–1713
Poems	The Poems of Jonathan Swift
PW	The Prose Writings of Jonathan Swift
Tale	"A Tale of a Tub" and Other Works
Williams	The Correspondence of Jonathan Swift

PREFACE

1. Swift to Charles Ford, 4 April 1720, in *Correspondence*, 2:327; Swift to Knightley Chetwode, 11 November 1721, in *Correspondence*, 2:403. All subsequent references to letters to and from Swift cite him by last name only. In dating letters throughout this study, I follow David Woolley's editorial lead for correspondence that straddles Old and New Style calendars. According to the Old Style (Julian) calendar still used in Britain during Swift's day, the new year began on March 25. So, a date of 7 February 1720–21, for example, would be 1720 in the Old Style calendar and 1721 in the New Style (Gregorian) calendar, which had been used in the rest of Europe since 1582 but was not adopted in Britain until 1752.
2. In my own references to Ménière and the disease that bears his name, I have kept the original accents *aigu* and *grave*. In citing various secondary sources, I follow the practices of the authors.

3. Swift to the Rev. Thomas Sheridan, 18 September 1728, in *Correspondence*, 3:194.
4. Swift to Alexander Pope, 1 November 1734, in *Correspondence*, 4:8; Swift to Alexander Pope, 23 June 1737, in *Correspondence*, 4:445; 6 July 1711, in *JS*, 239.
5. Swift to Knightley Chetwode, 30 January 1721-22, in *Correspondence*, 2:411.
6. Frank, *Will of the Body*, 13.

1. TAKING SWIFT BACK

1. *Verses on the Death of Dr. Swift, D.S.P.D. Occasioned by Reading a Maxim in Rochefoulcault*, lines 83–84, in *Poems*, 2:556, cited hereafter as *Verses on the Death*; "On His Own Deafness," line 1, in *Poems*, 2:673.
2. Ingram, *Swift, Pope and the Doctors*; Wilde, *Closing Years*.
3. Ehrenpreis, *Swift*, 3:319.
4. Among those few readers who have discussed these topics, see titles by Child, Creaser, LaCasce, Probyn, and Washington in the bibliography of secondary sources.
5. Orrery, *Remarks on the Life and Writings*, 270.
6. Quoted in Ehrenpreis, *Swift*, 3:915.
7. This study uses the word *madness* broadly to denote both the "lunacy" and "idiotism" (or "imbecility") from which Swift's biographers said he suffered. Despite the distinction that those such as Lord Orrery and John Locke make, I feel safe in following Johnson's own first, comprehensive definition of madness: "Distraction; loss of understanding; perturbation of the faculties." *Dictionary*, 2, s.v. "madness."
8. Johnson, "Swift," 207, 190.
9. Orrery, 275.
10. Wilde, iii.
11. The words *clinic* and *clinical*, which I invoke routinely in this study, require brief explication. In its basic sense, clinical medicine is that which arrives at its conclusions about a patient's health and illness by careful observation of "signs," detectable indications of a disease. Medical practitioners as early as Hippocrates had relied upon clinical signs to diagnose imbalances of the fluid humors that constituted the body. Such external signs could indicate invisible internal disorders otherwise inaccessible to the senses. As the sixteenth-century pathologist Jean Fernel wrote, "Diseases hidden in the innermost crevices of the body, that cannot be distinguished or perceived through the senses, are understood by signs. With these as

evidence, the mind is led by sound reasoning to penetrate into what is hidden" (*Pathologiae Libri Septem: De Morbis Eorumque Causis* [Venice, 1555], quoted in Laqueur, "Question of Judgment," 535). What modern medicine would call internists could diagnose diseases by looking at the signs that the body gave them about the inner workings and balances of that body. An eruption of painful pustules on the upper back, for example, could indicate an excess of the hot, acrid humor choler working its way out of the body; the doctor would see these as signs of shingles.

"Clinical Physicians," said Ephraim Chambers's 1728 *Cyclopædia*, "were those who visited their Patients a-bed, to examine their Cases.... In opposition to the Emperists, who sold their Medicines in the Streets" (2:809). The distinction between a confraternity of practitioners bound by an agreed-upon way of knowing the body and the ragtag crowd of "empiricists" who hawked their cure-all nostrums, miracle pills, potions, and drops to the unwary sick, defines the "professional." "Clinical Physicians" are bound by common epistemology and method to the responsible care of their patients. This shared way of knowing the body and disease increasingly structured the medical education that, in turn, determined who was a professional and who was not. By the early eighteenth century, the medical school at Leyden, where Swift's own Gulliver "studie[s] Physick two Years and seven Months," had marked itself as a progressive clinical school in which medical students made rounds, taking case notes and paying careful attention to symptomatology in making diagnoses (*GT*, 30). The students interviewed patients and recorded their symptoms, thereby acknowledging them as "subjective bodies." Even then, there was some movement at Leyden and other progressive medical schools toward a uniform systematizing of diagnoses based on signs common to what Michel Foucault calls "disease entities." This taxonomizing of disease was itself a notional structure by which the clinic that we know enforced its way of understanding and exerted its authority upon the body.

The modern clinic of Foucault's construction, which underpins the distinction that I make between clinical and humoral bodies here, is an ascendant epistemology that has institutionalized and imposed its ways of knowing and producing new knowledge about the body, of diagnosing disease, and of determining treatment. See Foucault, *Birth of the Clinic*.

12. "Dean Swift's Disease," 142.
13. Damrosch, *Jonathan Swift*, 68.
14. Ingram, xi.

15. Hawkesworth, *Works of Jonathan Swift, D.D.*, 1:55–56. In a useful discussion of the narrative about Swift's madness, Ingram quotes Hawkesworth's passage at greater length (17–18).
16. Gosse, *History of Eighteenth Century Literature*, 161; Delany, *Observations*, 102–3.
17. Ingram, xi.
18. Cunningham, "Identifying Disease in the Past," 17.
19. Anderson, *Physician Heal Thyself*, 55.
20. For the distinction between "ontological" and "physiological" notions of disease, see Temkin's classic "The Scientific Approach to Disease: Specific Entity and Individual Sickness."
21. Foucault.
22. Cunningham, 16.
23. Swift to Alexander Pope, 2 December 1736, in *Correspondence*, 4:365.
24. Swift and Mrs. Whiteway to the Earl of Orrery, 2 February 1737–38, in *Correspondence*, 4:494.
25. While the four-humor system is common knowledge, the explanation in this study benefits greatly from secondary sources such as Noga Arikha's superb intellectual history of the humors, which has appeal for both academic and popular readers: *Passions and Tempers: A History of the Humours*. Humoralism is invariably associated with "Hippocrates" or, more correctly, the Hippocratic corpus, the collection of sixty or so medical writings gathered under the name of Hippocrates of Cos, produced between the late fifth and mid-fourth centuries BCE. Helen King notes, though, that the "canonical" four humors are named in only one of the Hippocratic works, *On the Nature of Man*. It was Galen who systematized the model of four humors that persisted into the eighteenth century. "Female Fluids in the Hippocratic Corpus," 30–35.
26. Moyle, *Experienced Chirurgeon*, 3–4. While some conceptions of the body had five, three, or as few as two humors, the classic Galenic model had four, "concocted" (that is, processed) from food in the stomach. Because what Moyle calls the "Mass of Blood" *carried* the humors, the common practice of bleeding, to which Swift and most of his contemporaries submitted, was intended to remove a "plethora" of a given humor or to rid the body of a "corrupt" humor.
27. *Report of the Paris Medical Faculty*.
28. Moyle, 3–4. *Plethory*, said a dictionary of the day, is the "too great abounding with blood or laudable [natural] humours, which proves hurtful to the body"; *cacochymy* is the "abundance of corrupt humours in the body

caused by bad nourishment or ill digestion." Bailey, Gordon, and Miller, *Dictionarium Britannicum*, s.v. "plethory"; s.v. "cacochymy."

29. In his best-selling regimen books, George Cheyne speaks of his "own crazy Carcase" and of a "crazy Constitution." *Essay of Health*, xvi, 2. In 1734, Charles Jervas wrote to Swift that Pope had "a carkass so crazy." Jervas to Swift, 24 November 1734, in *Correspondence*, 4:22. And writing to Pope himself, William Wycherley hoped that his "great, Vigorous, and active Mind, will not be able to destroy, [his] little, tender, and crazy Carcase." 19 February 1708–9, in *Correspondence of Alexander Pope*, 1:55.
30. Swift to Charles Ford, 20 November 1733, in *Correspondence*, 3:707.
31. Sydenham, *Dr. Sydenham's Compleat Method*, 140.
32. Moyle, 3–4.
33. Swift, "Bec's Birth-Day. November 8th, M DCC XXVI," lines 11–16, in *Poems*, 2:761.
34. 4 November 1711, in *JS*, 316.
35. 26 August 1711, in *JS*, 268.
36. 28 April 1711, in *JS*, 195.
37. Radcliffe quoted in Macalpine and Hunter, *George III and the Mad-Business*, 221–22; Porter and Rousseau, *Gout*, 240–41.
38. The term *peccant* was routinely applied to characterize humoral corruptions. Alexander Pope, for example, wrote to Swift in 1728 of Bolingbroke, "Upon his return from the Bath, all peccant humours, he finds, are purg'd out of him." 28 June 1728, in *Correspondence*, 3:186.
39. Cheyne, *Essay of Health*, 172–73. Cheyne, a compatriot of Swift's London doctor, William Cockburn, and of his close friend John Arbuthnot, had emigrated from Scotland to London in 1701; he became an immensely popular practitioner in London and Bath. Swift likely knew him as one of the "parcel of Scots" who, he complained, seemed always to gang around Cockburn. 21 January 1710–11, in *JS*, 126. For a good biography of Cheyne, see Guerrini, *Obesity and Depression*.
40. The very etymology of the word *crisis*—from the Greek "to decide"—reminds us of the crucial value of the fever crisis to prognosis.
41. In the *Journal to Stella*, Swift reports in great detail about the onset and process of this painful disorder, which lasted some four months. This is one of the few instances in which Swift describes "clinically" his own illnesses, going into great detail about symptoms and diagnosis. See *JS*, 418–40.
42. 31 March to 8 April 1712, in *JS*, 420. The prognosis of a quick recovery following the skin eruptions is important in distinguishing Swift's and his doctors' understanding of outcome from that of the "vulgar." Speaking

of the common presentation of shingles around the waist, Peter Shaw stated that the disease is "quite painful, and often continues for two or three weeks" but noted with some disdain, "The vulgar think them dangerous, and pretend they are mortal if they go quite round." *New Practice of Physick*, 1:339. In the late eighteenth century, the surgeon John Pearson equivocated by condemning the "vulgar opinion" that shingles can be fatal, but at the same time admitting that he had never seen the eruptions form a complete circle: "A vulgar notion indeed prevails, that if the eruption forms a Circle round the body the termination will be certainly fatal. I never saw it encompass the body, but it is more than probable that this Prognosis is as well supported as the generality of vulgar opinions." *Principles of Surgery*, 196. In the different prognoses, we see claims for competing medical narratives.
43. Cook, *Anatomical and Mechanical Essay*, 2:45–46.
44. Sydenham, 120.
45. Cooper, *Thesaurus Linguae Romanæ & Britannicæ*, 265.
46. For a helpful discussion of the processes of concoction in humoral physiology, see Stolberg, "'You Have No Good Blood in Your Body': Oral Communication in Sixteenth-Century Physicians' Medical Practice."
47. An early eighteenth-century medical text written for a popular audience explains, "By Congestion a Tumour is gathered for want of the digestive Faculty in the Part, which is insufficient to concoct the Humour, or to expel it by insensible Transpiration: Sometimes the vicious Quality of the Matter designed for the Alimentation of that Part, gathers by degrees into a Tumour, as being not qualify'd to be converted into the Substance of said Part." Dubé, *Poor Man's Physician and Surgeon*, 334.
48. Paxton, *Directory Physico-Medical*, 169.
49. Weisser, *Ill Composed*, 7.
50. Ishizuka, "'Fibre Body,'" 563.
51. Harvey himself was wary of the mechanical view of the body. For him, the heart was an organic pump, part of the whole organism, rather than a mechanical one, a cog in a machine. Nonetheless, Harvey's discovery that the heart circulated the same blood in a continuous round dismantled the long-held Galenic belief that blood was continuously being brewed anew in the liver and then burned up in the body.
52. The prefix "iatro-" comes from the combining form of the Greek ἰατρός, "physician," and is used generally to designate "medical." *OED*, s.v. "iatro-."
53. Arikha, 196–97.
54. Shackelford, review of *"Divulging of Useful Truths in Physick,"* 256–57.

55. *Tale*, 107.
56. Cockburn (1669–1739), whom Swift consulted frequently in medical matters during his time in London between 1710 and 1714, was formerly a ship's doctor. He made a fortune selling a proprietary remedy for dysentery to the English fleet and died, says the *Oxford Dictionary of National Biography*, a "very rich quack" (Creighton, "Cockburn"). Arbuthnot (1667–1735), physician, satirist, mathematician, Scriblerian "brother" to Swift—and originator of John Bull—emigrated from Scotland to England around 1691. Swift met him in a London coffeehouse in 1711, first mentioning him in an entry in the *Journal to Stella* of March 19 of that year (*JS*, 166). Helsham (1683–1738), a Fellow of the Royal College of Physicians of Ireland (1710), was a natural philosopher and celebrated mathematician at Trinity College, Dublin. He was the first Erasmus Smith's Professor of Natural and Experimental Philosophy (1724–38) and Regius Professor of Physic (1733–38) at Trinity. He was also appointed an executor of Swift's will but predeceased the Dean by some seven years.
57. Arbuthnot, Γνῶθι σεαυτον: *Know Your Self*, lines 15–16, 10, 13. I am grateful to the anonymous external reviewer at the University of Virginia Press who drew my attention to this piece.
58. Swift, *A Discourse Concerning the Mechanical Operation of the Spirit, &c.*, in *Tale*, 173.
59. *GT*, 145. For an explication of this episode in its scientific contexts, see Lynall, *Swift and Science*, 46.
60. Temple, *Essay upon Health and Long Life*, 149. Swift himself owned a 1658 copy of Paracelsus's *Opera Omnia*, prefaced by an attack on the errors of the Galenists. *Tale*, 493n129.
61. In book 4 of the *Travels*, Gulliver describes the repulsive compositions of herbs, minerals, and animal parts used as emetics and clysters. *GT*, 378–80.
62. Swift, *The Battel of the Books*, in *Tale*, 156, 153. A "stink-pot," Marcus Walsh explains, is the doctor's or apothecary's gallipot, a jar used for holding medicines and ointments; it suggests also the vessels that physicians used when inspecting urine. *Tale*, 484n82.
63. Michael Gordin defines "vestigial doctrines" as "systems of thought that used to be considered sciences but that professional scientists have, over time, either gradually moved away from or actively excluded. The most well-known are astrology and alchemy, which during the Renaissance were largely synonymous with what would become by the end of the Enlightenment 'astronomy' and 'chemistry.'" "Problem with Pseudoscience,"

1483. For the persistence of humoralism beyond early modern medicine, see Arikha, passim.
64. Wear, "Medical Practice," 295.
65. Arikha, 199.
66. Orrery, 215.
67. Cheyne, *Essay on Regimen*, xxvii.
68. See, for example, Cheyne's *A New Theory of Continu'd Fevers*.
69. Wear, "Medical Practice," 295.
70. Paxton, 169.
71. Guerrini, 58.
72. Cheyne, *Essay of Health*, 3.
73. Wear, "Medical Practice," 301.
74. Ephraim Chambers's encyclopedia of 1728 explicates the term *humour* in both its classical and modern senses: "HUMOUR, in Medicine, is apply'd to any Juice, or fluid Part of the Body, as the *Chyle, Blood, Milk, Fat, Serum, Lymph, Spirits, Bile, Seed, Salival* and *Panchreatic* Juices *&c.* . . . The *four Humours* so much talk'd of by the ancient Physicians, are four liquid Substances which they suppose to moisten the whole Body of all Animals, and to be the Cause of the divers Temperaments thereof. . . . These are *Phlegm* . . . *Blood, Bile* [choler], and *Melancholly*. . . . But the Moderns do not allow of these Divisions. The *Humours* they rather chuse to distinguish into *Nutritious*, called also *Alimentary*, as *Chyle* and *Blood;* those separated from the Blood, as *Bile, Saliva, Urine*, &c. and those return'd into the Blood. *Humours*, again, are distinguish'd into *natural* or salutary, and *morbid*, or corrupted.—To the former Class belong all the Juices ordinarily secreted for the Uses of the Body. To the latter belong those compound *Humours*, which thicken, and grow putrid; causing Tumors, Abscesses, Obstructions, and most Diseases. . . . These are distinguish'd by various Names, *Malignant, Adust, Acrimonious, Corrosive, Crude, Peccant*, &c." *Cyclopædia*, 1:262.
75. Boyle, quoted in Lynall, 41. Cheyne tells us that "when a Machine is disordered, if we should see it righted by adjusting such a particular Part, we might without scruple affirm, that it was some injury done to that part, which had disorder'd the Machine; especially, if after the whole was taken to Peices, we should find them all sound, save that particular one. Thus, if we should see a Watchmaker, by adjusting only the Balance of a Watch, make her go right; we might say the distortion of the Axe thereof had occasion'd her going wrong; especially, if all the other parts be found as they should be." *New Theory of Continu'd Fevers*, 2.

2. STORIES OF ILLNESS AND RETROSPECTIVE DIAGNOSIS

1. Rosenberg, "Framing Disease," xiii. Rosenberg adopts the term *frame* from social psychologist Erving Goffman's *Frame Analysis: An Essay on the Organization of Experience*.
2. Cheyne, "Case of the Author," 359–60.
3. Shuttleton, *Smallpox and the Literary Imagination*, 46–48.
4. Defoe, *Robinson Crusoe*, 105.
5. Cheyne, "Case of the Author," 364.
6. Among the earliest uses of the term "*autopathography*—autobiographical narrative of illness or disability"—is Thomas Couser's, in *Recovering Bodies*, 5. For a good discussion of the designation, see Jeffrey K. Aronson, "Autopathography: The Patient's Tale." Besides Cheyne's "Case of the Author," another of the few examples from the eighteenth century is Frances Flood's *The Devonshire Woman; or, A Wonderful Narrative of Frances Flood*.
7. Hawkins, *Reconstructing Illness*, 18.
8. *Accounts*, 62.
9. Swift to Archbishop King, 6 January 1708–09, in *Correspondence*, 1:225.
10. 29 September 1710, in *JS*, 21. John Radcliffe (1650–1714), among the wealthiest and most famous London physicians of his day, openly sneered at academic medicine, remarking once of some vials of herbs and a skeleton in his study, "*This* is Radcliffe's library." That he should bequeath a substantial sum of money to Oxford for the founding of the Radcliffe Library, Samuel Garth reportedly scoffed, was as fitting "as if an eunuch was to found a seraglio." Aikin et al., *General Biography*, 8:438. Charles Bernard (ca. 1652–1710), surgeon to St. Bart's for twenty-five years and, for the last eight years of his life, Serjeant Surgeon to Queen Anne, was famous for his operating skills; like Cockburn and Radcliffe, he, too, accrued a great fortune in practice. Bernard died only two weeks after Swift's mention of him (Lyle, "Bernard").
11. Swift to Mrs. Whiteway, 26 July 1740, in *Correspondence*, 4:627.
12. *PW*, 4:88.
13. *Daily Post* [London], 23 October 1725. Swift had stayed with Thomas Sheridan and family at Quilca, in County Cavan, from about April 20 to the end of September 1725. Quilca was hardly a "Country Seat." In a poem written during his stay, Swift grumbled that he lived there in a "rotten Cabbin," with "Stools, Tables, Chairs, and Bed-steds broke," beset all around with "*Sloth, Dirt,* and *Theft*." "To Quilca, a Country House in No Very Good Repair, Where the Supposed Author, and Some of His Friends, Spent a Summer, in the Year 1725," lines 2, 4, 12, in *Poems*, 3:1035.
14. *Grub Street Journal* [London], 15 September 1737.

15. *Country Journal, or The Craftsman* [London], 26 September 1741; virtually the same notice appears in the *London Daily Post and General Advertiser* for 23 September 1741.
16. Pilkington, *Memoirs*, 1:33. Pilkington wrote the memoirs largely as self-vindication from what she claimed were the slanders of her husband Matthew, from whom she had been by this time ecclesiastically divorced. Long considered self-serving and unreliable, Pilkington's collective *Memoirs* have recently been reassessed more generously. See Elias, introduction to Pilkington, xv–lxii; and Cook, "Lord Orrery's *Remarks on Swift*," 62–63.
17. Orrery, *Remarks on the Life and Writings*, 81.
18. Orrery, 276, 215.
19. Orrery, 81.
20. For my use of *madness* as a term that comprehends both "lunacy" and "idiotism," see chapter 1, note 7.
21. Orrery, 272.
22. Orrery, 275–76. In the context of Orrery's discussion of cause, "absolute naturals" are not only those born "imbecile" but those, too, in whom the "state of idiotism" is permanent.
23. Orrery, 270–71.
24. Locke, *Essay Concerning Humane Understanding*, 94.
25. Swift to Lord Orrery, 16–17 July 1735, in *Correspondence*, 4:145–46.
26. Swift to George Faulkner, 13 July 1738, in *Correspondence*, 4:526.
27. Delany, *Observations*, 52.
28. Delany, 195. Although their friendship cooled in the late 1730s, Delany was witness to Swift's sad decline.
29. Johnson, "Swift," 207, 190.
30. Johnson, *Vanity of Human Wishes*, 25. Johnson seizes here upon the unsubstantiated story that Swift's servants exhibited the mute, pitiable old man for money. Such was the common acceptance of the tale about Swift's decline into imbecility that his case became a dismal comparison for others. In 1780, Thomas Alcock wrote of his own late brother Nathan's "old nervous disorder" and attendant "dizziness, giddiness, and stupor in the head," "He put me in mind of Dean Swift's case, who was troubled in the latter part of life with such a giddiness; and I was always apprehensive, that [Nathan's] disorder, like the Dean's, would terminate in a depravation, or deprivation of the mental faculties." *Some Memoirs*, 43–44.
31. Gosse, *History of Eighteenth Century Literature*, 161.
32. Thackeray, *English Humourists*, 41.

33. "[Phrenological Examination of Jonathan Swift's Skull]," 559. The phrenological examination is cited by Lorch, "Language and Memory Disorder," 3132. Charting the evolution of theories of insanity and other psychological disorders since the eighteenth century, Lorch surveys the various attempts to diagnose Swift's mental health in his final years. In my own discussion of retrospective diagnoses of Swift's mental debilities, I borrow liberally from her excellent survey. For a valuable essay on the phrenological examination of Swift's skull, see Deutsch, "'Alas, poor Yorick!'"
34. Scott, *Life of Swift*, 409n.
35. Lecky, *Leaders of Public Opinion*, 56, quoted in Lorch, 3131.
36. In 1888, the psychiatrist Julian Koch coined the term *psychopath* (*Psychopastiche*, or "suffering soul," in his original German) to distinguish a certain category of patients from others suffering from psychosis. While the psychotic loses contact with reality in delusions, hallucinations, and incoherent thoughts, the psychopath exhibits what Philippe Pinel saw as "moral insanity," a marked behavioral trait that occurs without confusions of mind and intellect. Kiehl and Lushing, "Psychopathy."
37. See, for instance, Ferenczi, "Gulliver's Phantasies" (1928); Karpman, "A Modern Gulliver: A Study in Coprophilia" (1949); Greenacre, "The Mutual Adventures of Jonathan Swift and Lemuel Gulliver" (1955); and Freedman, "Gulliver's Voyage to the Country of the Houyhnhnms" (1986). Chaim Melamed helpfully surveys the psychoanalytical diagnoses of Swift in his unpublished dissertation, "Gulliver and the *Other*: A Psychoanalytical Examination."
38. Wilson, "Mental and Physical Health," 177.
39. Wilde, *Closing Years*, iii; Dalrymple, "Greatest Torture," 777. Sir William was Oscar's father.
40. Beddoes, *Hygeia*, 3:189ff.; Mahony, *Jonathan Swift*, 66–67.
41. Wilde, 5. In our own day, other clinicians have similarly attributed Swift's late-life aphasia, memory loss, disorientation, and erratic behavior to neurodegenerative—that is, physiological—disorders. One has diagnosed Swift with Alzheimer's disease, another with Pick's disease (frontotemporal dementia); both are thought to be caused by protein "tangles" that interfere with nerve transmission. Lewis, "Jonathan Swift and Alzheimer's Disease"; Crichton, "Jonathan Swift and Alzheimer's Disease."
42. Wilde, 27.
43. Wilde, 70.
44. Wilde, 64.

45. Legg, "Swift's Giddy Fits."
46. Ménière, "Ménière's Original Papers," 14–15, quoted in Baloh, *Vertigo*, 13. See also Rubin, "Natural History."
47. Baloh, 13–14.
48. Bucknill, "Dean Swift's Disease."
49. Bucknill, 816.
50. Bucknill, 807–8, 809.
51. Bucknill, 807.
52. "Dean Swift's Deafness," 233.
53. There are rare exceptions. In 1908, for example, the American ophthalmologist George Gould challenged Bucknill's diagnosis, claiming that Swift's symptoms all indicated chronic migraines. "Bucknill's worthless article," sneered Gould, "is a good example of the easy slipshod acceptance of a diagnosis by the modern 'scientist,' who without any labor in gathering facts or ability to digest them, slides over all difficulties with that skill which gives the false satisfaction to the author and to the careless reader the erroneous impression of knowledge and observation." "Case of Jonathan Swift," 953n. In 1952, Philip Marshall Dale argued that Swift's giddiness and hearing disorders were symptoms of allergies rather than Ménière's disease. *Medical Biographies*, cited by Lorch, 3133. Few others have disagreed with Bucknill, even when they have refined his diagnosis some. In 1939, for example, the Irish surgeon T. G. Wilson elaborated upon Bucknill's conclusion by claiming that "the exciting cause" of Swift's Ménière's disease "was probably Eustachian obstruction caused by a badly deviated septum." "Swift's Deafness and His Last Illness." The deviated septum was apparent from a cast of his skull, unearthed in the 1830s when the crypt of St. Patrick's flooded.
54. James, *Asperger's Syndrome and High Achievement*, 45–52. For this lead, I am indebted to John Stubbs's fine recent biography: *Jonathan Swift: The Reluctant Rebel*, 656n71.
55. Bartley, "Blindness of John Milton," 399.
56. Mitchell, "Retrospective Diagnosis," 87.
57. Some clinicians speak of a tetrad of symptoms, to include aural fullness, comparable to Swift's own "stufft" ears.
58. 31 October 1710, in *JS*, 53–54.
59. Swift to William Richardson, 30 April 1737, in *Correspondence*, 4:427–28. In a comic poem to his friend Delany, Swift claims that his "Left Ear was deaf a Fortnight." "The Answer," line 42, in *Poems*, 2:367.
60. Swift to Knightley Chetwode, 11 November 1721, in *Correspondence*, 2:403.
61. Swift to John Barber, 31 March 1738, in *Correspondence*, 4:510.

NOTES TO PAGES 30-34   193

62. Kirby and Yardley, "Cognitions."
63. Swift to Knightley Chetwode, 27 May 1725, in *Correspondence*, 2:554.
64. Swift to Knightley Chetwode, 23 November 1727, in *Correspondence*, 3:139.
65. In her discussion of Swift's disorders, Wanda Creaser gives an especially good description of the Ménière's patient's physical and psychological experiences. "'Most Mortifying Malady.'" See also her unpublished dissertation, "Shifting Identities in the Life and Writings of Jonathan Swift," passim.
66. Karenberg, "Retrospective Diagnosis," 142.
67. Among those who engage the debate over retrospective diagnosis, see not only Karenberg, above, but also Cunningham, "Identifying Disease in the Past"; Arrizabalaga, "Problematizing Retrospective Diagnosis"; Muramoto, "Retrospective Diagnosis"; Foxhall, "Making Modern Migraine Medieval"; Green, "Value of Historical Perspective"; and Larner, "Retrospective Diagnosis." For a survey of retrospective diagnoses of Swift's psychological disorders specifically, see Lorch.
68. Some clinicians debate whether the disorder is rightly a "disease," a complex of symptoms with a common pathophysiology, or a "syndrome," a group of symptoms that occur together but have different causes. See Henry Williams, "Definition of Terms in Meniere's Disease."
69. Portmann, "Old and New in Meniere's Disease."
70. Because episodes strike irregularly and inexplicably, classifying the Ménière's sufferer as "disabled" or "impaired" is problematic. In America, the legal burden of proving functional disability under ADA standards rests with the patient. See Cohen, Ewell, and Jenkins, "Disability in Ménière's Disease."
71. Portmann, 567.
72. Stubbs, 391.

3. AS SWIFT WOULD HAVE IT

1. 28 March 1712, in *JS*, 418. In her Cambridge edition of the *Journal to Stella*, a remarkable editorial achievement, Abigail Williams reminds us that the letters that Swift sent back to Dublin in packets during his time in London between 1710 and 1713 were addressed not only to Esther Johnson but also to Rebecca Dingley. That this is the journal to *Stella* is the misdirection of its first editors, who accepted stories, however apocryphal, that Swift had married Johnson. Swift did not use the name Stella itself in his letters; he first used that for Johnson in 1719, years after the correspondence from which the "journal" takes its title. *JS*, xxxvi–xxxix.
2. 31 March–8 April 1712, in *JS*, 420; 30 March 1712, in *JS*, 419.

3. 31 March–8 April 1712, in *JS*, 420.
4. 31 March–8 April 1712, in *JS*, 420.
5. 17 July 1712, in *JS*, 437.
6. Couser, *Recovering Bodies*, 14.
7. Couser, 14.
8. Moyle, *Experienced Chirurgeon*, 4.
9. Swift to Dean Mossom, 14 February 1720–21, in *Correspondence*, 2:365.
10. Swift to Knightley Chetwode, 22 September 1724, in *Correspondence*, 2:522.
11. Swift to Charles Ford, 27 November 1724, in *Correspondence*, 2:531.
12. Swift to Edward Harley, Second Earl of Oxford, 16 February 1733–34, in *Correspondence*, 3:722.
13. Swift to the Rev. Thomas Sheridan, 12 August 1727, in *Correspondence*, 3:115.
14. *Verses on the Death*, lines 83–84, in *Poems*, 2:556.
15. Couser, 5.
16. "Family of Swift," in *PW*, 5:193.
17. Orrery, *Remarks on the Life and Writings*, 81.
18. Swift to Mrs. Howard, 19 August 1727, in *Correspondence*, 3:120. A pippin is a tart, full-sized apple. By this claim, Swift's appetite would have been prodigious. In an ironic historical turn, some modern clinicians claim that pectin, found in apples, reduces the endolymphatic hydrops of Ménière's disease. See, for example, Takeda et al., "Decompression Effects of Erythritol."
19. Swift to Mrs. Pendarves, 29 January 1735–36, in *Correspondence*, 4:256–57.
20. Swift to William Richardson, 30 April 1737, in *Correspondence*, 4:427.
21. 9 October 1712, in *JS*, 451.
22. Case, "Swift and Sir William Temple."
23. Case's argument would also solve the apparent discrepancy of locations. Swift's letter to Mrs. Howard states that he contracted his giddiness at Richmond—that is, the estate at Sheen that Temple had left before Swift came to him in Moor Park. Because, as Swift tells us in the autobiographical fragment, Temple's "Father had been a great Friend to the Family," it seems likely that Swift would have visited Sheen when he was younger and could then have gluttonized upon the pippins ("Family of Swift," in *PW*, 5:193). The language in the fragment is ambiguous, however, and it is difficult to say whether Swift means that he contracted his giddiness at Moor Park or was already suffering from it by the time that Temple employed him there.

24. 24 February 1713, in *JS*, 502.
25. *Family Physician*, 91.
26. Physician, *Treatise of Diseases*, 17. Although the author's "treatise" is a glorified advertisement for various proprietary medicines, including a "vertiginous spirit" of his own invention, his explanation of giddiness comes straight from humoralism. Because of the resiliency and pliancy of humoral explanations of pathogenesis, the same basic principle of humoral imbalance was adopted by nerve theories, which became ascendant in the mid-eighteenth century. In 1771, in a lecture on the "chronical Diseases of the Head," the physician Theophilus Lobb attributed vertigo to "too great a flux of nervous fluid, through the optic nerves, to the *tunica retina* of the eye; which humour perhaps has a kind of *circumgyration*, or motion, which may be the reason that external objects seem to the patient" "to be in a sort of circular motion, turning round." "Here it appears to me," says Lobb, "that the optic nerves are *too lax*, and the *influx of nervous fluid* too great." *Practice of Physick in General*, 2:162.
27. Physician, 18–19.
28. Delany, *Observations*, 102.
29. The quoted words are those of Swift's editor George Faulkner, who had his information about the postmortem examination from Lyon. "Life of the Reverend Jonathan Swift," n260. John Whiteway, the surgeon who performed the autopsy, was the son of Swift's cousin Martha Whiteway. In his final will, Swift bequeathed to John a hundred pounds, with an additional five pounds for purchasing "Physical or Chirurgical Books." *Correspondence*, 4:299n2.
30. Arikha, *Passions and Tempers*, 299.
31. By the doctrine of "contraries," popular and learned medical opinion alike recommended fruit for "hot," "dry" diseases like fevers and inflammations. In *An Essay upon Health and Long Life*, which Swift himself edited for publication, Sir William Temple advised eating fruit before and after meals for "all Illnesses of Stomach, or Indigestion, proceeding from hot and sharp Humours": "I have never found any thing of much or certain Effect, besides the eating of *Strawberries*, common *Cherries*, white *Figs*, soft *Peaches*, or *Grapes*, before every Meal during their Seasons; and when those are past, *Apples* after Meals." *Essay upon Health and Long Life*, 187.
32. Muffett, *Healths Improvement*, 197.
33. Lémery, *Treatise of Food*, 19.
34. 1 September 1711, in *JS*, 271.
35. Chomel, *Dictionaire Oeconomique*, vol. 1, s.v. "Deafness."

36. Verwaal, "Fluid Deafness," 367.
37. Shaw, *New Practice of Physick*, 1:77.
38. Papin, "Some Observations on the Mechanic Arts," 45.
39. Shaw, *New Practice of Physick*, 1:77.
40. Southwell, *Medical Essays and Observations*, 3:100.
41. Marryat, *New Practice of Physick*, 232. Swift's friend Matthew Prior attributed his own bouts of deafness to such deposits. He wrote to Swift, "I labour under the distemper you complain of, Deafness: especially upon the least Cold . . . but am now syrringing, and I hope to profit by it." 4 May 1720, in *Correspondence*, 2:332.
42. Verwaal, 372.
43. Quoted in Cockayne, "Experiences of the Deaf," 497. There were those who argued for the *efficacy* of cold in cases of deafness. The proponent of cold bathing Sir John Floyer claimed that "Cold Immersion" is "useful in all the Infirmities of the Head and Eyes: And I might add, That Deafness has been lately cured by the same, in the Cold Bath at *London*." *Ancient Psychrolousia Revived*, 81–82. See also Browne, *Account of the Wonderful Cures*, 11.
44. Wilson, *Treatise on Electricity*, 202–8. While Mary Smargins "continue[d] to hear very well" some two years later, Wilson confessed that his electrical experiments upon "six other persons, whose complaints were deafness," were unsuccessful, even though "three of them fancied themselves better for a few days" (207–8).
45. Arbuthnot, *John Bull*, 44.
46. In light of Thomas Beddoes's conjectures about Swift's chronic ailments, it is worth noting here that Samuel Tissot, in his notorious, widely read *Onanism: or, A Treatise upon the Disorders Produced by Masturbation; or, The Dangerous Effects of Secret and Excessive Venery*, cites the case of a man who, "deaf for several weeks, after a long cold," "when he had a nocturnal pollution, was much more deaf the next day" (62).
47. Swift to Lord Orrery, 9 March 1735–36, in *Correspondence*, 4:271.
48. Swift to Charles Ford, 20 November 1733, in *Correspondence*, 3:707.
49. "The Answer" [to Delany's complaint, "Sent by Dr. *Delany* to Dr. *S—t*, in Order to Be Admitted to Speak to Him"], lines 34, 38, 42–43, in *Poems*, 2:367.
50. Bickerton, *Accurate Disquisitions in Physick*, 34.
51. *OED*, s.v. "animal spirit." While the third-century BCE Alexandrian physicians who theorized the animal spirits saw them as superfine, invisible particles (*pneuma psychikon*), in the Cartesian iatromechanical model that

gained ascendancy after the middle of the seventeenth century, they were fluid, subject to laws of hydraulics, and expressible in quantifiable, mathematical terms. The iatromechanical model of sensation's being transmitted though hollow tubes by these spirits conformed with humoral logic: A healthy or impeded flow of fluid spirits through the nerves depended still upon the proper balance of the humoral matrix. Not long after Swift's death in 1745, the iatromechanical narrative of sensation was challenged by a new neurophysiology that saw the nerves as wires. In this model, the repurposed animal spirits communicated between the senses and the brain no longer by fluid conveyance but by electrical impulse. Porter, *Mind-Forg'd Manacles*, 45ff., 176–78.

52. Cockburn, *Sea Diseases*, 84–85.
53. Orrery, 276.
54. Cockburn, *Sea Diseases*, 85. In a sardonic comment upon the metrics of Dr. Joseph Brown's early eighteenth-century translation of Horace, a "Gentleman in Town" commented, "I am afraid the Reader will be apt to think the good Dr. has got a great Cold lately, which may have caus'd an unhappy obstruction in his Auditory Nerves; for no Mortal breathing, except he's as Deaf as a Door-Nail, can ever find Musick in this Verse." *Letter from a Gentleman*, 52.
55. Bickerton, 4.
56. Jonston, *Idea of Practical Physick*, 54–55.
57. Swift to Knightley Chetwode, 30 January 1721-22, in *Correspondence*, 2:411.
58. Swift to Lord Orrery, 26–31 March 1737, in *Correspondence*, 4:409.
59. John Allen is here citing the medical wisdom of the German physician Michael Ettmüller. *Synopsis Medicinæ*, 2:115.
60. Shaw, *New Practice of Physick*, 1:23–24.
61. Arbuthnot, *Essay Concerning the Nature of Aliments*, 364. There is historical irony here: Most modern biographers and medical writers agree that Swift likely suffered a stroke or a series of minor brain lesions in his last years; these events, they say, would explain his final aphasia and lethargy.
62. Swift to the Rev. Thomas Sheridan, 12 August 1727, in *Correspondence*, 3:115.
63. Swift to Knightley Chetwode, 11 November 1721, in *Correspondence*, 2:403.
64. Swift to Alexander Pope, 2 December 1736, in *Correspondence*, 4:365.
65. The Earl of Orrery to Deane Swift, 4 December 1742, in *Correspondence*, 4:664–65.

66. Deane Swift to the Earl of Orrery, 4 April 1744, in *Correspondence*, 4:669–70.
67. *OED*, s.v. "wits." Here the word *wits* has particular bearing on Cassinus's horrified response to his mistress Cælia's "Crime": "These Eyes, these Eyes beheld the fact. / . . . / Nor wonder how I lost my Wits; / Oh! *Cælia, Cælia, Cælia* sh—." Beholding the foul business of her humoral body has irrevocably disordered his wits; he has gone mad. "Cassinus and Peter. A Tragical Elegy," lines 68, 98, 117–18, in *Poems*, 2:595–97.
68. Miss Esther Vanhomrigh to Swift, [November/December] 1720, in *Correspondence*, 2:352.
69. Swift to Knightley Chetwode, 27 May 1725, in *Correspondence*, 2:554.
70. Swift to Charles Ford, 14 August 1725, in *Correspondence*, 2:585. *Tetter* is a "general term for any pustular herpetiform eruption of the skin, as eczema, herpes, impetigo, ringworm, etc." *OED*, s.v. "tetter."
71. Swift to Mrs. Howard, 19 August 1727, in *Correspondence*, 3:121.
72. The *OED* states that since the 1530s, the uses of the term *senses* to designate, variously, (1) the five physical senses, (2) reason or sanity, and (3) the combined faculties of perception and sensation have been "sometimes not easily distinguishable." *OED*, s.v. "sense."
73. Porter, *Flesh in the Age of Reason*, 67.
74. Berkeley, *Alciphron*, 1:134.
75. For the history of early modern theories of madness, I draw liberally from Porter's *Mind-Forg'd Manacles*, passim.
76. Blankaart, *Physical Dictionary*, 280. For this lead, I am indebted to the unpublished dissertation of Darren Neil Wagner. As Wagner says, "The sensorium was both an anatomical nexus for nerves and a metaphysical margin where reason and will became impressed onto the corporeal body." "Sex, Spirits, and Sensibility," 154. The processes by which the animal spirits carried sense data to the brain and the brain sent commands to the body were subject to much debate and speculation but never exactly understood.
77. Locke, *Essay Concerning Humane Understanding*, 85–86.
78. In *Mind-Forg'd Manacles*, Porter explains at length the importance of the imagination in definitions of *madness* in the long eighteenth century.
79. *Tale*, 110.
80. The term "nervous humour" is that of Thomas Willis, among the earliest to map out brain functions. He wrote that in obstructions "of the Nerves and nervous fibres," the "nervous humour" is "hindred in [its] courses, and compell'd to proceed slowly and to stagnate." *Pharmaceutice Rationalis*, 84.

81. Swift to John Barber, 30 March 1737, in *Correspondence*, 4:414.
82. Swift to Alexander Pope and Viscount Bolingbroke, 8[-24] August 1738, in *Correspondence*, 4:534-35.
83. Young, *Conjectures on Original Composition*, 64-65.
84. Harvey, *Third Edition*, 36.
85. Cheyne, *Philosophical Principles of Natural Religion*, 225; Cheyne, *New Theory of Continu'd Fevers*, 81.
86. Cheyne, *English Malady*, 78-79, 85.
87. Cheyne, *English Malady*, 241.
88. Porter, *Mind-Forg'd Manacles*, 177. In Swift's day the word *depression* did not denote the clinical psychiatric condition of our own day. But even before his birth, it designated a "condition of being depressed in spirits; dejection." OED, s.v. "depression."
89. Swift to Charles Ford, 4 April 1720, in *Correspondence*, 2:326; Swift to John Gay and the Duchess of Queensberry, 13 March 1730-31, in *Correspondence*, 3:368.
90. "Family of Swift," in *PW*, 5:193.
91. "Irel^d.," line 1, in *Poems*, 2:421.
92. See, for example, Flynn, *Body in Swift and Defoe*, 97-100.
93. 27 August 1711, in *JS*, 268.
94. Fabricant, *Swift's Landscape*, 64.
95. "Family of Swift," in *PW*, 5:190.
96. "Family of Swift," in *PW*, 5:187.
97. "Family of Swift," in *PW*, 5:188.
98. Yet another orchard thief was Augustine, who robbed a pear tree with his boyhood friends. Because "this fruit was not enticing, either in appearance or in flavor," he concluded that the theft was proof of his sinful nature: "I simply wanted to enjoy the theft for its own sake, and the sin.... [I] derived pleasure from the deed simply because it was forbidden." *Confessions*, 41. Olivia Weisser explains that sick persons in early modern Britain who blamed fruit for their illnesses often invoked Augustine's orchard theft as narrative trope to make sense of their own sufferings. *Ill Composed*, 46-47, 213.
99. Deane Swift, *An Essay*, 28.
100. Swift to Charles Ford, 20 November 1733, in *Correspondence*, 3:707.
101. Swift to Alexander Pope, 22 April 1736, in *Correspondence*, 4:283.

4. HELP FOR THE HUMORAL BODY

1. Porter and Rousseau quip that "*Chronicity* was the flip side of *crisis.*" *Gout,* 238.
2. Cheyne, *Essay of Health,* 173, 174. The conditional word "timeously" is a sort of disclaimer for the advising physician. Cheyne, like most doctors of the day, was careful to qualify any promises of recovery. Too often, he said, "the Failing is in the *Patient* himself, who will not, or cannot, *deny himself* for a Time sufficient to bring about the *Cure*" (174).
3. Swift to the Rev. Thomas Sheridan, 2 September 1727, in *Correspondence,* 3:124.
4. Swift to Alexander Pope, 11 August 1729, in *Correspondence,* 3:245.
5. Swift to John Gay, 26 February 1727-28, in *Correspondence,* 3:162; Swift to John Gay, 28 March 1728, in *Correspondence,* 3:169.
6. In *Swift, Pope and the Doctors* (169–201), Allan Ingram devotes a thoughtful chapter to discussing how Swift's and Pope's chronic illnesses evoked meditations on death.
7. Swift to William Pulteney, 8 March 1736-37, in *Correspondence,* 4:393; Swift to the Rev. Thomas Sheridan, 12 August 1727, in *Correspondence,* 3:115.
8. Swift to the Rev. Thomas Sheridan, 29 August 1727, in *Correspondence,* 3:122.
9. Swift to Charles Ford, 20 November 1733, in *Correspondence,* 3:707.
10. Beier, *Sufferers and Healers,* 4–5.
11. Jewson argues that, among doctors courting the patronage of well-to-do patients, both diagnosis and therapy were often collaborative. His thesis about social and economic power relations is that the doctor's reputation, social status, and income rested upon his willingness to bend to the expectations and therapeutic preferences of his patients. Jewson's argument fails to consider the greater social range of patients treated by a greater social range of practitioners. Nevertheless, his claim that the "bedside" model of medicine, which prevailed before hospital medicine became ascendant toward the end of the eighteenth century, privileged the patient's own understanding of the body and his or her narrative about that body helps us to understand that medicine of Swift's day was "patient-centered." "Medical Knowledge." See also Jewson, "Disappearance of the Sick-Man." For a brief but useful assessment of Jewson's important contributions to medical history, see Gillam, "Reappearance of the Sick Man."
12. Among Porter's many contributions to the discussion of medical literacy and medical consumerism, see *Health for Sale: Quackery in England,*

1660–1850; "The Patient's View: Doing Medical History from Below"; "Lay Medical Knowledge in the Eighteenth Century: The Evidence of the *Gentleman's Magazine*"; *Patient's Progress: Doctors and Doctoring in Eighteenth-Century England,* coauthored with Dorothy Porter; and his edited volumes, *Patients and Practitioners: Lay Perceptions of Medicine in Pre-Industrial Society* and *The Popularization of Medicine, 1650–1850.* For the consumption of vernacular medical works, see Fissell, "Marketplace of Print" and "Popular Medical Books."

13. Porter, "Lay Medical Knowledge."
14. Porter and Porter, *Patient's Progress,* 198.
15. *Catalogue of Books* [Swift].
16. While Gibson's best-selling *The Anatomy of Humane Bodies Epitomized* (first published in London, 1682) describes the entire body, Glisson's *Anatomia Hepatis* describes only the liver. (The latter work was published in London in 1654, although the sale catalogue of Swift's library lists an Amsterdam edition printed in 1650.)
17. In 1733, Swift wrote to Charles Ford of Fuller's *Pharmacopoeia,* "Although in the London Dispensatory approved by the Physicians there are Remedyes named both for Giddyness and deafness; none of them that I can find, were prescribed to me. I have the Book, but my books are so confused that I can not find it, nor would I value it if I did." 20 November 1733, in *Correspondence,* 3:707.
18. Swift to Theophilus Harrison, 25 March 1735, in *Correspondence,* 4:75. While Galen does not appear among the titles in the sale catalogue, a 1715 list of books in Swift's own hand includes "Galeni op. Lat. 3 Volines Froben 1549," presumably the three-volume edition he gave to Harrison. Le Fanu, "Catalogue of Dean Swift's Library." For more details on the medical texts that Swift owned, see Marcus Walsh's notes to *A Tale of a Tub* (487n92 and 493n129). Theo Harrison, the beneficiary of Swift's gift, died in February 1735–36, before realizing his ambitions of becoming a physician. However, his younger brother, John Whiteway, became a surgeon; it was he who performed Swift's autopsy. *Correspondence,* 4:76nn1–2.
19. See Passmann and Real, "Annotating J. S. Swift's Reading." In reconstructing Swift's reading at Moor Park, Passmann and Real discuss at length the thirty-seven volumes that Swift listed as having read from January 1696 to January 1697. While we need to be wary of making generalizations from this single year, notably absent are books of medical interest. This absence raises important questions about how Swift—or, for that matter, anyone who was not training for a medical career—"read" medical texts. He may

have read them systematically, from cover to cover. But as seems more likely from his comment to Ford, above, he used medical books primarily for reference, consulting sections of them either for advice about his own health or for literary purposes.

20. Deane Swift, *An Essay*, 271.
21. William Pulteney to Swift, 21 December 1736, in *Correspondence*, 4:372.
22. Swift to William Pulteney, 7 March 1736–37, in *Correspondence*, 4:391. Arbuthnot had died two years earlier, in February of 1734–35.
23. Temple, *Essay upon Health and Long Life*, 136.
24. Temple, 140.
25. Temple, 140.
26. Campbell, *London Tradesman*, 37–38.
27. As the axiom ascribed to Hippocrates held, doctors and sufferers themselves should trust the healing power of nature, *vis medicatrix naturae*.
28. Temple, 172.
29. Apperley, *Observations in Physick*, 142. Herman Boerhaave explained the importance of reading signs to medical diagnosis and treatment: "The third Part of Physic is termed SEMIOTICA, which shews the *Signs* distinguishing between Sickness and Health, Diseases, and their Causes in the human Body; it also imports the State and Degrees of Health and Diseases, and presages their future Events." *Dr. Boerhaave's Academical Lectures*, 1:78. The debate among Queen Anne's physicians during her final days, in late July 1714, gives us an instructive look into the importance of semiotics to medical authority. Attending the deathbed, the celebrated Richard Mead, for example, predicted that Anne would die within minutes, and he was frustrated and apparently professionally embarrassed when she seemed to recover, if only for a brief time. Her physician-in-ordinary Arbuthnot was more guarded in his opinion. Charles Ford, who was at Kensington during Anne's final days, reported to Swift on July 31, "Before I came away [Anne] had recover'd a warmth in her breast & one of her arms, & all the D^{rs} agreed she would in all probability hold out till to morrow, except Mead who pronounc'd several hours before she could not live two minutes, & seems uneasie it did not happen so. I did not care to talk much to A[rbuthnot] because I heard him cautious in his answers to other people, but by his manner I fancy he do's not yet absolutely despair." Ford to Swift, 31 July 1714, in *Correspondence*, 2:39–40. Anne died the next day.
30. 31 March to 8 April 1712, in *JS*, 420.
31. 31 March to 8 April 1712, in *JS*, 420.
32. Apperley, 142.

33. 28 March 1712, in *JS*, 418.
34. Porter and Rousseau, 14.
35. 24 April 1712, in *JS*, 421.
36. Lady Elisabeth Germain to Swift, 7 November 1734, in *Correspondence*, 4:13.
37. [Addison], *The Spectator*, no. 21, 24 March 1711, 1:117. In the same *Spectator* number, Addison cites Temple's claim that "Students in Physick" have caused a drop of population among Northern peoples.
38. "Ode to Dr. William Sancroft, Late Lord Archbishop of Canterbury," lines 253–54, in *Poems*, 1:42. For studies of Swift's satires of medicine, see LaCasce, "Swift on Medical Extremism"; and Child, "Jonathan Swift's Latin Quacks."
39. 10 July 1711, in *JS*, 241.
40. Swift knew well how the health of the nation was tied precariously to the queen's physical health. He wrote to Stella and Dingley in the summer of 1711, "Bank stock is fallen three or four *per cent.* by the whispers about the town of the queen's being ill, who is however very well." 14 July 1711, in *JS*, 243.
41. *GT*, 380.
42. 18 December 1710, in *JS*, 94.
43. 29 September 1710, in *JS*, 21; 31 October 1710, in *JS*, 54. The pills in question are unknown, but Cockburn would have given these to Swift during his first venture to London on behalf of the Irish Church, sometime between November 1707 and June 1709.
44. 26–30 January 1710–11, in *JS*, 130.
45. 21 April 1711, in *JS*, 189.
46. Swift to Charles Ford, 5 April 1733, in *Correspondence*, 3:618. "Deally" is thought to have been Charles Daly, "chirurgus." *Correspondence*, 3:620n2.
47. Swift to Charles Ford, 9 October 1733, in *Correspondence*, 3:692.
48. Swift to the Rev. John Blachford, 17 December 1734, in *Correspondence*, 4:27. Swift often uses the word *fence* in speaking of the measures that he takes against disease. In most cases, the context makes clear the denotation that he is warding off or protecting against disease. But there is also the tantalizing possibility of a dueling metaphor, that Swift as self-imagined aristocrat is parrying and thrusting against an inveterate and wily antagonist.
49. Swift to the Duke of Dorset, 30 December 1735, in *Correspondence*, 4:249.
50. "I have ever hated all Nations professions and Communityes and all my love is towards individualls," he wrote to Pope as he was readying

Gulliver's Travels for publication. "For instance I hate the tribe of Lawyers, but I love Councellor such a one, Judge such a one for so with Physicians (I will not Speak of my own Trade) Soldiers, English, Scotch, French; and the rest but principally I hate and detest that animal called man, although I hartily love John, Peter, Thomas and so forth." Swift to Alexander Pope, 29 September 1725, in *Correspondence*, 2:606–7.

51. Temple, 167–68. Some frail constitutions could not bear such violent interventions. On more than one occasion, Pope wrote that he could never visit Swift in Ireland because of his fears of sea-sickness and vomiting: "Why cannot I cross the Sea? The unhappiest Malady I have to complain of, the unhappiest Accident of my whole Life, is that Weakness of the Breast wh[i]^{ch} makes the Physicians of opinion that a strong Vomit w[oul]^d kill me: I have never taken one, nor had a natural Motion that way, in fifteen Years. I went some years agoe with Lord Peterborow ab[ou]^t 10 leagues at Sea, purely to try if I c[oul]^d sail without Seasickness, and with no other view than to make y^{r}self & Ld Bolingbroke a Visit before I dy'd. But the Experiment, tho almost all the way near the Coast, had almost ended all my Views at once." Alexander Pope to Swift, 17 May 1739, in *Correspondence*, 4:581–82.

52. Temple, 168.

53. Swift to the Rev. Thomas Sheridan, 5 June 1736, in *Correspondence*, 4:312.

54. 31 March–8 April 1712, in *JS*, 420.

55. Swift to Knightley Chetwode, 10 June 1721, in *Correspondence*, 2:382. The Jesuits' or Peruvian Bark "was the bark of various species of the Cinchona tree, from which quinine is procured, formerly ground into powder and taken as a febrifuge," especially in malarial cases. *OED*, s.v. "bark." The bark was dried and pulverized, then typically mixed for ingestion with a liquid, sometimes wine.

56. Cheyne, *Essay of Health*, 74.

57. *GT*, 378–80. Among these purgatives are both "Galenical" and "Chymical" preparations.

58. Swift to Charles Ford, 20 November 1733, in *Correspondence*, 3:707. In their editions of Swift's correspondence, both Harold Williams and David Woolley identify this "London Dispensatory" as Thomas Fuller's *Pharmacopoeia Extemporanea*, the 1708 (4th) edition of which appears in the sale catalogue of his books. It seems as likely that the book in question is the *Pharmacopeia Londinensis*, which bore the subtitle *The London Dispensatory* in editions going back as far as the mid-seventeenth century.

59. 15 September 1712, in *JS*, 444.

60. Swift to the Rev. Thomas Sheridan, 12 August 1727, in *Correspondence*, 3:115.
61. Swift, *Letter to a Young Gentleman*, 22.
62. *Accounts*, 178.
63. *Accounts*, 177, 182.
64. Arbuthnot wrote to Swift on October 14 and, says Harold Williams on the evidence of Arbuthnot's opening line here, Swift evidently responded. If so, his letter does not survive. Williams, 2:303n3.
65. John Arbuthnot to Swift, 11 December 1718, in *Correspondence*, 2:282. Quotations from the same letter follow in the next two paragraphs.
66. While it is uncertain whether Arbuthnot had met Helsham in person, in a letter to Swift of November 5, 1730, he notes, "I recommended Dr Helsham to be physician to the Lord Liewtenant [Lionel Sackville, First Duke of Dorset, who began as Lord Lieutenant of Ireland the following year]. I know not what effect it will have. My respects to him and Dr deLane [Swift's friend and early biographer Patrick Delany]." John Arbuthnot to Swift, in *Correspondence*, 3:331.
67. Browne, *Essay Towards the Forming a True Idea*, 133.
68. Lewis, *Edinburgh New Dispensatory*, 56, 166.
69. Strother, *Family Companion for Health*, 31.
70. Swift to Alexander Pope, 2 May 1730, in *Correspondence*, 3:308.
71. Swift to Edward Harley, Second Earl of Oxford, 28 August 1730, in *Correspondence*, 3:321.
72. John Arbuthnot to Swift, 5 November 1730, in *Correspondence*, 3:330.
73. *Correspondence*, 3:330n16, 3:331n1.
74. Arbuthnot's own collected correspondence is not particularly helpful here either, since his letters do not contain persistent complaints about any one disorder over many years. See *Correspondence of Dr. John Arbuthnot*.
75. Gould, "Case of Jonathan Swift," 952.
76. 10 May 1712, in *JS*, 422.
77. Swift to Charles Ford, 20 November 1733, in *Correspondence*, 3:707.
78. There are purging medicines such as ipecac, designed to rid the stomach of foul excess in preparation for the remedies that follow; "stomachics" such as Roman wormwood and Peruvian bark, used to encourage the appetite and strengthen digestion; and astringents, iron rust and the bitters drink, designed to constrict mucous membranes, thereby reducing the secretions that might otherwise accumulate in the head and toning the fibrous parts of the body. Some medicines, such as the iron rust, which had both astringent and aperient (gentle laxative) virtues, served more than one purpose. See the appendix to this study.

79. Alexander Pope and John Arbuthnot to Swift, 5 December 1732, in *Correspondence*, 3:562.
80. The full title of Goodall's work tells its own story of a beleaguered corporation trying to stake out and maintain a legal monopoly against all manner of economic and professional challenges: *The Royal College of Physicians of London, Founded and Established by Law; as Appears by Letters Patent, Acts of Parliament, Adjudged Cases, &c. and an Historical Account of the College's Proceedings against Empiricks and Unlicensed Practisers in Every Prince's Reign from the First Incorporation to the Murther of the Royal Martyr King Charles the First.*
81. H. Cook, *Decline of the Old Medical Regime*; Pelling, "Medical Practice in Early Modern England"; Pelling and Webster, "Medical Practitioners." These works are classics in an extensive literature that has convincingly challenged the narrative of Royal College hegemony and influence.
82. In her *Memoirs*, Lætitia Pilkington tells a story about having out-doctored the doctors when she cured her gravely ill father, himself a respected obstetrician and president of the College of Physicians of Ireland. The best Dublin medical men—"Dr. *Cope*, Dr. *Helsham*, Mr. *Nicholls*, and in all seven Physicians and three Surgeons (as [her] Father was universally esteemed)"—had attended him without success. Then in their absence, Pilkington administered a remedy of "Hock and Sack mix'd": "When the Physicians came in the Morning, they were agreeably surpriz'd to find my Father's Fever quite gone, and his Eyes look very lively; he told them, their merry Prescription had done him great Service. I wink'd at them not to undeceive him; they understood me, and Doctor *Helsham* call'd me aside, under Pretence of giving me some Directions, but, in Reality, to enquire of me, what I had administer'd. I told him, and he could not forbear smiling. He call'd the Gentlemen into the next Room to a Consultation, to which presently after I was summon'd. As both Doctor *Helsham* and Doctor *Cope* were Men of Wit and Pleasantry, they rallied me agreeably on presuming to practice Physick, having never taken my Degrees, and assur'd me, I should be call'd before the College of Physicians, and be prosecuted as an Empyrick. I rose up, and making a low Courtesy, I told them, as the best Part of the College of Physicians were then present, they would, I hop'd, have Candour enough to permit me to make my own Defence; to which they all assented by a gracious Nod, and bade me proceed; I then, making another Reverence, told them, that as to my Right of practising Physick, I held it *extra judice*, and smiling said, I suppos'd they all understood *Latin*—but as their proper Business was to destroy Life, I hop'd they

would not take it amiss, if I for once, in a Case which so nearly and deeply concern'd me, had, to the utmost of my Power, frustrated their Designs." Pilkington, *Memoirs*, 1:74–75. The story is another opportunity for Pilkington to strut her spunk and wit; it nevertheless exemplifies the contest for medical authority between professional and lay practitioners—and the acute awareness of this contest.

83. 29 December 1710, in *JS*, 102; 31 December 1710, in *JS*, 105.
84. 26–30 January 1710–11, in *JS*, 130. A *bitter* or *bitters* were "bitter medicines generally, as Peruvian bark, quinine, etc.; spec. alcoholic (or other) liquors, impregnated with the extract of gentian, quassia, wormwood, orange peel, etc. and used as stomachics, anthelmintics, etc." *OED*, s.v. "bitters." Bitters were thought to have astringent qualities, which would prevent secretions of mucus. At the same time, some argued, they promoted "insensible Perspiration," the imperceptible excretion of moisture as vapor. "And hence 'tis," wrote Thomas Short, "that some People cannot endure the Use of Bitters, because they occasion such a vast Dissipation of the Fluids thro' the Skin, that they are parched with a most intolerable Thirst." *Discourse*, 74.
85. 4 February 1710–11, in *JS*, 133.
86. 9 February 1710–11, in *JS*, 140.
87. 13 February 1710–11, in *JS*, 142.
88. 7 March 1713, in *JS*, 508.
89. 25 March 1712–13, in *JS*, 517–18.
90. 25 March 1713, in *JS*, 517–18. Hiera picra was commonly prescribed as a purgative electuary. But Nicholas Culpeper explicitly recommends hiera picra for "Vertigo, or Dizziness in the Head." *Pharmacopœia Londinensis*, 183.
91. 18 September 1712, in *JS*, 447. Ginger was used widely as a stomachic, carminative (that is, a medicine that expelled flatulence), and mild laxative.
92. Swift to Charles Ford, 31 December 1724, in *Correspondence*, 2:539.
93. 30 March 1712, in *JS*, 419.
94. Swift to Knightley Chetwode, 13 March 1721–22, in *Correspondence*, 2:415.
95. Wesley, *Primitive Physick*, 50. In her popular *Guide to the Female Sex*, an anonymous "Lady" recommended to those suffering from "Noise in the Head," "Take a Clove of Garlick, peel it, and prick three or four holes in the middle, dip it in Honey, and put it into your ear, stop it with black wooll; and so continue at times for a day or two, and the noise will cease." *Whole Duty of a Woman*, 114.
96. W. Lewis, 121.

97. Quincy, *Pharmacopoia Officinalis and Extemporanea,* 226.
98. For a classic discussion of the divide between "empiricism" and rational "systematism," see L. King, *Medical World of the Eighteenth Century.*

5. DISCIPLINING THE HUMORAL BODY

1. Cheyne, *Essay of Health,* 173.
2. Cheyne, *Essay of Health,* 174.
3. William Pulteney to Swift, 21 December 1736, in *Correspondence,* 4:372.
4. Swift to William Pulteney, 7 March 1736–37, in *Correspondence,* 4:391.
5. The literature of regimen is too extensive to review here. But among the Hippocratic writings, see *On Regimen;* Galen's best-known regimen work is *On Hygiene* (*De Sanitate Tuenda*).
6. A subtitle of one of many sixteenth-century English translations promises that this is a *Boke Teachinge All People to Governe Them in Helthe* (1530).
7. *Catalogue of Books* [Swift], 23, 18.
8. For discussions of the non-naturals in Swift's own day, see, among many others, Wainewright, *Mechanical Account of the Non-Naturals;* Burton, *Treatise of the Non-Naturals;* and Valangin, *Treatise on Diet.* For recent discussions of the term *non-naturals* in Galenic medicine, see Niebyl, "The Non-Naturals"; and Rather, "'Six Things Non-Natural.'"
9. Cheyne, *Essay of Health,* 3.
10. As Andrew Wear observes, early modern preventative medicine, manifest in regimen, was "one of the primary means whereby the principles and ethos of learned medicine were spread to the literate part of the population, thus helping to create a unified medical culture." *Knowledge and Practice,* 154. But the attention to the non-naturals was no less the oft-unspoken guiding principle behind household receipt books and the lore of folk medicine. A broad spectrum of social orders had faith in the regimen that had persisted since classical days.
11. 3 November 1711, in *JS,* 314.
12. The Rev. Thomas Sheridan to Swift, 3 April 1736, in *Correspondence,* 4:280. "Some of your eight Rules I follow," responded Swift, "some I reject, some I cannot compass, I mean merry Fellows." Swift and Mrs. Whiteway to the Rev. Thomas Sheridan, 24 April 1736, in *Correspondence,* 4:285. "Merry fellow" that Sheridan seems to have considered himself, he died two years later, not long after Swift and Whiteway hurtfully sent him away from the deanery, where he had overstayed his welcome.
13. 7 June 1711, in *JS,* 224.
14. Swift to Knightley Chetwode, 20 October 1714, in *Correspondence,* 2:89.

15. Swift to Matthew Prior, 28 April 1719, in *Correspondence*, 2:297.
16. Swift to the Rev. Thomas Sheridan, 29 August 1727, in *Correspondence*, 3:122. The physician in question is likely Arbuthnot.
17. Deane Swift, *An Essay*, 370.
18. 19 January 1710-11, in *JS*, 125. Nicholas Culpeper (1616-54) was the physician, botanist, astrologer, and author of the popular compendium of herbs, *The English Physician* (1652), which stresses the importance of rest in all sorts of disorders and recommends a number of herbal remedies for procuring it. Abigail Williams says that Swift most likely invented this jingle himself (*JS*, 125n11).
19. 20 October 1711, in *JS*, 302.
20. 9 October 1711, in *JS*, 296.
21. Swift to Archdeacon Walls, 18 June 1716, in *Correspondence*, 2:169-70.
22. Swift to Alexander Pope, 7 February 1735-36, in *Correspondence*, 4:259-60.
23. Brookes, *General Practice of Physic*, 1:52. For a thorough discussion of sleep and humoral health, see Handley, *Sleep in Early Modern England*, esp. chapter 1, "Sleep, Medicine and the Body."
24. Sanctorius, *Medicina Statica*, 220. (Swift himself owned the cited edition.) Insensible perspiration is that form in which the water of sweat evaporates before the body senses that the skin is moist; sensible perspiration is that which the body senses as moistness on the skin.
25. Sanctorius, 49.
26. Groeneveld, *Grounds of Physick*, 137.
27. Physician in London, *Two Letters*, 25.
28. 18 September 1712, in *JS*, 445.
29. Swift to Charles Ford, 16 February 1718-19, in *Correspondence*, 2:290.
30. Delany, *Observations*, 99.
31. Swift, "Thoughts on Various Subjects," 275.
32. Swift and Mrs. Whiteway to the Earl of Orrery, 2 February 1737-38, in *Correspondence*, 4:494.
33. Sanctorius, 141.
34. Sanctorius (1561-1636), who numbers among early iatrophysicists attempting to explain all physiological processes mathematically, built a special balance chair so that he could measure his own net weight after intake of food and excretion of waste. An illustration of Sanctorius in his chair appears on the frontispiece of the edition of his work that Swift owned.
35. In the fuller context, Lyttelton wrote, "The immortal Doctor Cheyney... desires his compliments to you, and bids me tell you that he shall live

at least two centuries by being a Real and practical Philosopher, while such Gluttonous Pretenders to Philosophy as You, Dr Swift and My Lord Bolingbroke die of Eating and Drinking at fourscore." George Lyttelton to Alexander Pope, 4 December 1736, in *Correspondence of Alexander Pope*, 4:46. Given Lyttelton's obvious tongue-in-cheek tone, George Sherburn's emphatic remark in notes to the correspondence that this "description is additional evidence of Pope's reputation for overeating!" seems peculiar (4:46n4).

36. Cheyne tells the story in "The Author's Case," the third section of his popular *The English Malady*.
37. 19 October 1711, in JS, 302. Later Swift wrote, "I have a sad vulgar appetite. . . . I cannot endure above one dish; nor could since I was a Boy and loved stuffing." 12 March 1713, in JS, 511. Reading this comment, David Nokes suggests that Swift's "childhood of relative poverty left a taste for simple dishes that all the acquired tastes of the town could not alter." *Jonathan Swift, a Hypocrite Reversed*, 170. Nokes does not acknowledge Swift's more practical dietary concerns here.
38. 26–30 January 1710–11, in JS, 130. While he does not specify, we presume that the advice on diet has come from William Cockburn, whose "drops" he reported taking at the same time.
39. 21 April 1711, in JS, 189.
40. Swift to Alexander Pope, 23–31 March 1733, in *Correspondence*, 3:616.
41. Speaking in the character of his friend Tom Ashe, "the most eternal unwearied punster that perhaps ever lived," Swift quipped that "in our *dieting*, we may be said to *die eating*." "To the Earl of Pembroke. The Dying Speech of Tom Ashe," in *PW*, 4:263, 264.
42. 31 March–8 April 1712, in JS, 420.
43. Swift to Charles Ford, 2 April 1724, in *Correspondence*, 2:493.
44. Cheyne, *Essay of Health*, 225.
45. 15 May 1711, in JS, 208.
46. Robinson, *New Theory of Physick and Diseases*, 205.
47. Swift routinely diluted his wine with water and even composed a "good receipt for sobriety": "Drink little at a time; / Put water with your wine; / Miss your glass when you can; / And go off the first man." 21 April 1711, in JS, 189. While it is a myth that no one drank water in early modern Britain, even in dirty cities, Swift himself rarely drank water by itself. When he and others spoke of "drinking the waters," they were referring to mineral waters from Wexford, Bath, or one of many other spas. Swift's friends—Gay, Ford, Bolingbroke, Arbuthnot, Mary Barber—often enjoined him to drink

various spa waters for his health. Mrs. Barber extolled the virtues of the Bath waters specifically for "disorders ... occasion'd by a cold stomach": "I believe there is not anything in this World so likely to cure that disorder as the Bath Waters which are daily found to be a soverain remedy for disorders of *that kind*[.] I know Sir you have no opinion of Drugs and why will you not try so agreable a medicine prepared by providence alone if you wou'd not try for *your own sake*, why will you not in pity to your Country." Mrs. Barber to Swift, 3 November 1736, in *Correspondence*, 4:359-60. Swift's one experiment in drinking mineral water for giddiness, in early 1712-13, ended badly: "I have drank Spaw Waters this 2 or 3 days; but they do not pass, and make me very giddy: I an't well fais—I'll take them no more." 30 January 1712-13, in *JS*, 490.

48. John Barber to Swift, 27 July 1738, in *Correspondence*, 4:529-30. A "specifick" is a remedy "specially or exclusively efficacious for, or acting upon, a particular ailment or part of the body." *OED*, s.v. "specific."

49. Doläus, *Dolæus*, 147. Pope wrote to Swift, "The D[octo]r puts me into Asses Milk, and I must neither use Study nor Exercise." Viscount Bolingbroke and Pope to Swift, 20 March 1730-31, in *Correspondence*, 3:374. Ass's milk was also recommended by some for preserving one's memory in old age. See, for example, Floyer, *Medicina Gerocomica*, 95.

50. Swieten, *Commentaries*, 1:60.

51. Lord Bathurst to Swift, 19 April 1731, in *Correspondence*, 3:379. Drinking human milk was a fashionable practice of the day. Lady Orrery, whose own newborn rejected her milk, wrote to Martha Whiteway in 1742, "Mr Cleland who attended [the infant] said, as Milk was a Windy Food, the Child must not suck, I have consented, and he is to be brought up by Hand, he feels very well, and will not want my Breast. I may therefore go and suckle her Grace of Marlborough, who lives entirely upon Breast Milk." Lady Orrery to Mrs. Whiteway, 29 December 1742, in *Correspondence*, 4:666. Sarah, Duchess of Marlborough, was then eighty-two and infirm.

52. Swift to Lord Bathurst, 17 July 1731, in *Correspondence*, 3:405, 3:406.

53. Pope to Alexander Pope, 20 April 1731, in *Correspondence*, 3:382, 3:383.

54. Swift to Alexander Pope, 23-31 March 1733, in *Correspondence*, 3:616. As a younger man, Bolingbroke had hardly been abstemious, but in 1728 Pope reported a newfound "great Temperance" after a "return from Bath," where "all peccant humours, he finds, are purg'd out of him." Alexander Pope to Swift, 28 June 1728, in *Correspondence*, 3:186. In a letter to Ford, Swift argued by inversion for the health benefits of wine: "When I was

much younger than You, not above 32 years old, I had by my drinking water, and hating wine, got a swelling in my left Leg." Swift to Charles Ford, 22 June 1736, in *Correspondence*, 4:316. One might be unhealthy by *not* drinking wine or not drinking enough of it: "I fear you are too temperate in drinking, and not strict enough in avoyding to eat what is improper in your Disorder," Swift wrote to Lord Orrery (11 June 1737, in *Correspondence*, 4:436).

55. Swift to John Arbuthnot, ca. 12–15 November 1734, in *Correspondence*, 4:15.
56. Swift to Alexander Pope, 1 May 1733, in *Correspondence*, 3:638.
57. Swift to John Barber, 21 March 1734–35, in *Correspondence*, 4:62.
58. Swift to John Barber, 3 September 1735, in *Correspondence*, 4:172. Quoting Galen, the Royal Collegian Peter Shaw argued that "sweet Wines are excellent in Diseases arising from a cold Cause, because they heat, tho' in a mild and gentle Manner." *Juice of the Grape*, 15n.
59. Swift to Charles Wogan, 1735–36, in *Correspondence*, 4:273.
60. Swift to the Rev. John Towers, ca. August 1735, in *Correspondence*, 4:155.
61. Temple, *Essay upon Health and Long Life*, 199.
62. 30 July 1711, in *JS*, 251. Friends testified to Swift's moderation in drinking. Lætitia Pilkington recalled, for example, that when Swift drank, "strict Temperance [was] preserved, for the Doctor never drank above half a Pint of Wine, in every Glass of which, he mix'd Water and Sugar" (*Memoirs* 1:23).
63. Swift to Alexander Pope, 1 June 1728, in *Correspondence*, 3:185. Pope himself wrote that "Between Excess and Famine lies a mean, / Plain, but not sordid, tho' not splendid, clean." "The Second Satire of the Second Book of Horace Paraphrased," lines 47–48, in *Poetry and Prose of Alexander Pope*, 220.
64. Swift to Charles Ford, 9 December 1732, in *Correspondence*, 3:566.
65. Swift to Charles Ford, 22 June 1736, in *Correspondence*, 4:316.
66. 1 September 1711, in *JS*, 271.
67. Swift to the Rev. Thomas Sheridan, 12 August 1727, in *Correspondence*, 3:115.
68. 6 July 1711, in *JS*, 239.
69. 15 September 1712, in *JS*, 444.
70. Swift to the Rev. Thomas Sheridan, 1 July 1727, in *Correspondence*, 3:103.
71. Flynn sees Swift's vows to avoid fruit as emblematic of his attempts to contain disordering desire. Fruit is surrogate for sexual desire. Desire is embodied in "an appetite both physical and sexual." And only by denying his appetite can Swift contain the disordering materiality of the body.

Flynn says that in attributing his giddiness to forbidden fruit, Swift "links his 'bad' head to his 'bad' desires." *Body in Swift and Defoe*, 97. Leo Damrosch responds that "what really horrified Swift about the body was not physicality in itself, but decay." *Jonathan Swift*, 368.

72. Deane Swift, 100.
73. Deane Swift, 271–72.
74. Pilkington, 1:35. To "troll" is to "move or walk about or to and fro; to ramble, saunter, stroll." *OED*, s.v. "troll."
75. 21 February 1710–11, in *JS*, 148. Throughout his life, Swift spoke of losing weight by exercising vigorously. In later years, he complained of having "not an ounce of flesh between the skin and bone; yet I often walk four or five miles, and ride ten or a dozen." Swift to Alexander Pope, 7 February 1735–36, in *Correspondence*, 4:259–60.
76. 1 May 1711, in *JS*, 199.
77. 10 November 1711, in *JS*, 321.
78. Swift to Archbishop King, 28 September 1721, in *Correspondence*, 2:399.
79. Swift to John Barber, 8 August 1738, in *Correspondence*, 4:533.
80. Pilkington, 1:36.
81. Swift to Alexander Pope, 2 December 1736, in *Correspondence*, 4:365.
82. 31 May 1712, in *JS*, 428.
83. Sanctorius, 76.
84. Sydenham, *Dr. Sydenham's Compleat Method*, 134.
85. Blankaart, *Physical Dictionary*, 132.
86. Fuller, *Medicina Gymnastica*, [xiii].
87. Swift to Charles Ford, 16 February 1718–19, in *Correspondence*, 2:290. Not long after this letter, Swift's friend Prior wrote to him, "I hope there is a little Spleen mixt with yor Distemper [giddiness], in wch case y^{or} Horse may be your Physician, and your Physician [Helsham] may have the happiness of being your Companion (an honor wch Many here would envy him)." Matthew Prior to Swift, 5 May 1719, in *Correspondence*, 2:303.
88. *PW*, 1:xxxvii.
89. 23 May 1711, in *JS*, 212; 3 November 1711, in *JS*, 315. "Pattens" are thick-soled shoes, suitable for walking. In the "little language"—"ourrichar Gangridge"—that Swift slips in and out of in his letters to Stella and Dingley, "Ppt." likely means "poppet," one of his pet names for Stella. 11 March 1712, in *JS*, 406. A poppet, says the *OED*, is a "small or dainty person. In later use frequently as a term of endearment, esp. for a child or young woman: darling, pet." *OED*, s.v. "poppet."
90. Swift to Miss Anne Long, 18 December 1711, in *Correspondence*, 1:401.

91. Swift to Archbishop King, 29 March 1712, *Correspondence*, 1:421.
92. Swift to Edward Harley, Second Earl of Oxford, 28 August 1730, in *Correspondence*, 3:322.
93. Lady Elisabeth Germain to Swift, 7 September 1731, in *Correspondence*, 3:432.
94. John Gay and the Duchess of Queensberry to Swift, 8 November 1730, in *Correspondence*, 3:333.
95. Temple, 199.
96. The Rev. Thomas Sheridan to Swift, 3 April 1736, in *Correspondence*, 4:280.
97. Charles Ford to Swift, 14 April 1733, in *Correspondence*, 3:625.
98. Delany, 100–101. Among the several Grattan brothers who were friends of Swift, James (1673–1747) was one of his Dublin physicians.
99. Cockburn, *Nature and Cure of Fluxes*, 142.
100. Robinson, 65.
101. Swift to Alexander Pope, 20 April 1731, in *Correspondence*, 3:382.
102. Delany, 100–101.
103. Swift to Robert Cope, 1 June 1723, in *Correspondence*, 2:459.
104. Swift to Knightley Chetwode, 24 June 1730, in *Correspondence*, 3:314.
105. Mrs. Whiteway to the Earl of Orrery, 22 November 1742, in *Correspondence*, 4:663.
106. *GT*, 378.
107. Swift to John Barber, 3 September 1735, in *Correspondence*, 4:172.

6. THE DISORDERED SOCIAL BODY AND HUMORAL IDENTITY

1. Swift to the Rev. John Blachford, 17 December 1734, in *Correspondence*, 4:26–27.
2. Swift to the Rev. Thomas Sheridan, 2 September 1727, in *Correspondence*, 3:123.
3. Swift to Knightley Chetwode, October 1724, in *Correspondence*, 2:524; Swift to Mrs. Howard, 19 August 1727, in *Correspondence*, 3:121.
4. *Accounts*, 63.
5. Swift to Alexander Pope, 20 April 1731, in *Correspondence*, 3:382.
6. Swift to Knightley Chetwode, 17 May 1729, in *Correspondence*, 3:235.
7. Swift to the Rev. Thomas Sheridan, 15 and 16 June 1735, in *Correspondence*, 4:122.
8. Swift to Edward Harley, Second Earl of Oxford, 27 November 1724, in *Correspondence*, 2:529.

9. *"Doctor Swift,"* said Lætitia Pilkington, "very well observes, that many Persons have done a *just*, many a *generous*, but few a *grateful* Act" (*Memoirs* 1:265).
10. Swift to Archbishop King, 16 July 1713, in *Correspondence*, 1:517; the Earl of Orrery to Deane Swift, 4 December 1742, in *Correspondence*, 4:665.
11. 30 March 1712, in *JS*, 419.
12. "Family of Swift," in *PW*, 5:193.
13. Swift to Charles Ford, 29 August 1714, in *Correspondence*, 2:76. With the French *anéantissement*—"annihilation" or "devastation"—Swift seems to mean psychological exhaustion.
14. Swift to Knightley Chetwode, 28 June 1715, in *Correspondence*, 2:131.
15. Swift to Knightley Chetwode, 28 June 1715, in *Correspondence*, 2:131.
16. Swift to Knightley Chetwode, 27 September 1714, in *Correspondence*, 2:82–83.
17. Swift to Miss Esther Vanhomrigh, December 1714, in *Correspondence*, 2:102.
18. Swift to Knightley Chetwode, 20 October 1714, in *Correspondence*, 2:89. For his riding injury, see Swift to Archdeacon Walls, 6 May 1716, in *Correspondence*, 2:163. Swift, "In Sickness: Written Soon After the Author's Coming to Live in Ireland, upon the Queen's Death, October 1714," line 5, in *Poems*, 1:203.
19. Swift speaks only obliquely of his own giddiness, writing to Chetwode, "You surprise me with the Acc[oun]t of a Disorder in y^r head; I know what it is too well." 28 June 1715, in *Correspondence*, 2:131. Swift himself did not say much about his illnesses during these years, but his friends nevertheless worried about him. In May 1715, the Duke of Ormonde enquired, "How is your health, how the giddiness of your head? I can see no body that can tell me those minute Circumstances that are so necessary to our quiet." 3 May 1715, in *Correspondence*, 2:121.
20. Swift to Archdeacon Walls, 22 May 1715, in *Correspondence*, 2:127. We know from a number of his letters that Swift spent his early days in Ireland searching for a reliable horse for riding.
21. *Accounts*, 178.
22. Swift to Knightley Chetwode, 25 November 1718, in *Correspondence*, 2:280. The trouble with his eyes, of which Swift occasionally complained, has led some to diagnose his disorders retrospectively as symptoms of migraine. See Gould, "Case of Jonathan Swift." Swift did not like to wear reading spectacles.
23. John Arbuthnot to Swift, 11 December 1718, in *Correspondence*, 2:282. I explicate Arbuthnot's prescription letter in an appendix to this study.
24. Swift to Matthew Prior, January 1719–20, in *Correspondence*, 2:320–21.

25. Swift to William Pulteney, 8 March 1736-37, in *Correspondence*, 4:393.
26. Swift to John Barber, 3 September 1735, in *Correspondence*, 4:172.
27. Swift to John Barber, 17[-28] January 1737-38, in *Correspondence*, 4:490-91.
28. Swift to Charles Ford, 4 April 1720, in *Correspondence*, 2:326-27.
29. Swift to Edward Harley, Second Earl of Oxford, 27 November 1724, in *Correspondence*, 2:529.
30. Swift to Knightley Chetwode, 11 November 1721, in *Correspondence*, 2:403.
31. Swift to Knightley Chetwode, 30 January 1721-22, in *Correspondence*, 2:411.
32. Swift to the Earl of Orrery, 21 November 1738, in *Correspondence*, 4:547.
33. Ehrenpreis, *Swift*, 3:872.
34. Swift to Mrs. Pendarves, 29 January 1735-36, in *Correspondence*, 4:257.
35. Swift to Alexander Pope, 9 February 1736-37, in *Correspondence*, 4:386.
36. Swift to the Rev. Thomas Sheridan, 2 March 1735[-36], in *Correspondence*, 4:269.
37. Swift to Edward Harley, Second Earl of Oxford, 14 August 1725, in *Correspondence*, 2:583. Swift's absence was noticeable enough that the newspapers picked up on it, reporting after his return to Dublin in late September "that he was arrived in that City from his Country Seat."
38. Swift to Charles Ford, 14 August 1725, in *Correspondence*, 2:585.
39. Interestingly, Sheridan owned a copy of *Philocophus, or, The Deafe and Dumbe Mans Friend* (1648), attributed to John Bulwer, physician and early disciple of Francis Bacon. In this fascinating work, the author talks at length about "Lip-Grammar," that is, lip-reading, citing the case of a man "that had an Ear in his Eye." Bulwer, *Philocophus*, [x], 69. Swift himself never spoke of lip-reading, and we cannot know if Sheridan availed himself of Bulwer's work while communicating with his own friend. For Sheridan's ownership of the work, see the sale catalog of his own books, page 18.
40. Swift to Charles Ford, 18 March 1728-29, in *Correspondence*, 3:221.
41. Swift to Mrs. Pendarves, 29 January 1735-36, in *Correspondence*, 4:256.
42. Swift to William Richardson, 9 April 1737, in *Correspondence*, 4:421.
43. Swift to Miss Katharine Richardson, 28 January 1737-38, in *Correspondence*, 4:492, 494n3.
44. Swift to John Barber, 12 July 1735, in *Correspondence*, 4:139.
45. Swift to Alexander Pope, 12 May 1735, in *Correspondence*, 4:104.
46. Turner, *Disability in Eighteenth-Century England*, 111, 123.
47. Swift to Knightley Chetwode, 23 November 1727, in *Correspondence*, 3:139.
48. Swift to Alexander Pope, 13 February 1728-29, in *Correspondence*, 3:209.

49. Swift to Francis Grant, 23 March 1733–34, in *Correspondence*, 3:730; Swift to Alexander Pope, 3 September 1735, in *Correspondence*, 4:175.
50. After Swift slipped into senility in 1742, Deane Swift wrote to Orrery, "His old Friend Mrs Ridgeway still continues in his House, is very faithful to her Trust, and treats the Dean with great Care and Tenderness. His Butler is kept to attend him constantly, and his Butler's Mother [Mrs. Barnard] is his Nurse-keeper. Their Wages are high, and it is their Interest to preserve him. The Dean is always clean and decent, as if twenty People were employed about him." Deane Swift to the Earl of Orrery, 17 December 1743, in *Correspondence*, 4:667.
51. Swift to Alexander Pope, 20 April 1731, in *Correspondence*, 3:382.
52. John Gay and Alexander Pope to Swift, 1 December 1731, in *Correspondence*, 3:448.
53. Swift to Alexander Pope, 23–31 March 1733, in *Correspondence*, 3:616.
54. Swift to John Gay, 4 May 1732, in *Correspondence*, 3:468, 469.
55. Swift to Edward Harley, Second Earl of Oxford, 31 May 1733, in *Correspondence*, 3:650.
56. Cheyne, *Essay of Health*, 106. Cheyne continued, "*House* Exercises are never to be allow'd, but when the *Weather* or some Bodily *Infirmity* will not permit going abroad; for *Air* contributes mightily to the Benefit of *Exercise*" (106–7). We recall here Pilkington's memory of the alarming energy with which Swift bounded up and down the stairs of the deanery on rainy days and Martha Whiteway's sad picture of him in his final years, tramping through the house for ten hours a day.
57. Turner, *Disability in Eighteenth-Century England*, 110. See also Turner, "Disability Humor," 63.
58. Swift to Charles Ford, 8 December 1719, in *Correspondence*, 2:310.
59. Swift to Alexander Pope, 9 February 1736–37, in *Correspondence*, 4:386.
60. Swift, "To Stella, Visiting Me in My Sickness," lines 88–113, in *Poems*, 2:726–27. For Swift's representations of Stella's masculine virtues, see Jaffe, *Poet Swift*, 89–90.
61. Swift to Archbishop King, 20 May 1712, in *Correspondence*, 1:422.
62. Swift, "To Stella ... Written on the Day of Her Birth, But Not on the Subject, When I Was Sick in Bed," lines 10–18, in *Poems*, 2:754.
63. Swift, "To Stella ... Written on the Day of Her Birth, But Not on the Subject, When I Was Sick in Bed," lines 7–8, in *Poems*, 2:754.
64. Swift, "When I Come to Be Old," in *PW*, 1:xxxvii.
65. Swift to Mrs. Pendarves, 22 February 1734–35, in *Correspondence*, 4:58.
66. Swift to Alexander Pope, 7 February 1735–36, in *Correspondence*, 4:259–60.

67. Swift to Alexander Pope, 19 July 1725, in *Correspondence*, 2:576.
68. 10 November 1711, in *JS*, 321.
69. 4 January 1710–11, in *JS*, 112. That Swift should imagine that "MD had been by" as he was undressing is sexually suggestive.
70. Swift to Knightley Chetwode, 10 June 1721, in *Correspondence*, 2:383; Swift to the Rev. Thomas Sheridan, 12 August 1727, in *Correspondence*, 3:115.
71. Swift to Charles Ford, 4 April 1720, in *Correspondence*, 2:328.
72. Stubbs, *Jonathan Swift*, 164.
73. Swift to Knightley Chetwode, October 1724, in *Correspondence*, 2:523, 524.
74. Swift to Benjamin Motte, 28 December 1727, in *Correspondence*, 3:149.
75. Swift to Alexander Pope, 7 February 1735–36, in *Correspondence*, 4:259–60.
76. Swift to Mrs. Whiteway, 26 July 1740, in *Correspondence*, 4:628.
77. Samuel Johnson to Mrs. Thrale, 12 November 1773, in *Letters to and from the Late Samuel Johnson*, 1:144; Johnson to James Boswell, 27 October 1779, in Boswell, *Life of Samuel Johnson, LL.D.*, 2:308. Johnson claimed that he himself had been "mad all [his] life, at least not sober." Quoted in Porter, *Mind-Forg'd Manacles*, 59. In a long letter to Deane Swift, Lord Orrery suggested that Swift's late-life decline was due in part to his bachelorhood: "Men in years ought always to secure a friend to take care of declining life, and watch narrowly as they fall the last minute particles of the hour glass. A batchelor will seldom find, among all his kindred, so true a nurse, so faithful a friend, so disinterested a companion, as one tied to him by the double chain of duty and affection." The Earl of Orrery to Deane Swift, 4 December 1742, in *Correspondence*, 4:665.
78. Johnson, "Swift," 207.
79. Prout, *Reliques of Father Prout*, 127. For a history of what is now St. Patrick's University Hospital, see Malcolm, *Swift's Hospital*.
80. Swift to Lord Carteret, 18 January 1727–28, in *Correspondence*, 3:152.
81. Pilkington, 1:23.
82. B. Hammond, *Jonathan Swift*, 24.
83. Rawson, *Swift's Angers*, 146, 228.
84. Child, "Swift's 'Carefull' Nurse and Sick Relations," 133–35.
85. Damrosch, *Jonathan Swift*, 2.
86. Orrery, *Remarks on the Life and Writings*, 176.
87. Deane Swift, *An Essay*, 359.
88. McMinn, "Swift and the Formation"; Reilly, "Displaced Person," 71.
89. Fox, *Cambridge Companion to Jonathan Swift*, 36.

90. Yunck, "Skeptical Faith of Jonathan Swift," 533.
91. Orwell wrote, "We are right to think of Swift as a rebel and iconoclast, but except in certain secondary matters, such as his insistence that women should receive the same education as men, he cannot be labelled 'Left.' He is a Tory anarchist, despising authority while disbelieving in liberty, and preserving the aristocratic outlook while seeing clearly that the existing aristocracy is degenerate and contemptible." "Politics vs. Literature," 209.
92. Orrery, 138, 256.
93. Reilly, *Jonathan Swift*, vii.
94. McKeon, *Origins of the English Novel 1600–1740*, 61; Deane, "Swift and the Anglo-Irish Intellect."
95. Berkeley, *Three Dialogues Between Hylas and Philonous*, 148–49.
96. Swift to the Rev. Thomas Sheridan, 18 September 1728, in *Correspondence*, 3:194.
97. Swift to Edward Harley, Second Earl of Oxford, 14 June 1737, in *Correspondence*, 4:440.
98. "Written by the Reverend Dr. Swift. On His Own Deafness," line 1, in *Poems*, 2:673; "In Sickness: Written Soon After the Author's Coming to Live in Ireland, upon the Queen's Death, October 1714," line 3, in *Poems*, 1:203.
99. Swift to Alexander Pope, 26 February 1729–30, in *Correspondence*, 3:285.
100. Deane Swift, who first published the fragment in 1755, stated that it had been "writ ... about six or eight and twenty years ago" (7n). Disputing this dating, Irvin Ehrenpreis argues that Swift wrote the piece sometime after 1736 (1:30n). For a thoughtful discussion of the fragment, see E. Hammond, *Jonathan Swift: Irish Blow-In*, 17–23. In her popular biography of Swift, Glendinning gives a very fine reading of the piece.
101. Deane Swift, 7n.
102. "Family of Swift," in *PW*, 5:187.
103. Johnston, *In Search of Swift*, 14.
104. 10 May 1712, in *JS*, 422.

7. SWIFT IN THE SICK ROLE

1. Illich, *Limits to Medicine*.
2. Parsons, *Social System*.
3. Swift to the Duke of Dorset, 30 December 1735, in *Correspondence*, 4:249.
4. Swift, "Dean of St. Patricks Petition to the H. of Lords, against the Lord Blaney," in *PW*, 5:199–200.
5. Lord Howth to Swift, 6 July 1735, in *Correspondence*, 4:135.

6. Charles Ford to Swift, 8 July 1736, in *Correspondence*, 4:329.
7. Mrs. Pendarves to Swift, 24 October 1733, in *Correspondence*, 3:695. There are significant gaps in Swift's correspondence with Pendarves (later wife to his friend and biographer Delany) because some of his letters to her were destroyed before she died (Williams, 4:179n3). We have neither the earlier complaint about which she speaks here nor any other letters to her until October 7, 1734.
8. Swift to Miss Jane Waring, 4 May 1700, in *Correspondence*, 1:140. Swift met Waring, memorialized as "Varina," when he was a prebendary in Kilroot in Northern Ireland, in 1695–96. He returned to Sir William Temple's employ not long after she disappointed his hopes for marriage. David Nokes writes that Swift's Latinizing of Waring's name fit into a pattern of his romantic relations: Varina, Stella, and Vanessa. "The device was a common enough feature of the amatory lyrics of the time," says Nokes, "but in Swift's case his habit of renaming these fatherless girls is a distancing process that both elevates them to mock divinities and reduces them to pets. At all events, it stops him from having to confront them as women." *Jonathan Swift, a Hypocrite Reversed*, 31.
9. 21 October 1710, in *JS*, 44; 5 February 1712–13, in *JS*, 493. Abigail Williams notes that Johnson's chronic "eye problems and headaches may have been the after-effects of facial palsy that she suffered as a child" (*JS*, 44n7).
10. Swift to Alexander Pope, 7 February 1735–36, in *Correspondence*, 4:260.
11. Swift to Charles Ford, 13 February 1723–24, in *Correspondence*, 2:489.
12. Swift to Mrs. Caesar, 30 July 1733, in *Correspondence*, 3:677.
13. Archbishop King to Swift, 29 May 1712, in *Correspondence*, 1:426.
14. The Rev. Marmaduke Phillips to Swift, 2 November 1734, in *Correspondence*, 4:12. In the same sentence, Phillips adds of Swift's illness, "I am in hopes your usual *medicina gymnastica* will carry it off."
15. Edward Harley, Second Earl of Oxford, to Swift, 12 October 1727, in *Correspondence*, 3:133; Charles Ford to Swift, 14 April 1733, in *Correspondence*, 3:625.
16. Miss Katharine Richardson to Swift, 23 February 1737–38, in *Correspondence*, 4:498–99.
17. "The Life and Character of Dean Swift. Upon a Maxim in Rochefoucault," lines 58–61, in *Poems*, 2:546.
18. Womersley, "'now deaf 1740,'" 168.
19. Swift to Archdeacon Walls, 3 July 1714, in *Correspondence*, 1:633. After the collapse of the Tory ministry, Anne's death, and the accession of the Whigs under the new Hanoverian regime in the same year, Oxford and Bolingbroke faced prosecution for alleged Jacobitism. Bolingbroke fled to

France, where he remained until his pardon in 1723; Oxford was imprisoned in the Tower of London for two years until he was acquitted by the House of Lords and released in 1717. In 1721, Matthew Prior, himself in custody between 1715 and 1717, wrote to Swift that Oxford "has been in the Country these two years, very ill in his health, and has not for many Months been out of his Chamber; yet what You observe of him is so true, that his Sickness is all counted for Policy, that He will not come up till the Public distractions force Some body or other (whom God knows) who will oblige some body else to send for Him in open triumph, and sett him in statu quo prius." 25 April 1721, in *Correspondence*, 2:373–74. Several years later, on the prospect of Swift's return to visit his friends in England, Bolingbroke wrote to him, "Remember this solemn Renewal of y^r Engagements, Remember that tho' you are a Dean, you are not great enough to despise the reproach of breaking y^r word. y^r deafness must not be a hackney excuse to you as it was to Oxford. what matter if you are deaf, what matter if you cannot hear what we say? you are not dumb, & we shall hear you, and that's enough." Viscount Bolingbroke to Swift, 17 February 1726–27, in *Correspondence*, 3:74–75.

20. Swift to the Rev. Thomas Wallis, 13 May 1721, in *Correspondence*, 2:379.
21. Swift to Eaton Stannard, 12 December 1733, in *Correspondence*, 3:713. Stannard was by this time Recorder of the City of Dublin; in 1740, he was appointed an executor of Swift's will and in 1742 served on the Dublin Commission of Lunacy that found Swift "unsound" of "mind and memory." *Correspondence*, 3:713n.
22. Swift to Archbishop Hoadly, 1 June 1737, in *Correspondence*, 4:434.
23. Swift to Knightley Chetwode, 23 November 1727, in *Correspondence*, 3:139.
24. In the allegorical *John Bull Still in His Senses* (1712), Arbuthnot's character Nicholas Frog (representing Holland) uses various sicknesses as a "shuffling Excuse" to avoid meeting Bull (England) and Lewis Baboon (France) for talk of an "agreement" (the Treaty of Utrecht, proposed to end the War of the Spanish Succession). One of Frog's excuses, that "he got a great Cold, that had struck him deaf of one Ear," comically memorializes Swift's own illness (43–44).
25. John Arbuthnot to Swift, 17 October 1725, in *Correspondence*, 2:615.
26. Alexander Pope to Swift, 14 September 1725, in *Correspondence*, 2:597–98.
27. Swift to Charles Ford, 27 November 1724, in *Correspondence*, 2:531. Between the time of this letter and Swift's previous one to Ford, in June 1724, no intervening correspondence from Ford survives, so we cannot know what his complaint was or how it was communicated to Swift.
28. Swift to Bishop Evans, 5 June 1721, in *Correspondence*, 2:381.

29. "A Dialogue Between an Eminent Lawyer and Dr. Swift Dean of St. Patrick's, Being an Allusion to the First Satire of the Second Book of Horace," lines 1–2, in *Poems*, 2:489.
30. Swift to Alexander Pope, 26 November 1725, in *Correspondence*, 2:623. Pope responded, "I wish as warmly as you, for the Hospital to lodge the *Despisers of the world* in, only I fear it would be fill'd wholly like Chelsea with Maim'd Soldiers, and such as had been dis-abled in *its* Service. And I wou'd rather have those that out of such generous principles as you and I, despise it, Fly in its face, than Retire from it. Not that I have much Anger against the Great, my Spleen is at the little rogues of it." Alexander Pope and Viscount Bolingbroke to Swift, 14 December 1725, in *Correspondence*, 2:626.
31. Swift, *Verses on the Death*, line 456, in *Poems*, 2:571.
32. Swift to Alexander Pope, 26 February 1729–30, in *Correspondence*, 3:283.
33. Swift to John Barber, 17[–28] January 1737–38, in *Correspondence*, 4:491.
34. Swift to the Rev. Thomas Sheridan, 9 April 1737, in *Correspondence*, 4:419.
35. Viscount Bolingbroke, to Swift, 28 July N.S. 1721, in *Correspondence*, 2:389.
36. Swift to Mrs. Howard, 19 August 1727, in *Correspondence*, 3:121.
37. Harold Williams explains these allusions in notes to this letter (Williams, 3:233n2, 233n3).
38. We recall Swift's condition that he be allowed "to talk nonsense when [he pleased]" if he visited the Duchess of Queensberry in 1731. The Duchess parried, "As for talking nonsence provided you do it on purpose she [that is, herself] has no objection there's some sence in nonsense when it does not come by Chance." The Duchess of Queensberry and John Gay to Swift, 18 July 1731, in *Correspondence*, 3:408.
39. Weisser, *Ill Composed*, 106.
40. 6 March 1713, in *JS*, 508. For a discussion of the Scriblerus Club, as it inspired *Gulliver's Travels*, see chapter 8.
41. Swift to Adrian Drift, 3 February 1721–22, in *Correspondence*, 2:412.
42. Swift to John Barber, 12 July 1735, in *Correspondence*, 4:138–39.
43. "I find that you and I are fellow-sufferers almost equally in our healths, although I am more than twenty years older," Swift wrote to Martha Whiteway late in life. 29 April 1740, in *Correspondence*, 4:615. Theorists such as Tobin Siebers speak of disability communities, which are based on the common identities of disabled persons. *Disability Theory*. In Swift's day, disability was not an identity; it was dysfunction. David Turner points to "the problem of writing disability history before 'disability' existed in its modern sense." *Disability in Eighteenth-Century England*, 11. Chris Mounsey's 2014 volume of essays, *The Idea of Disability in the Eighteenth*

Century, makes important contributions to this discussion of disability during Swift's day.

44. Swift to Charles Ford, 4 April 1720, in *Correspondence*, 2:326; Swift to Charles Ford, 2 April 1724, in *Correspondence*, 2:493. Only years later, as Ford aged and became ill, Swift wrote, "I am uneasy about your health." And again: "[I have] lately been made very uneasy at hearing how little care you take of your Health." Swift to Charles Ford, 14 October 1732, in *Correspondence*, 3:546; 9 December 1732, in *Correspondence*, 3:565. He urged temperance and exercise. Fifteen years his junior, Ford died four years earlier than Swift.
45. Swift, "To Stella ... Written on the Day of Her Birth, But Not on the Subject, When I Was Sick in Bed," lines 9–18, in *Poems*, 2:754.
46. Swift to Alexander Pope, 4 August 1726, in *Correspondence*, 3:5.
47. Alexander Pope to Swift, 28 November 1729, in *Correspondence*, 3:272. Pope was forty-one at the time of this letter, Swift on the eve of his sixty-second birthday.
48. Swift to Alexander Pope, 15 January 1730–31, in *Correspondence*, 3:355–56. "Sir W. Temple said that the loss of Friends was a Tax upon long life," Swift wrote in a later letter to Pope. 22 April 1736, in *Correspondence*, 4:284.
49. Swift to Alexander Pope, 19 July 1725, in *Correspondence*, 2:576.
50. Alexander Pope to Swift, 14 September 1725, in *Correspondence*, 2:597. Pope's mother, who lived into her nineties, was by this time quite ill; his old nurse, Mary Beach, died only two months after this letter.
51. Swift to the Rev. Thomas Sheridan, 12 August 1727, in *Correspondence*, 3:115. Pope wrote to Oxford's son a few days later, "The Dean is so much out of order, & withall so deaf, that he has conversd with no body, & fled all Company. Dr Arbuthnot comes to him to day or to morrow." Alexander Pope to Edward Harley, Second Earl of Oxford, 15 August 1727, in *Correspondence of Alexander Pope*, 2:443.
52. Ehrenpreis, *Swift*, 3:535.
53. Swift to the Rev. Thomas Sheridan, 12 August 1727, in *Correspondence*, 3:115. The complaint that Pope is too *complaisant* suggests that Swift found his deference and willingness to please cloying or unnatural. The context here also suggests Pope's passivity or lethargy.
54. Damrosch, *Jonathan Swift*, 389–90.
55. Swift to the Rev. Thomas Sheridan, 12 August 1727, in *Correspondence*, 3:115.
56. Alexander Pope to the Rev. Thomas Sheridan, 6 September 1727, in *Correspondence of Alexander Pope*, 2:445. In the same letter to Sheridan, Pope

claims that he visits Swift in London "as often as he will let [him]." There is no record of his having done so in fact.

57. Alexander Pope to Swift, 2 October 1727, in *Correspondence*, 3:130.
58. Swift to Alexander Pope, 12 October 1727, in *Correspondence*, 3:131–32.
59. Porter, *English Society in the Eighteenth Century*, 48ff.
60. Swift to Viscount Bolingbroke and Alexander Pope, 5 April 1729, in *Correspondence*, 3:231.
61. Swift to Viscount Bolingbroke, 31 October 1729, in *Correspondence*, 3:261.
62. Swift to Alexander Pope, 9 February 1736–37, in *Correspondence*, 4:386.
63. Williams, "Appendix XXX: Swift's Friends Classed by Their Characters," 5:270–71.
64. Swift to Edward Harley, Second Earl of Oxford, 27 November 1724, in *Correspondence*, 2:529.
65. Swift to Alexander Pope, 9 February 1736–37, in *Correspondence*, 4:386. Scorning Dublin as "the most disagreeable Place in Europe," he wrote to Knightley Chetwode that if he "had a home a hundred miles off [he] never would see this Town again" and that, in comparison with that city, he "suppose[d] a Jayl might be tolerable." 23 November 1727, in *Correspondence*, 3:139.
66. Swift to Edward Harley, Second Earl of Oxford, 3 April 1738, in *Correspondence*, 4:511–12.
67. 7 May 1711, in *JS*, 202.
68. Swift to Lord Orrery, 9 March 1735–36, in *Correspondence*, 4:271.
69. 13 February 1710–11, in *JS*, 142. To "conn" is to study or learn (*OED*, s.v. "conn"). There is also the sense of considering thoroughly, in comparison to something else.
70. 1 February 1710–11, in *JS*, 132.
71. 9 October 1712, in *JS*, 448. At another time, he wrote of a lingering cold that "is not yet off," "Did I tell y: that I believe it is Ldy Masham's hot room that gives it me; I never knew such a Stove; and in my Conscience, I believe, both my L^d [Masham] & she; my Ld Treas^r, Mr Secr^{ty} & my self, have all sufferd by it." 25 February 1711–12, in *JS*, 396. Henry St. John ("Mr Secr^{ty}") had not yet been elevated to his viscountcy as Bolingbroke, but he was the son of Henry St. John, Fourth Baronet. Swift again is the odd man out among the elite here.
72. 7 September 1711, in *JS*, 274.
73. Swift to Edward Harley, Second Earl of Oxford, 27 November 1724, in *Correspondence*, 2:529.

74. 7 September 1711, in *JS*, 274. In book 3 of *Gulliver's Travels*, Swift comically represents Oxford's and his own hearing disorders in the flapper episode, which I discuss in the next chapter.
75. Swift to John Gay and the Duchess of Queensberry, 19 November 1730, in *Correspondence*, 3:339.
76. Swift to Edward Harley, Second Earl of Oxford, 14 August 1725, in *Correspondence*, 2:583.
77. Swift to Alexander Pope, 12 October 1727, in *Correspondence*, 3:132.
78. Swift to Alexander Pope, 8 July 1733, in *Correspondence*, 3:662-63.
79. Swift to John Gay and the Duchess of Queensberry, 19 November 1730, in *Correspondence*, 3:339.
80. Swift to Alexander Pope, 10 May 1728, in *Correspondence*, 3:180. In *Verses on the Death*, Swift wrote that in his Irish "Exile with a steady Heart, / He spent his Life's declining Part: / . . . / His Friendship there to few confin'd, / Were always of the middling Kind: / No Fools of Rank, a mungril Breed, / Who fain would pass for Lords indeed." Lines 431-38, in *Poems*, 2:570.
81. Swift to Alexander Pope, 20 April 1731, in *Correspondence*, 3:383.
82. Swift to Alexander Pope, 20 April 1731, in *Correspondence*, 3:383. In the same passage, he writes, "The old Lord Sunderland was never without one or more of these [compliant folks], Lord Sommers had a humdrum Parson with whom he used to forget himself for three pence at Backgammon, and our friend Addison had a young fellow (now of figure in your Court) whom he made to dangle after him, to go where, and to do whatever he was bid." David Woolley conjectures that the compliant fellow who tagged after Addison was Edward Young (*Correspondence*, 3:386n8).
83. Swift to John Gay and the Duchess of Queensberry, 29 June 1731, in *Correspondence*, 3:402-4.
84. The Duchess of Queensberry and John Gay to Swift, 18 July 1731, in *Correspondence*, 3:408.
85. Swift to Lady Orrery, September 1739, in *Correspondence*, 4:595.
86. 26 October 1710, in *JS*, 49; 24 January 1710-11, in *JS*, 128.
87. 30 November 1710, in *JS*, 76. Anthony Raymond and James (Jemmey) Leigh were Irish friends in London at the same time as Swift. Williams, "Appendix F: Biographical Appendix," in *JS*, 664-65, 642-43. Smyth is unidentified.
88. 12 December 1712, in *JS*, 464. "Tp^t" is a variation of the more-frequent "Pp^t."
89. 17 September 1710, in *JS*, 13.

90. 25 February 1710–11, in *JS*, 150.
91. 9 October 1712, in *JS*, 451.
92. 1 May 1711, in *JS*, 199.
93. 7 March 1710–11, in *JS*, 156, 158. The "lass" Dingley would have been about forty-four at this time, a year older than Swift himself. Palsy water was a scented infusion of spices and flowers like lavender, drunk or applied topically, to relieve nervous disorders (*JS*, 26n21).
94. 23 May 1711, in *JS*, 213.
95. Even in verse homage to Dingley on her birthday, Swift writes that "she, tho' over-run with care, / Continues healthy, fat, and fair." In the lines that follow, he develops an elaborate humoral metaphor, which likens any cares that Dingley may have to gouty humors, driven from her brain to her extremities; she is healthy and bustling but witless:

> Rebecca thus I gladly greet,
> Who drives her cares to hands and feet;
> For, tho' philosophers maintain
> The limbs are guided by the brain,
> Quite contrary Rebecca's led,
> Her hands and feet conduct her head,
> By arbitrary pow'r convey her
> She ne'er considers why, or where:
> Her hands may meddle, feet may wander,
> Her head is but a mere by-stander:
> And all her bustling but supplies
> The part of wholesome exercise.
>   "Bec's Birthday," lines 9–10, 17–28, in *Poems*, 2:761.

96. 12 August 1711, in *JS*, 257. Swift's self-epithet "pdfr" has been taken variously to mean "poor dear fond rogue" and "poor dear fellow."
97. 26 June 1711, in *JS*, 230. For information on the Wexford waters, recommended for their chalybeate qualities, see Kelly, "'Drinking the Waters.'"
98. 24 August 1711, in *JS*, 263.
99. Swift, "The Blunders, Deficiencies, Distresses, and Misfortunes of Quilca," in *PW*, 5:220–21.
100. 1 February 1710–11, in *JS*, 132.
101. While she had not yet ascended to her title when Swift wrote to her, Howard was from the upper ranks, the daughter of Sir Henry Hobart, Fourth Baronet. When her father was killed in a duel, Howard became the ward of the Fifth Earl of Suffolk, Henry Howard. She married his son Charles,

unhappily. Although the two separated, they did not divorce, and when Charles succeeded to his father's earldom in 1731, she became Countess of Suffolk.
102. Alexander Pope to Swift, 14 September 1725, in *Correspondence*, 2:597.
103. Swift to Alexander Pope, 29 September 1725, in *Correspondence*, 2:607.
104. Alexander Pope to Swift, 14 September 1725, in *Correspondence*, 2:597. For a recent biography of Howard, see Borman, *King's Mistress, Queen's Servant*.
105. Despite Swift's hopes, Howard was never able to help him to a preferment in the English Church. Long after her time as George's mistress, Lord Hervey wrote of her, "After twenty years' duration [in 1734], ended the nominal favour and enervate reign of poor Lady Suffolk, who never had power enough to do good to those to whom she wished well, though, by working on the susceptible passions of him whom she often endeavoured to irritate [that is, George], she had just influence enough, by watching her opportunities, to distress those sometimes to whom she wished ill." *Lord Hervey's Memoirs*, 75.
106. Swift to Mrs. Howard, October 1726, in *Correspondence*, 3:42.
107. In 1778, James Boswell wrote, "*We Hypochondriacks* may ... console ourselves in the hour of gloomy distress, by thinking that our sufferings mark our superiority." "On Hypochondria," in Boswell, *Hypochondriack*, 1:135.
108. Swift to Mrs. Howard, 14 August 1727, in *Correspondence*, 3:116.
109. Swift used this expression in sick talk with another correspondent. Worried that his friend Stopford had no one to nurse him in his illness, he wrote, "[Stella and Dingley] tell me you are in an Ague; and what is worse, have no Creature to take Care of you, for God sake have some understanding Body about you." Swift to the Rev. James Stopford, 11 December 1724, in *Correspondence*, 2:534.
110. Swift to Mrs. Howard, 14 August 1727, in *Correspondence*, 3:116–17. George I died in Hanover on June 11, 1727, barely two months before this letter; his son George was crowned in October of that same year. George II's wife Caroline of Ansbach, dubbed "Caroline the Illustrious," was a vivacious, brilliant intellectual. She was well aware of Howard's relationship with her husband but, preferring to keep his mistresses in close view, appointed Howard as one of her own Women of the Bedchamber.
111. Mrs. Howard to Swift, 16 August 1727, in *Correspondence*, 3:117–18.
112. Hervey, 10. Frustrated perhaps because she had been unable to help his final bid for preferment in England, Swift later wrote the ambivalent "Character of Mrs. Howard." *PW*, 5:213–15.

113. Swift to Mrs. Howard, 17 August 1727, in *Correspondence*, 3:118. Arbuthnot had written to Swift a few years earlier that "Lord whitworth our plenipotentiary had this disease [vertigo] (which by the way is a little disqualifying for that imployment) he was so bad, that he was often forc'd to catch hold of any thing to keep him from falling." John Arbuthnot to Swift, 7 November 1723, in *Correspondence*, 2:475.
114. Swift to Mrs. Howard, 17 August 1727, in *Correspondence*, 3:118–19. Woolley states that Swift is not tottering *in fact* but is, rather, likening himself to a precariously balanced man of power (*Correspondence*, 3:119n1). The medical context of Swift's comment, however, conflates the ever-tenuous position of power and the giddiness that staggered him.
115. Swift to Mrs. Howard, 19 August 1727, in *Correspondence*, 3:120.
116. Mrs. Howard to Swift, 18 August 1727, in *Correspondence*, 3:119.
117. Mrs. Howard to Swift, 18 August 1727, in *Correspondence*, 3:119.
118. Swift to Mrs. Howard, 19 August 1727, in *Correspondence*, 3:120–21.

8. GULLIVER'S TRAVELS AND SWIFT'S TRAVAILS

1. Washington, "Swift's Menière's Syndrome and *Gulliver's Travels*."
2. Cotter, "Hundred Oceans of Jonathan Swift," 133.
3. Probyn, "Swift and the Physicians," 255. Probyn is talking about the poem "The Answer to Dr Delany," in which Swift cites Galen's *De Partium Usu*, which discusses the auditory nerves. Even though Abigail Williams is remarkably careful in historicizing Swift's experiences in her edition of the *Journal to Stella*, she notes that "Swift mistakenly attributed his attacks of Ménière's disease to the consumption of fruit" (*JS*, 54n). Almost all modern biographers and even the otherwise scrupulous editors of his correspondence, Harold Williams and David Woolley, accept the retrospective diagnosis.
4. Washington, "Swift's Menière's Syndrome and *Gulliver's Travels*," 105.
5. Hoskison, "Gulliver's Vertigo."
6. For the rich debate about how we are to read Swift's "personae," especially in the *Travels*, see Christopher Fox's valuable "Critical History of *Gulliver's Travels*."
7. Rawson, *Jonathan Swift*, 14.
8. Rawson, "Gulliver and the Gentle Reader"; Rawson, *Gulliver and the Gentle Reader*, viii; Fox, "Critical History of *Gulliver's Travels*," 290–91.
9. *Tale*, 27.
10. Spence, *Observations, Anecdotes, and Characters*, 1:56. For discussions of the composition of the *Travels*, see David Womersley's excellent introduction

to the authoritative Cambridge edition of the work (*GT*, xliv–l) and Charles Kerby-Miller's older but still creditable introduction to the *Memoirs of Martinus Scriblerus* (1–77), from which Womersley draws.
11. For the history of composition, I draw from Ehrenpreis, *Swift*, 3:442–47, and from Womersley's introduction to *Gulliver's Travels* (*GT*, xliv–l).
12. Swift to Charles Ford, 15 April 1721, in *Correspondence*, 2:372.
13. Swift to Mrs. Pendarves, 7 October 1734, in *Correspondence*, 4:5.
14. Swift to Mrs. Howard, October 1726, in *Correspondence*, 3:42.
15. Swift to Edward Harley, Second Earl of Oxford, 27 November 1724, in *Correspondence*, 2:529; Swift to Knightley Chetwode, 30 January 1721–22, in *Correspondence*, 2:411.
16. *GT*, 127.
17. Swift to Knightley Chetwode, October 1724, in *Correspondence*, 2:524.
18. *GT*, 65. Because Gulliver is twelve times the size of a Lilliputian, the emperor's mathematicians determine the amount of food that he will need by cubing his estimated volume: 12 × 12 × 12. David Womersley points out that this figure falls short of the correct product, 1,728. The "prudent and exact Oeconomy" of the Lilliputian emperor, about which Gulliver marvels, says Womersley, "is in fact simply parsimony" (*GT*, 65n24).
19. *GT*, 38. In this context, we should also consider Gulliver as "urinary fireman" who quenches the flames that would otherwise have destroyed the Lilliputian empress's apartment (*GT*, 79–80). While the picture of a giant urinating on tiny people has its literary source in Rabelais, himself a doctor, Christopher Fox has historicized the episode by reading it in the contexts of early modern medical literature. "Of Logic and Lycanthropy," 105–7. Psychoanalyst Sándor Ferenczi (1928) reads this episode as evidence of Swift's own sexual inadequacy. But Gulliver's three minutes of urinating, provoked by the heat that "a most delicious" "diuretick" wine has made, is, literally, prolific humoral evacuation.
20. *GT*, 43–44.
21. *GT*, 36. For further explication of such scenes in the *Travels*, see Benedict, "Body [in Swift]."
22. *GT*, 149. The queen herself is amused to watch Gulliver "eat in Miniature" (*GT*, 149). A hogshead was a "large cask . . . for storing liquids," its volume determined by the commodity that it held. *OED*, s.v. "hogshead." A hogshead of wine would have been somewhere around fifty-five imperial gallons.
23. *GT*, 168. Like the hogshead, a tun was a large barrel; it held about four hogsheads (*GT*, 168n23). Three tuns would be approximately 660 imperial gallons.

24. *GT*, 167. With wry irony, Swift has Gulliver protest of his Lilliputian friend's complaint about his smell that he is "as little faulty that way as most of [his] Sex." Speaking of Swift's "fixt persuasion, that a certain degree of exercise was absolutely necessary, not only to health, but also to cleanliness" because it kept the pores open for evacuating "the great and important discharges of our frame," Patrick Delany insists that the Dean himself "was in his person, one of the cleanliest men that ever lived": "cleanly in every character and circumstance of that personal virtue, to the utmost exactness, and even feminine nicety. His hands were not only washed . . . with the utmost care, but his nails were kept pared to the quick, to guard against the least appearance of a speck upon them. And as he walked much, he rarely dressed himself, without a bason of water by his side, in which he dipt a towel, and cleansed his feet with the utmost exactness." Delany, *Observations*, 118–19.
25. *GT*, 343.
26. *GT*, 125.
27. *GT*, 127.
28. *GT*, 172–73.
29. *GT*, 173.
30. *GT*, 34.
31. *GT*, 46.
32. *GT*, 123.
33. *GT*, 211.
34. Swift to Alexander Pope, 1 November 1734, in *Correspondence*, 4:9.
35. *GT*, 228, 227–28.
36. *GT*, 127–30.
37. Swift to Lord Orrery, 26–31 March 1737, in *Correspondence*, 4:409.
38. *GT*, 34–35.
39. *GT*, 205.
40. *GT*, 47, 66.
41. *GT*, 126.
42. *GT*, 139–40.
43. *GT*, 145.
44. *GT*, 336.
45. *GT*, 351.
46. *GT*, 226.
47. Swift to John Barber, 3 September 1735, in *Correspondence*, 4:172.
48. *GT*, 127–28. In notes to the Cambridge edition of *Gulliver's Travels*, David Womersley suggests that *surprize* in this context denotes "alarm, terror, or

perplexity" (*GT*, 128n68); all of these meanings characterize Swift's own experiences while giddy.
49. Swift to the Rev. Thomas Sheridan, 2 September 1727, in *Correspondence*, 3:123.
50. Swift to Knightley Chetwode, October 1724, in *Correspondence*, 2:524; Swift to Edward Harley, Second Earl of Oxford, 21 September 1728, in *Correspondence*, 3:197.
51. *GT*, 35–36.
52. *GT*, 125.
53. *GT*, 138.
54. *GT*, 35.
55. *GT*, 123.
56. *GT*, 336.
57. *GT*, 224.
58. *GT*, 37, 138, 345, 308. Gulliver himself translates the last of these, "My Tongue is in the Mouth of my Friend" (*GT*, 308). There is some debate about whether words like these mean anything or are merely antic nonsense. In an admirably Scriblerian study of language in the *Travels*, "A Gulliver Dictionary," Paul Odell Clark ventures translations of all Lilliputian, Brobdingnagian, Laputan, and Houyhnhnm words. For further discussion of "ourrichar Gangridge," see Williams's notes to *JS*, passim; Ehrenpreis, "Swift's 'Little Language'"; and Whitley, "Contextual Analysis."
59. 11 March 1712, in *JS*, 406.
60. *GT*, 13.
61. *GT*, 409.
62. *GT*, 138. Later the Brobdingnagian queen has her own cabinetmaker build a roomier, more elaborate "Box that might serve [him] for a Bedchamber" (*GT*, 148); it is nevertheless still a little box.
63. *GT*, 136. Some readers suggest that Glumdalclitch is Stella, saintly in nursing Swift during his episodes of giddiness and deafness. But others also caringly watched over him.
64. *GT*, 172. This episode echoes the story that Swift tells in the autobiographical fragment about having himself been abducted as an infant and taken to England by his loving wet-nurse. While Swift told this story in different ways to different people, this nameless nurse is the only woman in his childhood spoken of with any affection. Doody, "Swift and Women," 89.
65. *GT*, 173; Clark, 597.
66. *GT*, 48.
67. Swift to Francis Grant, 23 March 1733–34, in *Correspondence*, 3:730.

68. *GT*, 433.
69. *GT*, 158.
70. *GT*, 163–64. After another of the dwarf's mischiefs, Gulliver is less merciful: "The Dwarf at my Entreaty had no other Punishment than a sound Whipping" (*GT*, 152).
71. *GT*, 167.
72. *GT*, 123. Gulliver is here describing the stride of a Brobdingnagian. But because he is Brobdingnagian-sized in Lilliput, we can safely make the transference.
73. *GT*, 77.
74. *GT*, 169–70.
75. *GT*, 170.
76. *GT*, 170.
77. *GT*, 152.
78. *GT*, 174–75.
79. Swift to the Rev. John Worrall, 14 September 1721, in *Correspondence*, 2:396.
80. Swift to Charles Ford, 16 February 1718–19, in *Correspondence*, 2:290. To "founder," as applied to horses and riders, means to "stumble violently, fall helplessly to the ground, collapse; to fall lame." *OED*, s.v. "founder."
81. *GT*, 64.
82. *GT*, 138.
83. *GT*, 356.
84. Swift to John Gay, 10 November 1730, in *Correspondence*, 3:334.
85. Swift to Alexander Pope, 1 November 1734, in *Correspondence*, 4:8.
86. *GT*, 139.
87. *GT*, 126.
88. *GT*, 171.
89. *GT*, 154.
90. *GT*, 132–33.
91. *GT*, 61–62. Fittingly, Gulliver ends his paragraph with that word *Admiration*.
92. *GT*, 166–67.
93. *GT*, 168.
94. While he often advises that his female friends walk for their health, only rarely does Swift suggest that they ride. In one of his earliest letters to Stella and Dingley, he enjoins Stella to "ride little Johnson, who must needs be now in good Case [health]." 9 [September] 1710, in *JS*, 7. For want of a comma, the advice is ambiguous; it is unclear whether she should "ride, little Johnson" or "ride little, Johnson." A year later, in a rare instance of

ceding the reins to a woman, Swift speaks of Stella's riding for exercise but makes of it an elaborate comic production: "I am glad at heart MD rides, and rides, and rides.... Now, madam Ppt, what say you? you ride every day; I know that already, sirrah; and if you rid every day for a twelvemonth, you would be still better and better.... O Lord, how hasty we are, Ppt can't stay writing and writing; she must go a cock-horse, pray now. Well; but the horses are not come to the door; the fellow can't find the bridle; your stirrup is broken; where did you put the whips, Dd [Dingley]? Marg'et, where have you laid Mrs. Johnson's ribband to tie about her? reach me my mask: sup up this before you go. So, so, a gallop, a gallop: sit fast, sirrah, and don't ride hard upon the stones.—Well, now Ppt is gone, tell me, Dd, is she a good girl?" Swift moves on from there to discuss London news and business. But he cannot let the image of Stella's riding go and returns to it several lines later: "O madam Ppt, welcome home; was it pleasant riding? did your horse stumble? how often did the man light to settle your stirrup? ride nine miles? faith you have galloped indeed." 30 June 1711, in *JS*, 232–33. Because none of the letters from Stella and Dingley survive, we cannot know what prompted this particular comic narrative; the context suggests that Swift was bruised when Stella had to hurry off to ride while she and Dingley were writing to him. *Sirrah*, says the *OED*, was a "term of address used to men or boys, expressing contempt, reprimand, or assumption of authority on the part of the speaker." It was used jestingly or less seriously in speaking to children and women (s.v., "sirrah"). While Swift often addresses both Stella and Dingley as "sirrahs," calling Stella "sirrah" in this context comically masculinizes her in her riding.

95. *GT*, 168.
96. Swift to Alexander Pope, 7 February 1735–36, in *Correspondence*, 4:260.
97. Scholars have picked up on the suggestion that the Brobdingnagian girls use Gulliver as sex toy. See, for example, Boucé, "Gulliver Phallophorus"; and Armintor, "Sexual Politics of Microscopy."
98. *GT*, 400–401.
99. *GT*, 434.
100. *GT*, 434.
101. *GT*, 411.

9. GULLIVER'S ORDEALS AS SWIFT'S ORDER

1. Turner, "Disability Humor," 61–62.
2. Todd, *Imagining Monsters*, 153–61.

3. But rascally beggars might perform disability to hoodwink unwary charity-givers. Thomas Sheridan tells the story of his own grandfather, egged on by Swift himself to play a "blind fidler" at a beggar's wedding; Swift disguised himself, too, as the blind man's guide. Singing, dancing, and feasting, the wedding party were so pleased with the prankster's playing that they rewarded him "very handsomely." The next day, in their clerical garbs, Swift and Sheridan came across the same beggars. They "found some upon crutches, who had danced very nimbly at the wedding; others stone blind, who were perfectly clear sighted at the feast." Sheridan charitably doled out among these beggars the same money that they had given him the night before. Swift, however, outraged that they would perpetrate such "roguery," "rated them soundly" and threatened to "have them taken up, and sent to jail." Miraculously, "the lame once more recovered their legs, and the blind their eyes." Sheridan, *The Life*, 399–400.
4. Delany, *Observations*, 90, 91, 92n. This list of beggar women has its correlative in Brobdingnag, when tiny Gulliver encounters the street beggars, who shock him as "the most horrible Spectacles that ever an *European* Eye beheld. There was a Woman with a Cancer in her Breast, swelled to a monstrous Size, full of Holes, in two or three of which [he] could have easily crept, and covered [his] whole Body. There was a Fellow with a Wen in his Neck, larger than five Woolpacks; and another with a couple of wooden Legs, each about twenty Foot high" (*GT*, 158–59).
5. *Verses on the Death*, lines 467–68, in *Poems*, 2:572.
6. Dickie, "Hilarity and Pitilessness," 2. Trying to get at the psychology of such callous jokes, Dickie suggests, among other impulses, that "any physical peculiarity; any disability or incapacity; any stutter, lameness, or blindness simply made one a standing joke—a reminder, perhaps, of the hilarious intransigence of nature, of the physicality that lay behind all attempts at human dignity" (17).
7. *GT*, 172.
8. Swift to William Pulteney, 8 March 1734–35, in *Correspondence*, 4:66; Swift to Edward Harley, Second Earl of Oxford, 21 September 1728, in *Correspondence*, 3:197.
9. Swift might laugh at others; he might laugh at himself. If reports are true, however, he did not like being laughed at by his social inferiors. Pilkington tells the story of a plan by the Dean and his friends to hold an annual dinner, "in imitation of the *Saturnalia*," in which "the Servants personated their Masters, and the Masters waited as Servants": "The first Time they put this Scheme in Practice, was at the Deanery House. When all the

Servants were seated, and every Gentleman placed behind his own Man, the Dean's Servant took an Opportunity of finding Fault with some Meat that was not done to his Taste, and taking it up in his Hand, he threw it in his Master's Face, and mimick'd him in every other Foible which he had ever discover'd in him. At this the Dean flew in a violent Rage, beat the Fellow, and put every Thing into such Disorder, that the Servants affrighted, fled the Room; and here ended the Feast of *Saturnalia*" (*Memoirs* 1:280).

10. Todd, 82.
11. GT, 137.
12. GT, 138.
13. GT, 145–46.
14. Orrery, *Remarks on the Life and Writings*, 256; GT, 145–46.
15. GT, 94–95.
16. GT, 172.
17. GT, 349.
18. GT, 350.
19. GT, 398–99.
20. In Aesop's fable about the bird in borrowed plumage, a jackdaw puts on the fallen feathers of a peacock and assumes superiority over his fellow daws. When the truth is discovered, the other jackdaws jeer, peck out both the peacock feathers and many of his own, and drive him away.
21. Todd, 147.
22. Todd, 156.
23. GT, 334.
24. GT, 393.
25. GT, 393.
26. GT, 420.
27. GT, 437, 7–8.
28. GT, 43–44.
29. GT, 399.
30. GT, 13. In the same letter, Gulliver's use of the word *Jabber* to characterize human language echoes Swift's own desire that denotations of English words be fixed. Gulliver complains in his final retirement "near *Newark*, in *Nottinghamshire*," that both "Sea-*Yahoos*" (mariners) and "Land ones" have "become new fangled in their Words; which the latter change every Year; insomuch, as I remember upon each Return to mine own Country, their old Dialect was so altered, that I could hardly understand the new. And I observe, when any *Yahoo* comes from *London* out of Curiosity to visit me at mine own House, we neither of us are able to deliver our

Conceptions [ideas] in a Manner intelligible to the other" (*GT*, 15, 12–13). Womersley reminds us of the *Proposal for Correcting, Improving and Ascertaining the English Tongue* (1712), in which Swift himself proposed the founding of an academy for fixing the meanings of English words permanently (*GT*, 12n41).

31. *GT*, 351.
32. *GT*, 348.
33. *GT*, 351.
34. *GT*, 352.
35. Young, *Conjectures on Original Composition*, 62, 65; Fox, "Critical History of *Gulliver's Travels*," 275.
36. Delany, 198. In response to psychoanalytical critics who diagnosed Swift's apparent preoccupation with excremental matters as psychopathy, Norman O. Brown argued along the same lines. What the psychoanalysts saw as Swift's "obsessive preoccupation with anality" was diagnosis of their own "neurotic" denial of our common excremental natures. Readers' objections and the psychoanalysts' diagnoses of Swift's "anality," "coprophilia," and like psychopathic disorders, says Brown, are evidence of our "universal human neuroses." "Excremental Vision."
37. *GT*, 335.
38. *GT*, 393–94.
39. *GT*, 394.
40. William Salmon included dozens of excremental cures in annotations to his translation of Thomas Sydenham's *Praxis Medica*, which sat on Swift's own bookshelf. For a discussion of Swift and "excremental medicine," see Child, "Once More into the Breech."
41. *GT*, 344.
42. *GT*, 405.
43. *GT*, 405–6. We recall here not only Deane Swift's image of his cousin's running up and down a hill when taking breaks from his studious work for Temple but also the parodic version of Swift's own swimming when Gulliver, dropped by the Queen's dwarf in Brobdingnag, falls "over Head and Ears" "into a large Silver Bowl of Cream" and has to swim for his life. Deane Swift, *An Essay*, 271–72; *GT*, 152.
44. *GT*, 350. In making his case for revealed religion, George Cheyne asks in wonder, "What is more admirable, than the fitness of ev'ry Creature for the use we make of him?" He goes on to speak of the "Cleanness, Beauty, Strength, and Swiftness of the Horse, whose Breath, Foam, and ev'n Excrements are sweet, and thereby so well fitted for our Use and

Service." *Philosophical Principles of Natural Religion*, 280–81. Swift might well have lifted his Houyhnhnms' virtues ("*Temperance, Industry, Exercise* and *Cleanliness*") and the principles upon which they mate (strength and comeliness) from this very list (*GT*, 405, 404).

45. *GT*, 412. While they never get sick, the Houyhnhnms do occasionally suffer "accidental Bruises and Cuts in the Pastern or Frog of the Foot by sharp Stones, as well as other Maims and Hurts in the several Parts of the Body"; for such accidents, "they have excellent Medicines composed of Herbs" to induce healing (*GT*, 412).
46. *GT*, 345–46.
47. *GT*, 420.
48. *GT*, 345.
49. *GT*, 417.
50. Swift to the Rev. Thomas Sheridan, 18 September 1728, in *Correspondence*, 3:194.
51. Swift to William Pulteney, 7 March 1736–37, in *Correspondence*, 4:391.

10. VOYAGES OUT AND VOYAGES BACK

1. *GT*, 320.
2. Swift to Alexander Pope, 1 November 1734, in *Correspondence*, 4:8.
3. *GT*, 310.
4. *GT*, 310, 313.
5. *GT*, 317. Swift wrote to John Barber, "I have a constant Giddyness in my head, and what is more vexatious, as constant a Deafness: I forget every thing but old Friendships and old Opinions." 31 March 1738, in *Correspondence*, 4:510. Pope wrote consolingly the same year: "You lose little by *not hearing* such things as this idle and base generation has to tell you: You lose not much by *forgetting* most of what *now* passes in it." 12 October 1738, in *Correspondence*, 4:545.
6. *GT*, 318.
7. Mrs. Whiteway and Swift to William Richardson, 13 May 1740, in *Correspondence*, 4:621.
8. *Verses on the Death*, lines 85–90, in *Poems*, 2:556.
9. Pilkington, *Memoirs*, 1:314, 1:313.
10. Orrery, *Remarks on the Life and Writings*, 207.
11. Orrery, 271. Certainly, taking his cue from Orrery, Johnson linked the enemies Marlborough and Swift syntactically in a tableaux of pathetic shared idiocy: "From *Marlb'rough's* Eyes the Streams of Dotage flow, / And *Swift* expires a Driv'ler and a Show." *Vanity of Human Wishes*, 25. Marlborough

spent the last six years of his life paralyzed by strokes; for the popular story of Swift's being exhibited for money in his final years, see chapter 2, note 30.
12. Deane Swift, *An Essay*, 218.
13. Orrery, 81.
14. Orrery, 216.
15. Johnson, "Swift," 213.
16. Orrery, 215.
17. Gosse, *History of Eighteenth Century Literature*, 161. Gosse charts Swift's decline into madness in the *Travels*, saying that while book 4 is proof of madness, the voyages to Lilliput and Brobdingnag "belong to the period [that is, terminus] of his mental health" (160).
18. Thackeray, *English Humourists*, 40.
19. Stone, "Swift and the Horses," 369.
20. Seidel, "*Gulliver's Travels*," 80.
21. DePorte, "Teaching the Third Voyage"; Fox, "Of Logic and Lycanthropy."
22. *GT*, 111.
23. *GT*, 208, 210, 212.
24. *GT*, 214.
25. *GT*, 31.
26. *GT*, 57, 100.
27. *GT*, 188.
28. *GT*, 312, 311.
29. *GT*, 417.
30. *GT*, 403.
31. Swift to Viscount Bolingbroke, May 1719, in *Correspondence*, 2:298.
32. *GT*, 189.
33. *GT*, 112.
34. *GT*, 214.
35. *GT*, 218.
36. *GT*, 329–30.
37. *GT*, 431.
38. *GT*, 13.
39. *GT*, 433.
40. *GT*, 330, 434.
41. *GT*, 435. A stone-horse, that is, one with "stones" (testes), is a stallion, an uncastrated male. This is ironic reversal of the Houyhnhnms' plan to exterminate the Yahoo race by castrating them, an idea suggested to them by Gulliver himself. In this context, we can consider his own "Shame,

Confusion and Horror" upon reflecting "that by copulating with one of the *Yahoo*-Species, [he] had become a Parent of more" (*GT,* 434).

42. *GT,* 443.
43. Desperate for cure in a violent "Fit of Ague," Robinson Crusoe remembers "that the *Brasilians* take no Physick but their Tobacco, for almost all Distempers." He tries chewing it, infusing it in rum, and breathing in its smoke. Over several days, he experiments with tobacco "all the three Ways" and comes to believe that it helps cure him. Defoe, *Robinson Crusoe,* 105–12.
44. Culpeper, *English Physician Enlarged,* 284.
45. *GT,* 443–44.
46. *GT,* 438.
47. Swift to the Rev. Thomas Sheridan, 9 April 1737, in *Correspondence,* 4:419; Swift to Sir John Stanley, 30 October 1736, in *Correspondence,* 4:356.
48. Swift to Knightley Chetwode, 11 November 1721, in *Correspondence,* 2:403.
49. Swift to Mrs. Pendarves, 29 January 1735–36, in *Correspondence,* 4:257.
50. Swift to Alexander Pope, 13 February 1728–29, in *Correspondence,* 3:209; Swift to Charles Ford, 31 December 1724, in *Correspondence,* 2:540.
51. Swift to Knightley Chetwode, 30 January 1721–22, in *Correspondence,* 2:411.
52. Patrick Delany, "Sent by Dr. *Delany* to Dr. S—t, in Order to Be Admitted to Speak to Him," lines 1–2, 5–6, in *Poems,* 2:365.
53. We recall Swift's characterization of his deafness and giddyness in 1727 as "two friends," who, "being old acquaintance have now thought fit to come togeth[e]r." Swift to Mrs. Howard, 19 August 1727, in *Correspondence,* 3:120.
54. The full quotation reads, "The great direction which Burton has left to men disordered like you, *Be not solitary, be not idle:* which I would thus modify;—If you are idle, be not solitary; if you are solitary, be not idle." Johnson to James Boswell, 27 October 1779, in Boswell, *Life of Samuel Johnson, LL.D.,* 2:308. Robert Burton concludes the monumental *Anatomy of Melancholy* thus: "Only take this for a corollary and conclusion, as thou tenderest thine owne welfare in this, and all other melancholy, thy good health of body and mind, observe this short precept, give not way to solitarinesse and idlenesse. *Be not solitary, be not idle*" (723).
55. Johnson, "Swift," 207. Johnson added that because of "some ridiculous resolution or vow . . . never to wear spectacles," Swift had also stopped reading and had thus cut himself off from any meaningful improvement that this might bring (207). Swift likened reading to conversation: "When

I am reading a Book, whether wise or silly, it seemeth to me to be alive and talking to me." "Thoughts on Various Subjects," in *PW*, 4:253. Reading little or nothing was the same, then, as the withdrawal from company forced by his "unconversible Disorder."
56. Swift to the Rev. Thomas Sheridan, 29 August 1727, in *Correspondence*, 3:122.
57. Swift to Viscount Bolingbroke, 21 March 1729–30, in *Correspondence*, 3:295. Swift writes this oft-quoted statement in the context of complaining that he has been abandoned and forgotten in Ireland.
58. Brady, *Twentieth-Century Interpretations*, 1; Rawson, *Jonathan Swift*, 13; Fox, "Critical History of *Gulliver's Travels*," 291.

CONCLUSION

1. Dryden, *Absalom and Achitophel*, 4.
2. Dryden, 4–5.
3. Dryden, 5.
4. Only a few lines later comes Dryden's oft-quoted couplet "Great Wits are sure to Madness near alli'd; / And thin Partitions do their Bounds divide" (5).
5. Sterne, *Tristram Shandy*, 4:219.
6. *GT*, 276–77.
7. Swift to Alexander Pope, 29 September 1725, in *Correspondence*, 2:606.
8. "Family of Swift," in *PW*, 5:187.
9. "Family of Swift," in *PW*, 5:189.
10. "Family of Swift," in *PW*, 5:193.
11. "Family of Swift," in *PW*, 5:193–94.
12. Boswell, *Life of Samuel Johnson, LL.D.*, 2:400.
13. "Ppt [Stella] is a good girl for not being angry when I tell her of spelling," he wrote in the *Journal to Stella*. "I see none wrong in this." 8 January 1711–12, in *JS*, 363. Years later, he wrote to Mary Pendarves, "A woman of quality, who had excellent good sense, was formerly my correspondent, but she scrawled and spelt like a Wapping wench, having been brought up in a Court at a time before reading was thought of any use to a female; and I knew several others of very high quality with the same defect." Swift to Mrs. Pendarves, 29 January 1735–36, in *Correspondence*, 4:257. Woolley suggests that the lady in question is the Countess of Orkney, who, Swift wrote in 1713, "has neither Orthography, Grammar, nor choice of proper Words," although she is "a person of as much good naturall Sense and Judgment as I have ever known" (*Correspondence*, 4:258n3). Swift's own spelling, notes Damrosch, "was erratic at times." *Jonathan Swift*, 229. In this, he was like most others of his day.

14. Swift, *A Complete Collection of Genteel and Ingenious Conversation, According to the Most Polite Mode and Method Now Used at Court, and in the Best Companies of England. In Three Dialogues,* in *PW,* 4:97–201.
15. *GT,* 368–69.
16. *PW,* 4:3–21.
17. *PW,* 4:14. Inspired by the Académie Française, this institution would "be made of such Persons, as are generally allowed to be best qualified for such a Work, without any regard to Quality, Party, or Profession" (13–14).
18. Delany, *Observations,* 140.
19. Swift, *Letter to a Young Gentleman,* 6.
20. Deane Swift, *An Essay,* 366.
21. Deane Swift, 361–62.
22. Deane Swift, 361.
23. Deane Swift, 360.
24. This report from Orrery comes in a handwritten note in a copy of his book; quoted in Damrosch, 275. In *Directions to Servants,* first published in 1731 but begun much earlier, Swift gives comically cynical instructions to various members of a domestic staff, all of them designed to curry favor with their masters and mistresses.
25. Ross, *Shakespeare's Tremor and Orwell's Cough,* 60–61.
26. Rawson, *Gulliver and the Gentle Reader,* 109.
27. McMinn, "Swift and the Formation," 103.
28. [Carteret], *By the Lord Lieutenant.* Walter Scott attributed the "whole chain of paradoxes" in Swift's life and works to the "the humour of stubborn independence, which influenced the Dean's whole character." *Life of Swift,* 418.
29. "A Dialogue Between an Eminent Lawyer and Dr. Swift Dean of St. Patrick's, Being an Allusion to the First Satire of the Second Book of Horace," lines 1–6, in *Poems,* 2:489.
30. Pilkington, *Memoirs,* 1:317. Quoting Dryden's famous lines, "Great Wit to Madness sure is near allied, / And thin Partitions do their Bounds divide," Pilkington sees this insult as an early sign of Swift's lunacy.
31. Boswell, *Life of Samuel Johnson, LL.D.,* 1:374.
32. Johnson, "Swift," 212.
33. B. Hammond, "Scriblerian Self-Fashioning," 108.
34. Swift's sobriquet for the passionate Esther Vanhomrigh, "Vanessa" was an inversion of the prefix of her last name, "Van," and "Essa," a pet name for "Esther."
35. Of Sheridan, Swift wrote to the Earl of Orrery, "He writes me English latinized, and Latin Englyfyed, but neither of them equal to mine, as my

very enemyes allow. It is true indeed, I am gone so far in this Science that I can hardly write common English, I am so apt to mingle it with Latin. For instance instead of writing, *my Enemyes* I was going to spell it *mi en emis.*" Swift to Lord Orrery, 25 September 1735, in *Correspondence*, 4:189. Aside from his clever exchanges with Sheridan, Swift used the Latino-Anglicus form to satirize learned medicine of his day. See Child, "Jonathan Swift's Latin Quacks."

36. Faulkner, quoted in Nichols, *Supplement to Dr. Swift's Works*, 758–59. Nichols says that Faulkner's character was unimpeachable "but that his credulity might [have been] imposed upon"—by Swift himself, we presume (758n).
37. Sheridan, *The Life*, 396.
38. Pilkington, 1:28.
39. Rawson, *Jonathan Swift*, 7.
40. Swift to the Rev. William Tisdall, 16 December 1703, in *Correspondence*, 1:148. Swift abruptly ended communications with Tisdall not long after, when he realized that Tisdall sought Stella's hand in marriage.
41. Swift to Viscount Bolingbroke, 21 March 1729–30, in *Correspondence*, 3:295.
42. McKeon, *Origins of the English Novel*, 61. Deane, "Swift and the Anglo-Irish Intellect."
43. Swift to Thomas Tickell, 3 August 1724, in *Correspondence*, 2:511; Swift to Alexander Pope, 29 September 1725, in *Correspondence*, 2:606.
44. Rawson, *Jonathan Swift*, 13.
45. Orrery, *Remarks on the Life and Writings*, 125.
46. The limits of this study do not permit an extensive review of the continuing debate over Swift's "excremental vision," which goes back even to his own day. For an illuminating survey of the various responses to his apparent preoccupation with excremental matters, see Rushdy, "New Emetics of Interpretation."
47. Flynn, *Body in Swift and Defoe*, 88.
48. H. King, "Female Fluids in the Hippocratic Corpus"; and Duden, "Fluxes and Stagnations."
49. "The Lady's Dressing Room," line 4, in *Poems*, 2:525.
50. Deutsch, "Health and Sickness [in Swift]," 20; "Strephon and Chloe," line 16, in *Poems*, 2:584. Some of the men speak of their own bodily functions indirectly. Trying to rouse the "Swain" Cassinus from his doldrums, his friend Peter says, "And, I have heard thee oft salute / *Aurora* with thy early Flute," lines that sound suspiciously euphemistic of Cassy's urinating

upon waking or suggestive of an erection. "Cassinus and Peter. A Tragical Elegy," lines 33–34, in *Poems*, 2:594.
51. Deutsch, "Health and Sickness [in Swift]," 20.
52. "The Lady's Dressing Room," line 109, in *Poems*, 2:529.
53. "Strephon and Chloe," lines 11–20, in *Poems*, 2:584.
54. "The Lady's Dressing Room," lines 143–44, in *Poems*, 2:530.
55. "A Beautiful Young Nymph Going to Bed," lines 68–70, in *Poems*, 2:583.
56. "A Beautiful Young Nymph Going to Bed," line 34, in *Poems*, 2:582.
57. "The Progress of Beauty," lines 81–84, in *Poems*, 1:228.
58. Lynall, *Swift and Science*, 144.
59. Swift to John Gay, 8 January 1722–23, in *Correspondence*, 2:443.
60. See among other discussions, Smith, *Genres of "Gulliver's Travels"*; and Weinbrot, *Menippean Satire Reconsidered*. Menippean satire, usually written in prose, is a hybrid of generic forms that characteristically attacks ideas and attitudes rather than specific institutions and people.
61. Fabricant, *Swift's Landscape*; San Juan, "Anti-Poetry of Jonathan Swift."
62. Swift to the Rev. John Kendall, 11 February 1691–92, in *Correspondence*, 1:104.
63. Swift to Alexander Pope, 1 November 1734, in *Correspondence*, 4:8.

APPENDIX

1. John Arbuthnot to Swift, 11 December 1718, in *Correspondence*, 2:282.
2. Chambers, *Cyclopædia*, 1:219. For the uses of cinnabar of antimony in cases of vertigo and epilepsy, commonly classed as "cephalick" disorders, see, among many, the following: Lower, *Eminent Physicians Receipts*, 112; Salmon, *Medicina Practica*, 79; Woodman, *Medicus Novissimus*, 17, 139ff.
3. Browne, *Essay Towards the Forming a True Idea*, 133.
4. Lewis, *Edinburgh New Dispensatory*, 56, 166. Despite the late date of this work (1790), I draw from it because of its generally acknowledged authority in the long eighteenth century.
5. Strother, *Family Companion for Health*, 31. In the 1727 version of *The Dispensatory of the Royal College of Physicians of Edinburgh*, tinctura sacra is a compound of hiera picra, the purgative medicine that Swift himself declared "devilish Stuff"; cochineal, the dried and powdered bodies of the insect *Coccus cacti*, used as an antispasmodic; and Spanish white wine. Shaw, *Dispensatory*, 91.
6. John Arbuthnot to Swift, 5 November 1730, in *Correspondence*, 3:330.
7. Letter and enclosure from John Arbuthnot to Swift, 5 November 1730, in *Correspondence*, 3:330–31.

8. Lewis, 115.
9. Alleyne, *New English Dispensatory*, 34.
10. Lewis, 518. While the "bark" was touted primarily as a febrifuge, Swift, like many others of his day, resorted to it for a variety of ills, including attacks of giddiness and deafness. "I am still under the discipline of the bark to prevent relapses," he wrote to Robert Cope after a recent episode of deafness in 1720. 26 May 1720, in *Correspondence*, 2:334.
11. Lewis, 215.
12. Iron and steel were both considered chalybeates, both of them used widely in British pharmacopoeias. But eighteenth-century physicians preferred the use of iron (as Arbuthnot specifies here), as opposed to the alloy steel, because the former was softer and rusted more easily.
13. Lewis, 187.
14. Swift to Archbishop King, 21 October 1712, in *Correspondence*, 1:445.
15. 17 February 1712–13, in *JS*, 499.
16. 3 March 1712–13, in *JS*, 506.
17. Lewis, 137. Swift was well familiar with asafoetida, writing to Stella and Dingley, "I left [our Society meeting] at seven, and sat this evening with poor Mrs. Wesley, who has been mightily ill to-day with a fainting fit: she has often convulsions too; she takes a mixture with *assa fœtida*, which I have now in my nose; and every thing smells of it. I never smelt it before, 'tis abominable." 26 January 1711–12, in *JS*, 376. The physician Richard Brookes wrote that asafoetida "powerfully procures a Diaphoresis and Sweating; it drives malignant Humours from the Center [of the body] to the Circumference." *General Dispensatory*, 7.
18. Lewis, 218.

BIBLIOGRAPHY

EARLY MODERN SOURCES

Addison, Joseph, and Richard Steele. *The Spectator*. 8 vols. London, 1712–15.

Alcock, Thomas. *Some Memoirs of the Life of Dr. Nathan Alcock, Lately Deceased*. London, 1780.

Allen, John. *Synopsis Medicinæ: or, A Summary View of the Whole Practice of Physick* [. . .]. 2 vols. London, 1733.

Alleyne, James. *A New English Dispensatory, in Four Parts*. London, 1733.

Apperley, Thomas, *Observations in Physick, Both Rational and Practical: With a Treatise of the Small-Pox*. London, 1731.

Arbuthnot, John. *The Correspondence of Dr. John Arbuthnot*. Edited by Angus Ross. Munich: Wilhelm Fink, 2006.

Arbuthnot, John. *An Essay Concerning the Effects of Air on Human Bodies*. London, 1733.

Arbuthnot, John. *An Essay Concerning the Nature of Aliments, and the Choice of Them, According to the Different Constitutions of Human Bodies*. London, 1731.

Arbuthnot, John. *John Bull Still in His Senses: Being the Third Part of Law Is a Bottomless Pit*. London, 1712.

Arbuthnot, John. *Γνῶθι σέαυτον: Know Your Self; An Excellent Poem*. London, 1734.

Augustine of Hippo. *The Confessions*. Translated by Maria Boulding, edited by David Vincent Meconi. San Francisco: Ignatius Press, 1997.

Bailey, Nathan, George Gordon, and Philip Miller. *Dictionarium Britannicum* [. . .]. London, 1736.

Beddoes, Thomas. *Hygeia: or, Essays Moral and Medical; or, The Causes Affecting the Personal State of Our Middling and Affluent Classes*. 3 vols. Bristol, 1803.

Berkeley, George. *Alciphron: or, The Minute Philosopher* [. . .]. 2 vols. Dublin, 1732.

Berkeley, George. *Three Dialogues Between Hylas and Philonous* [. . .]. 2nd ed. London, 1725.

Bickerton, G. *Accurate Disquisitions in Physick*. London, 1719.

Blankaart, Steven. *The Physical Dictionary: Wherein the Terms of Anatomy, the Names and Causes of Diseases, Chyrurgical Instruments, and Their Use Are Accurately Describ'd*. 4th ed. London, 1702.

Boerhaave, Herman. *Dr. Boerhaave's Academical Lectures on the Theory of Physic* [. . .]. Anonymous translation. 6 vols. London, 1742–46.

Boswell, James. *The Hypochondriack: Being the Seventy Essays by the Celebrated Biographer, James Boswell*. Edited by Margery Bailey. 2 vols. Stanford, CA: Stanford University Press, 1928.

Boswell, James. *The Life of Samuel Johnson, LL.D.* 2 vols. London, 1791.

Brookes, Richard. *The General Dispensatory, Containing a Translation of the Pharmacopœias of the Royal Colleges of Physicians of London and Edinburgh*. London, 1753.

Brookes, Richard. *The General Practice of Physic; Extracted Chiefly from the Writings of the Most Celebrated Practical Physicians* [. . .]. 2nd ed. 2 vols. London, 1754.

Browne, Joseph. *An Account of the Wonderful Cures Perform'd by Cold Baths*. London, [1707?].

Browne, Joseph. *An Essay Towards the Forming a True Idea of Fundamentals in Physick, upon the Mechanism and Structure of the Blood*. London, 1709.

Bulwer, John [attributed]. *Philocophus, or, The Deafe and Dumbe Mans Friend*. London, 1648.

Burton, John. *A Treatise of the Non-Naturals*. York, 1738.

Burton, Robert. *The Anatomy of Melancholy: What It Is; With All the Kinds Causes Symptomes Prognostickes and Severall Cures of It* [. . .]. 2nd ed. London, 1638.

Campbell, R[obert]. *The London Tradesman* [. . .]. London, 1747.

[Carteret, John]. *By the Lord Lieutenant and Council of Ireland, a Proclamation*. Dublin, 1724.

A Catalogue of Books [. . .]: *The Library of the Late Rev. Dr. Swift, Dean of St. Patrick's, Dublin*. Dublin, 1745.

A Catalogue of Books: The Library of the Rev. Dr. Thomas Sheridan, Deceased. Dublin, 1739.

Chambers, Ephraim. *Cyclopædia: or, An Universal Dictionary of Arts and Sciences; Containing the Definitions of the Terms and Accounts of the Things Signify'd Thereby*. 2 vols. London, 1728.

Cheyne, George. "The Case of the Author." In *The English Malady*, 325–64. London, 1733.

Cheyne, George. *The English Malady.* London, 1733.
Cheyne, George. *An Essay of Health and Long Life.* London, 1724.
Cheyne, George. *An Essay on Regimen.* London, 1740.
Cheyne, George. *A New Theory of Continu'd Fevers* [. . .]. Edinburgh, 1701.
Cheyne, George. *Philosophical Principles of Natural Religion: Containing the Elements of Natural Philosophy, and the Proofs for Natural Religion, Arising from Them.* London, 1705.
Chomel, Noel. *Dictionaire Oeconomique: or, The Family Dictionary.* Rev. ed. 2 vols. Dublin, 1727.
Cockburn, William. *The Nature and Cure of Fluxes.* 3rd ed. London, 1724.
Cockburn, William. *Sea Diseases.* 2nd ed. London, 1706.
Cook, John. *An Anatomical and Mechanical Essay on the Whole Animal Œconomy in One View.* 2 vols. London, 1730.
Cooper, Thomas. *Thesaurus Linguae Romanæ & Britannicæ.* 2nd ed. London, 1578.
Culpeper, Nicholas. *The English Physician Enlarged.* London, 1708.
Culpeper, Nicholas. *The English Physician: or, An Astrologo-Physical Discourse of the Vulgar Herbs of This Nation.* London, 1652.
Culpeper, Nicholas. *Pharmacopœia Londinensis; or, The London Dispensatory.* London, 1683.
Defoe, Daniel. *The Life and Surprizing Adventures of Robinson Crusoe, of York, Mariner.* London, 1719.
Delany, Patrick. *Observations upon Lord Orrery's "Remarks on the Life and Writings of Dr. Jonathan Swift."* Dublin, 1754.
Doläus, Johann. *Dolæus upon the Cure of the Gout by Milk-Diet: To Which Is Prefixed, an Essay upon Diet; By William Stephens, M.D.F.R.S.* London, 1732.
Dryden, John. *Absalom and Achitophel: A Poem.* London, 1681.
Dubé, Paul. *The Poor Man's Physician and Surgeon* [. . .]. London, 1704.
The Family Physician; or, A Safe and Easy Method of Curing Most Diseases, Incident to Human Bodies. London, [1750?].
Faulkner, George. "The Life of the Reverend Jonathan Swift, D.D. Dean of St. Patrick's, Dublin." In *The Works of the Reverend Dr. Jonathan Swift, Dean of St. Patrick's: With an Account of His Life and Writings,* edited by George Faulkner, vol. 11, 190–280. Dublin, 1762.
Flood, Frances. *The Devonshire Woman; or, A Wonderful Narrative of Frances Flood.* London, [1723?].
Floyer, Sir John. *The Ancient Psychrolousia Revived: or, An Essay to Prove Cold Bathing Both Safe and Useful* [. . .]. London, 1702.
Floyer, Sir John. *Medicina Gerocomica: or, The Galenic Art of Preserving Old Men's Health, Explain'd* [. . .]. London, 1724.

Fuller, Francis. *Medicina Gymnastica: or, A Treatise Concerning the Power of Exercise, with Respect to the Animal Oeconomy; and the Great Necessity of It in the Cure of Several Distempers.* London, 1705.

Goodall, Charles. *The Royal College of Physicians of London, Founded and Established by Law; as Appears by Letters Patent, Acts of Parliament, Adjudged Cases, &c. and an Historical Account of the College's Proceedings against Empiricks and Unlicensed Practisers in Every Prince's Reign from the First Incorporation to the Murther of the Royal Martyr King Charles the First.* London, 1684.

Groeneveld, Johannes [John Greenfield]. *The Grounds of Physick, Containing So Much of Philosophy, Anatomy, Chimistry, and the Mechanical Construction of a Humane Body, as Is Necessary to the Accomplishment of a Physitian: With the Method of Practice in Common Distempers.* London, 1715.

Harvey, Gideon. *The Third Edition of the Vanities of Philosophy and Physick.* London, 1702.

Hawkesworth, John, ed. *The Works of Jonathan Swift, D.D. [. . .]: With Some Account of the Author's Life.* 12 vols. London, 1755.

Hervey, John. *Lord Hervey's Memoirs: His Witty and Malicious Account of the Personalities, Politics and Intrigues of the Royal Household 1727–37.* Edited by Romney Sedgwick. Harmondsworth: Penguin Books, 1963.

Johnson, Samuel. *A Dictionary of the English Language.* 2 vols. London, 1755.

Johnson, Samuel. *Letters to and from the Late Samuel Johnson, LL.D.: To Which Are Added, Some Poems Never Before Printed.* 2 vols. Dublin, 1788.

Johnson, Samuel. "Swift." In *The Lives of the Most Eminent English Poets: With Critical Observations on Their Works*, edited and with an introduction and notes by Roger Lonsdale, vol. 3, 189–214. Oxford: Clarendon Press, 2006.

Johnson, Samuel. *The Vanity of Human Wishes: The Tenth Satire of Juvenal, Imitated by Samuel Johnson.* London, 1749.

Jonston, John. *The Idea of Practical Physick in Twelve Books [. . .]: Written in Latin by John Johnston.* Translated by Nicholas Culpeper. London, 1657.

Kerby-Miller, Charles, ed. *Memoirs of the Extraordinary Life, Works, and Discoveries of Martinus Scriblerus.* By John Arbuthnot, John Gay, Robert Harley, Thomas Parnell, Alexander Pope, and Jonathan Swift. New York: Oxford University Press, 1988.

Lady. *The Whole Duty of a Woman: or, A Guide to the Female Sex. From the Age of Sixteen to Sixty.* 3rd ed. London, 1701.

Lémery, Louis. *A Treatise of Food, in General.* London, 1706.

A Letter from a Gentleman in Town to His Friend in the Country, Concerning Dr. Joseph Brown's New Translation of Horace, with Some Remarks on the Same. London, 1705.

Lewis, William. *The Edinburgh New Dispensatory.* 2nd ed. Edinburgh, 1790.
Lobb, Theophilus. *The Practice of Physick in General* [...]. 2 vols. London, 1771.
Locke, John. *An Essay Concerning Humane Understanding: In Four Books.* 5th ed. London, 1706.
Lower, Richard. *Dr. Lower's, and Several Other Eminent Physicians Receipts* [...]. 2nd ed. London, 1701.
Marryat, Thomas. *The New Practice of Physick, Founded on Irrefragable Principles and Confirmed by Long and Painful Experience.* Dublin, 1764.
Moyle, John. *The Experienced Chirurgeon.* London, 1703.
Muffett, Thomas. *Healths Improvement: or, Rules Comprizing and Discovering the Nature, Method, and Manner of Preparing All Sorts of Food Used in This Nation.* London, 1655.
Nichols, John, ed. *A Supplement to Dr. Swift's Works* [...]. London, 1779.
Orrery, 5th Earl of (John Boyle). *Remarks on the Life and Writings of Dr. Jonathan Swift.* Edited and with an introduction and notes by João Fróes. Newark: University of Delaware Press, 2000.
Papin, F. "Some Observations on the Mechanic Arts, and Physic of the Indians in 1709." In *Memoirs of the Royal Society: Being a New Abridgment of the "Philosophical Transactions,"* vol. 2, edited by Benjamin Baddam, 43–46. London, [1738]–41.
Paxton, Peter. *A Directory Physico-Medical, Compos'd for the Use and Benefit of All Such as Design to Study and Practice the Art of Physick.* London, 1707.
Pearson, John. *Principles of Surgery, for the Use of Chirurgical Students.* London, 1788.
Physician. *A Treatise of Diseases of the Head, Brain, and Nerves.* London, 1711.
Physician in London. *Two Letters from a Physician in London, to a Gentleman at Bath.* London, 1749.
Pilkington, Lætitia. *Memoirs of Laetitia Pilkington.* Edited and with an introduction and notes by A. C. Elias Jr. 2 vols. Athens: University of Georgia Press, 1997.
Pope, Alexander. *The Correspondence of Alexander Pope.* Edited by George Sherburn. 5 vols. Oxford: Clarendon Press, 1956.
Pope, Alexander. *Poetry and Prose of Alexander Pope.* Edited by Aubrey Williams. New York: Houghton Mifflin, 1969.
Quincy, John. *Pharmacopoia Officinalis and Extemporanea: or, A Compleat English Dispensatory, in Four Parts.* London, 1718.
The Report of the Paris Medical Faculty, October 1348. Translated by Rosemary Horrox. Manchester: Manchester University Press, 1994.
Robinson, Nicholas. *A New Theory of Physick and Diseases, Founded on the Principles of the Newtonian Philosophy.* London, 1725.

Salmon, William. *Medicina Practica: or, The Practical Physician*. London, 1707.
Sanctorius [Santorio Santorio]. *Medicina Statica: Being the Aphorisms of Sanctorius*. Translated and annotated by John Quincy. 2nd ed. London, 1720.
Shaw, Peter, trans. *The Dispensatory of the Royal College of Physicians of Edinburgh*. London, 1727.
Shaw, Peter. *The Juice of the Grape: or, Wine Preferable to Water* [. . .]. London, 1724.
Shaw, Peter. *A New Practice of Physick* [. . .]. 2 vols. London, 1726.
Sheridan, Thomas. *The Life of the Rev. Dr. Jonathan Swift, Dean of St. Patrick's, Dublin*. London, 1784.
Short, Thomas. *A Discourse Concerning the Causes and Effects of Corpulency: Together with the Method for Its Prevention and Cure*. London, 1728.
Southwell, Thomas. *Medical Essays and Observations, Abridged from the Memoirs of the Royal Academy* [Académie Royale des Sciences]. 4 vols. London, 1764.
Sterne, Laurence. *The Life and Opinions of Tristram Shandy, Gentleman*. 9 vols. London, 1759–67.
Strother, Edward. *The Family Companion for Health: or, Plain, Easy, and Certain Rules, Which Being Punctually Observ'd and Follow'd, Will Infallibly Keep Families Free from Disease, and Procure Them a Long Life*. London, 1729.
Swieten, Gerard van. *The Commentaries upon the Aphorisms of Dr Herman Boerhaave* [. . .]. Anonymous translation. 2 vols. London, 1744–47.
Swift, Deane. *An Essay upon the Life, Writings, and Character, of Dr. Jonathan Swift*. London, 1755.
Swift, Jonathan. *The Account Books of Jonathan Swift*. Edited and with an introduction by Paul V. Thompson and Dorothy J. Thompson. Newark: University of Delaware Press, 1984.
Swift, Jonathan. *The Correspondence of Jonathan Swift*. Edited and with an introduction and notes by Harold Williams. 5 vols. Oxford: Clarendon, 1963–65.
Swift, Jonathan. *The Correspondence of Jonathan Swift, D.D.* Edited and with a preface and notes by David Woolley. Indexed by Hermann J. Real and Dirk F. Passmann. 5 vols. Frankfurt am Main: Peter Lang, 1999-2014.
Swift, Jonathan. *Directions to Servants*. Foreword by Colm Tóibín. London: Hesperus Press Limited, 2003.
Swift, Jonathan. *Gulliver's Travels*. Edited and with an introduction and notes by David Womersley. Cambridge: Cambridge University Press, 2012.
Swift, Jonathan. *Journal to Stella: Letters to Esther Johnson and Rebecca Dingley, 1710-1713*. Edited and with an introduction and notes by Abigail Williams. Cambridge: Cambridge University Press, 2013.

Swift, Jonathan. *A Letter to a Young Gentleman, Lately Enter'd into Holy Orders.* London, 1721.

Swift, Jonathan. *The Poems of Jonathan Swift.* 2nd ed. Edited and with an introduction and notes by Harold Williams. 3 vols. Oxford: Clarendon Press, 1958.

Swift, Jonathan. *The Prose Writings of Jonathan Swift.* Edited by Herbert Davis et al. 16 vols. Oxford: Basil Blackwell, 1939–74.

Swift, Jonathan. *"A Tale of a Tub" and Other Works.* Edited and with an introduction and notes by Marcus Walsh. Cambridge: Cambridge University Press, 2010.

Swift, Jonathan. "Thoughts on Various Subjects." In *Miscellanies: The Second Volume,* 273–88. London, 1731.

Sydenham, Thomas. *Dr. Sydenham's Compleat Method of Curing Almost All Diseases, and Description of Their Symptoms* [. . .]. Anonymous translator. 4th ed. London, 1710.

Temple, Sir William. *An Essay upon Health and Long Life.* In *Miscellanea: The Third Part,* edited by Jonathan Swift, 99–200. London, 1701.

Tissot, Samuel. *Onanism: or, A Treatise upon the Disorders Produced by Masturbation; or, The Dangerous Effects of Secret and Excessive Venery.* Translated by A. Hume. London, 1766.

Valangin, François Joseph Pahud de. *A Treatise on Diet, or the Management of Human Life: By Physicians Called the Six Non-Naturals.* London, 1768.

Wainewright, Jeremiah. *A Mechanical Account of the Non-Naturals.* London, 1707.

Wesley, John. *Primitive Physick: or, An Easy and Natural Method of Curing Most Diseases.* London, 1747.

Willis, Thomas. *Pharmaceutice Rationalis: or, An Exercitation of the Operations of Medicines in Humane Bodies* [. . .]. 2nd ed. London, 1679.

Wilson, Benjamin. *A Treatise on Electricity.* London, 1750.

Woodman, Philip. *Medicus Novissimus: or, The Modern Physician; Shewing the Principal Signs, Causes, and Most Material Prognosticks.* London, 1712.

Young, Edward. *Conjectures on Original Composition: In a Letter to the Author of "Sir Charles Grandison."* London, 1759.

SECONDARY SOURCES

Aikin, John, et al. *General Biography; or, Lives Critical and Historical, of the Most Eminent Persons of All Ages, Countries, Conditions, and Professions, Arranged According to Alphabetical Order.* 10 vols. London: John Stockdale et al., 1813.

Anderson, Marynita. *Physician Heal Thyself: Medical Practitioners of Eighteenth-Century New York.* New York: Peter Lang, 2004.

Arikha, Noga. *Passions and Tempers: A History of the Humours.* New York: HarperCollins, 2007.

Armintor, Deborah. "The Sexual Politics of Microscopy in Brobdingnag." *SEL: Studies in English Literature* 47, no. 3 (2007): 619–40.

Aronson, Jeffrey K. "Autopathography: The Patient's Tale." *BMJ* 321, no. 7276 (23 December 2000): 1599–602.

Arrizabalaga, Jon. "Problematizing Retrospective Diagnosis in the History of Disease." *Asclepio* 54, no. 1 (2002): 51–70.

Baloh, Robert William. *Vertigo: Five Physician Scientists and the Quest for a Cure.* New York: Oxford University Press, 2017.

Bartley, George B. "The Blindness of John Milton." *Mayo Clinic Proceedings* 68, no. 4 (1 April 1993): 395–99.

Beier, Lucinda McCray. *Sufferers and Healers.* New York: Routledge, 1987.

Benedict, Leah. "The Body [in Swift]." In *Jonathan Swift in Context*, edited by Joseph Hone and Pat Rogers, 327–34. Cambridge: Cambridge University Press, 2024.

Bewley, Thomas H. "The Health of Jonathan Swift." *Journal of the Royal Society of Medicine* 91, no. 11 (November 1998): 602–5.

Borman, Tracy. *King's Mistress, Queen's Servant: The Life and Times of Henrietta Howard.* London: Jonathan Cape, 2007.

Boucé, Paul-Gabriel. "Gulliver Phallophorus and the Maids of Honour in Brobdingnag." *Revue de la Société d'Études Anglo-Américaines des XVIIe et XVIIIe Siècles*, no. 53 (2001): 81–98.

Brady, Frank, ed. *Twentieth-Century Interpretations of "Gulliver's Travels": A Collection of Critical Essays.* Englewood Cliffs, NJ: Prentice, 1968.

Brain, Walter Russell. "The Illness of Dean Swift." *Irish Journal of Medical Science*, 6th series, nos. 320–21 (1952): 337–45.

Brown, Norman O. "The Excremental Vision." In *Life Against Death*, 179–201. Middletown: Wesleyan University Press, 1959. Reprinted in *Swift: A Collection of Critical Essays*, edited by Ernest Tuveson, 31–54. Englewood Cliffs, NJ: Prentice-Hall, 1964.

Bucknill, J[ohn] C[harles]. "Dean Swift's Disease." *Brain: A Journal of Neurology* 4, no. 4 (January 1882): 493–506. Reprinted in *Popular Science Monthly* 20 (April 1882): 806–17. Page numbers refer to the reprint.

Case, Arthur. "Swift and Sir William Temple—A Conjecture." *Modern Language Notes* 60, no. 4 (April 1945): 259–65.

Child, Paul William. "Jonathan Swift's Latin Quacks: 'A Consultation of Four Physicians upon a Lord That Was Dying.'" *Cambridge Quarterly* 40, no. 1 (March 2011): 21–35.

Child, Paul William. "Once More into the Breech: Jonathan Swift and Excremental Medicine." *Swift Studies*, no. 20 (2005): 82–101.

Child, Paul William. "Swift's 'Carefull' Nurse and Sick Relations." In *From Enlightenment to Rebellion: Essays in Honor of Christopher Fox*, edited by James Buickerood, 133–49. Lewisburg, PA: Bucknell University Press, 2018.

Clark, Paul Odell. "A *Gulliver* Dictionary." *Studies in Philology* 50, no. 4 (October 1953): 592–624.

Cockayne, Emily. "Experiences of the Deaf in Early Modern England." *Historical Journal* 46, no. 3 (2003): 493–510.

Cohen, Helen, Lana R. Ewell, and Herman A. Jenkins. "Disability in Ménière's Disease." *Archives of Otolaryngology—Head and Neck Surgery* 121 (January 1995): 29–33.

Cook, Daniel. "Lord Orrery's *Remarks on Swift* and Literary Biography after 1750." *Eighteenth-Century Ireland / Iris an dá Chultúr*, no. 28 (2013): 62–77.

Cook, Harold J. *The Decline of the Old Medical Regime in Stuart London*. Ithaca, NY: Cornell University Press, 1986.

Cotter, John. "The Hundred Oceans of Jonathan Swift." *Raritan* 39, no. 4 (2020): 128–50.

Couser, Thomas. *Recovering Bodies: Illness, Disability, and Life Writing*. Madison: University of Wisconsin Press, 1997.

Creaser, Wanda. "'The Most Mortifying Malady': Jonathan Swift's World and Dublin's Mentally Ill." *Swift Studies*, no. 19 (2004): 27–48.

Creaser, Wanda. "Shifting Identities in the Life and Writings of Jonathan Swift." PhD diss., Arizona State University, 2000.

Creighton, Charles. "Cockburn, William (1669–1739)." In *Oxford Dictionary of National Biography*, revised by Anita Guerrini. Oxford University Press. Article published 2004; last modified 2021. https://doi-org.shsu.idm.oclc.org/10.1093/ref:odnb/5777.

Crichton, Paul. "Jonathan Swift and Alzheimer's Disease." *Lancet* 342, no. 8875 (2 October 1993): 874.

Cunningham, Andrew. "Identifying Disease in the Past: Cutting the Gordian Knot." *Asclepio* 54, no. 1 (2002): 13–34.

Dale, Philip Marshall. *Medical Biographies: The Ailments of Thirty-Three Famous Persons*. Norman: University of Oklahoma Press, 1952.

Dalrymple, Theodore. "The Greatest Torture." *British Medical Journal* 338, no. 7697 (28 March 2009): 777.

Damrosch, Leo. *Jonathan Swift: His Life and His World*. New Haven, CT: Yale University Press, 2013.

"Dean Swift's Deafness." *British Medical Journal* 2, no. 4154 (17 August 1940): 233.

"Dean Swift's Disease." *Medical Press and Circular* [Dublin], 15 February 1882, 142.

Deane, Seamus. "Swift and the Anglo-Irish Intellect." *Eighteenth-Century Ireland / Iris an dá Chultúr*, no. 1 (1986): 9–22.

DePorte, Michael. "Teaching the Third Voyage." In *Approaches to Teaching Swift's "Gulliver's Travels,"* edited by Edward J. Rielly, 57–62. New York: Modern Language Association, 1988.

Deutsch, Helen. "'Alas, poor Yorick!': Jonathan Swift, Madness and Fashionable Science." In *Disease and Death in Eighteenth-Century Literature and Culture: Fashioning the Unfashionable*, edited by Allan Ingram and Leigh Wetherall Dickson, 225–45. London: Palgrave Macmillan, 2016.

Deutsch, Helen. "Health and Sickness [in Swift]." In *Jonathan Swift in Context*, edited by Joseph Hone and Pat Rogers, 18–25. Cambridge: Cambridge University Press, 2024.

Dickie, Simon. "Hilarity and Pitilessness in the Mid-Eighteenth Century: English Jestbook Humor." *Eighteenth-Century Studies* 37, no. 1 (Fall 2003): 1–22.

Doody, Margaret Anne. "Swift and Women." In *The Cambridge Companion to Jonathan Swift*, edited by Christopher Fox, 87–111. Cambridge: Cambridge University Press, 2003.

Duden, Barbara. "Fluxes and Stagnations: A Physician's Perception and Treatment of Humours in Baroque Ladies." In *The Body in Balance: Humoral Medicines in Practice*, edited by Peregrine Horden and Elisabeth Hsu, 53–68. New York: Berghahn, 2013.

Ehrenpreis, Irvin. *Swift: The Man, His Works, and the Age*. 3 vols. Cambridge, MA: Harvard University Press, 1962–83.

Ehrenpreis, Irvin. "Swift's 'Little Language' in the 'Journal to Stella.'" *Studies in Philology* 45, no. 1 (January 1948): 80–88.

Fabricant, Carole. *Swift's Landscape*. Baltimore, MD: Johns Hopkins University Press, 1982.

Ferenczi, Sandor. "Gulliver's Phantasies." *International Journal of Psychoanalysis*, no. 9 (1928): 283–300.

Fissell, Mary E. "The Marketplace of Print." In *Medicine and the Market in England and Its Colonies, c. 1450–c. 1850*, edited by Mark S. R. Jenner and Patrick Wallis, 108–32. London: Palgrave Macmillan, 2007.

Fissell, Mary E. "Popular Medical Books." In *Oxford History of Popular Print Culture, Volume 1: Beginning to 1660*, edited by Joad Raymond, 418–31. New York: Oxford University Press, 2011.

Flynn, Carol Houlihan. *The Body in Swift and Defoe*. Cambridge: Cambridge University Press, 1990.

Foucault, Michel. *The Birth of the Clinic: An Archaeology of Medical Perception.* Translated by A. M. Sheridan. London: Routledge, 1989.

Fox, Christopher, ed. *The Cambridge Companion to Jonathan Swift.* Cambridge: Cambridge University Press, 2003.

Fox, Christopher. "A Critical History of *Gulliver's Travels.*" In *"Gulliver's Travels": Complete, Authoritative Text with Biographical and Historical Contexts, Critical History, and Essays from Five Contemporary Critical Perspectives,* edited by Christopher Fox, 269–304. Boston: Bedford Books of St. Martin's Press, 1995.

Fox, Christopher. "Of Logic and Lycanthropy: Gulliver and the Faculties of the Mind." In *Literature and Medicine During the Eighteenth Century,* edited by Marie Mulvey Roberts and Roy Porter, 101–17. London: Routledge, 1993.

Foxhall, Katherine. "Making Modern Migraine Medieval: Men of Science, Hildegard of Bingen and the Life of a Retrospective Diagnosis." *Medical History* 58, no. 3 (2014): 354–74.

Frank, Arthur. *At the Will of the Body: Reflections on Illness.* Boston: Houghton Mifflin, 1991.

Freedman, William. "Gulliver's Voyage to the Country of the Houyhnhnms: Adolescence and the Resurgence of the Instincts." *International Review of Psychoanalysis* 13, no. 4 (1986): 473–87.

Gillam, Stephen. "The Reappearance of the Sick Man: A Landmark Publication Revisited." *British Journal of General Practice* 66, no. 653 (2016): 616–17.

Glendinning, Victoria. *Jonathan Swift: A Portrait.* New York: Henry Holt & Company, 1998.

Goffman, Erving. *Frame Analysis: An Essay on the Organization of Experience.* Cambridge, MA: Harvard University Press, 1974.

Gordin, Michael D. "The Problem with Pseudoscience: Pseudoscience Is Not the Antithesis of Professional Science but Thrives in Science's Shadow." *EMBO Reports* 18, no. 9 (September 2017): 1482–85.

Gosse, Edmund. *A History of Eighteenth-Century Literature (1660–1780).* London: Macmillan and Co., 1889.

Gould, George. "The Case of Jonathan Swift." *Interstate Medical Journal* 15, nos. 11–12 (1908): 878–90, 943–59.

Green, Monica. "The Value of Historical Perspective." In *The Ashgate Research Companion to the Globalization of Health,* edited by Ted Schrecker, 17–38. Farnham: Ashgate, 2012.

Greenacre, Phyllis. "The Mutual Adventures of Jonathan Swift and Lemuel Gulliver." *Psychoanalytic Quarterly,* no. 24 (1955): 20–62.

Guerrini, Anita. *Obesity and Depression in the Enlightenment: The Life and Times of George Cheyne.* Norman: University of Oklahoma Press, 2000.

Hammond, Brean. *Jonathan Swift*. Newbridge, County Kildare: Irish Academic Press, 2010.

Hammond, Brean. "Scriblerian Self-Fashioning." *Yearbook of English Studies*, no. 18 (1988): 108–24.

Hammond, Eugene. *Jonathan Swift: Irish Blow-In*. Newark: University of Delaware Press, 2016.

Hammond, Eugene. *Jonathan Swift: Our Dean*. Newark: University of Delaware Press, 2016.

Handley, Sasha. *Sleep in Early Modern England*. New Haven, CT: Yale University Press, 2016.

Hawkins, Anne Hunsaker. *Reconstructing Illness: Studies in Pathography*. Lafayette, IN: Purdue University Press, 1999.

Hoskison, Emma. "Gulliver's Vertigo." Paper presented at the Annual Meeting of the British Society of the History of ENT, London, 3 December 2015.

Illich, Ivan. *Limits to Medicine. Medical Nemesis: The Expropriation of Health*. London: Marion Boyars, 1975.

Ingram, Allan. *Swift, Pope and the Doctors: Medicine and Writing in the Early Eighteenth Century*. Paderborn: Brill Fink, 2022.

Ishizuka, Hisao. "'Fibre Body': The Concept of Fibre in Eighteenth-Century Medicine, c. 1700–40." *Medical History* 56, no. 4 (2012): 562–84.

Jaffe, Nora Crow. *The Poet Swift*. Hanover, NH: University Press of New England, 1977.

James, Ioan. *Asperger's Syndrome and High Achievement: Some Very Remarkable People*. London: Jessica Kingsley Publishers, 2006.

Jewson, Nicholas D. "The Disappearance of the Sick-Man from Medical Cosmology, 1770–1870." *Sociology* 10, no. 2 (1976): 225–44.

Jewson, Nicholas D. "Medical Knowledge and the Patronage System in 18th Century England." *Sociology* 8, no. 3 (1974): 369–85.

Johnston, Denis. *In Search of Swift*. Dublin: Hodges Figgis & Co., 1959.

Karenberg, Axel. "Retrospective Diagnosis: Use and Abuse in Medical Historiography." *Prague Medical Report* 110, no. 2 (2009): 140–45.

Karpman, Ben. "A Modern Gulliver: A Study in Coprophilia." *Psychoanalytic Review* 36, nos. 2–3 (April and July 1949): 162–85, 260–82.

Kelly, James. "'Drinking the Waters': Balneotherapeutic Medicine in Ireland, 1660–1850." *Studia Hibernica* 35 (January 2008): 99–146.

Kiehl, Kent, and Julian Lushing. "Psychopathy." *Scholarpedia, the Peer-Reviewed Open Access Encyclopedia*. Last modified May 14, 2014. http://www.scholarpedia.org/article/Psychopathy.

King, Helen. "Female Fluids in the Hippocratic Corpus: How Solid Was the Humoral Body?" In *The Body in Balance: Humoral Medicines in Practice*, edited by Peregrine Horden and Elisabeth Hsu, 25–52. New York: Berghahn, 2013.

King, Lester S. *The Medical World of the Eighteenth Century.* Chicago: University of Chicago Press, 1958.

Kirby, Sarah E., and Lucy Yardley. "Cognitions Associated with Anxiety in Ménière's Disease." *Journal of Psychosomatic Research* 66, no. 2 (February 2009): 111–18.

LaCasce, Steward. "Swift on Medical Extremism." *Journal of the History of Ideas*, no. 31 (1970): 599–606.

Laqueur, Walter. "The Question of Judgment: Intelligence and Medicine." *Journal of Contemporary History* 18, no. 4 (1983): 533–48.

Larner, A. J. "Retrospective Diagnosis: Pitfalls and Purposes [Editorial]." *Journal of Medical Biography* 27, no. 3 (2019): 127–28.

Lecky, William. *The Leaders of Public Opinion in Ireland.* London: Saunders, Ottley, 1861.

Le Fanu, T. P. "The Catalogue of Dean Swift's Library in 1715, with an Inventory of His Personal Property in 1742." *Proceedings of the Royal Irish Academy* 37, sect. C, no. 13 (1927): 263–75.

Legg, J. Wickham. "Swift's Giddy Fits." *The Academy* 19, no. 477 (25 June 1881): 475.

Lewis, John M. "Jonathan Swift and Alzheimer's Disease." *Lancet* 342, no. 8869 (21 August 1993): 504.

Lorch, Marjorie Perlman. "Language and Memory Disorder in the Case of Jonathan Swift: Considerations on Retrospective Diagnosis." *Brain* 129, no. 11 (2006): 3127–37.

Lyle, Ian. "Bernard, Charles (bap. 1652, d. 1710)." In *Oxford Dictionary of National Biography.* Oxford University Press. Published 2004; last modified 2004. https://doi-org.shsu.idm.oclc.org/10.1093/ref:odnb/2238.

Lynall, Gregory. *Swift and Science: The Satire, Politics, and Theology of Natural Knowledge, 1690–1730.* London: Palgrave Macmillan, 2012.

Macalpine, Ida, and Richard Hunter. *George III and the Mad-Business.* London: Allen Lane, 1969.

Mahony, Robert. *Jonathan Swift: The Irish Identity.* New Haven, CT: Yale University Press, 1995.

Malcolm, Elizabeth. *Swift's Hospital: A History of St. Patrick's Hospital, Dublin, 1746–1989.* Dublin: Gill and Macmillan, 1989.

McKeon, Michael. *The Origins of the English Novel 1600–1740.* Baltimore, MD: Johns Hopkins University Press, 1987.

McMinn, Joseph. "Swift and the Formation of an Anglo-Irish Identity." *Eighteenth-Century Ireland / Iris an dá Chultúr*, no. 2 (1987): 103–13.

Melamed, Chaim. "Gulliver and the *Other*: A Psychoanalytical Examination." PhD diss., University of Montreal, 1995.

Ménière, Prosper. "Ménière's Original Papers." Translated by M. Atkinson. *Acta Otolaryngolica*, no. 162 (1961): 1–78.

Mitchell, Piers. "Retrospective Diagnosis and the Use of Historical Texts for Investigating Disease in the Past." *International Journal of Paleopathology*, no. 1 (2011): 81–88.

Mounsey, Chris, ed. *The Idea of Disability in the Eighteenth Century*. Lewisburg, PA: Bucknell University Press, 2014.

Muramoto, Osamu. "Retrospective Diagnosis of a Famous Historical Figure: Ontological, Epistemic, and Ethical Considerations." *Philosophy, Ethics, and Humanities in Medicine* 9, no. 10 (2014): 1–15. https://doi.org/10.1186/1747-5341-9-10.

Niebyl, Peter. "The Non-Naturals." *Bulletin of the History of Medicine*, no. 45 (1971): 486–92.

Nokes, David. *Jonathan Swift, a Hypocrite Reversed: A Critical Biography*. New York: Oxford University Press, 1985.

Ober, William. *Boswell's Clap and Other Essays: Medical Analyses of Literary Men's Afflictions*. Carbondale: Southern Illinois University Press, 1979.

Orwell, George. "Politics vs. Literature: An Examination of *Gulliver's Travels*." In *The Collected Essays, Journalism, and Letters of George Orwell*, edited by Sonia Orwell and Ian Angus, vol. 4, 205–23. New York: Harcourt, Brace & World, 1968.

Parsons, Talcott. *The Social System*. London: Free Press of Glencoe, 1951.

Passmann, Dirk F., and Hermann J. Real. "Annotating J. S. Swift's Reading at Moor Park in 1697/8." In *Reading Swift: Papers from the Seventh Münster Symposium on Jonathan Swift*, edited by Janika Bischof, Kirsten Juhas, and Hermann J. Real, 101–24. Munich: Wilhelm Fink, 2019.

Pelling, Margaret. "Medical Practice in Early Modern England: Trade or Profession?" In *The Professions in Early Modern England*, edited by Wilfrid Prest, 90–128. London: Croom Helm, 1987.

Pelling, Margaret, and Charles Webster. "Medical Practitioners." In *Health, Medicine, and Mortality in the Sixteenth Century*, edited by Charles Webster, 165–235. Cambridge: Cambridge University Press, 1979.

"[Phrenological Examination of Jonathan Swift's Skull]. Article XIII. Dublin Phrenological Society." *Phrenological Journal and Miscellany*, no. 9 (September 1834–March 1836): 558–90.

Porter, Roy. *English Society in the Eighteenth Century*. Rev. ed. London: Penguin Books, 1982.

Porter, Roy. *Flesh in the Age of Reason*. New York: W. W. Norton & Company, 2003.

Porter, Roy. *Health for Sale: Quackery in England, 1660–1850*. Manchester: Manchester University Press, 1989.

Porter, Roy. "Lay Medical Knowledge in the Eighteenth Century: The Evidence of the *Gentleman's Magazine*." *Medical History*, no. 29 (1985): 138–68.

Porter, Roy. *Mind-Forg'd Manacles: A History of Madness in England from the Restoration to the Regency*. London: Penguin Books, 1987.

Porter, Roy, ed. *Patients and Practitioners: Lay Perceptions of Medicine in Pre-Industrial Society*. Cambridge: Cambridge University Press, 1985.

Porter, Roy. "The Patient's View: Doing Medical History from Below." *Theory and Society* 14, no. 2 (March 1985): 175–98.

Porter, Roy, ed. *The Popularization of Medicine, 1650–1850*. London: Routledge, 1992.

Porter, Roy, and Dorothy Porter. *Patient's Progress: Doctors and Doctoring in Eighteenth-Century England*. Stanford, CA: Stanford University Press, 1989.

Porter, Roy, and G. S. Rousseau. *Gout: The Patrician Malady*. New Haven, CT: Yale University Press, 1998.

Portmann, Georges. "The Old and New in Meniere's Disease—Over 60 Years in Retrospect and a Look to the Future." In "Symposium on Meniere's Disease," edited by I. Kaufman Arenberg, 567–75. Special issue, *Otolaryngologic Clinics of North America* 13, no. 4 (November 1980): 565–787.

Probyn, Clive. "Swift and the Physicians: Aspects of Satire and Status." *Medical History* 18, no. 3 (July 1974): 249–61.

Prout, Andrew. *The Reliques of Father Prout, Late P.P. of Watergrasshill, in the County of Cork, Ireland*. Edited by Oliver Yorke (Francis Sylvester Mahony). London: H. G. Bohn, 1860.

Rather, L. J. "The 'Six Things Non-Natural': A Note on the Origins and Fate of a Doctrine and a Phrase." *Clio Medica*, no. 3 (1968): 337–47.

Rawson, Claude. "Gulliver and the Gentle Reader." In *Imagined Worlds: Essays on Some English Novels and Novelists in Honour of John Butt*, edited by Maynard Mack and Ian Gregor, 51–90. London: Methuen, 1968.

Rawson, Claude. *Gulliver and the Gentle Reader: Studies in Swift and Our Time*. London: Routledge & Kegan Paul, 1973.

Rawson, Claude, ed. *Jonathan Swift: A Collection of Critical Essays*. Englewood Cliffs, NJ: Prentice Hall, 1995.

Rawson, Claude. *Swift's Angers*. Cambridge: Cambridge University Press, 2014.

Reilly, Patrick. "The Displaced Person: Swift and Ireland." *Swift Studies*, no. 8 (1993): 68–82.

Reilly, Patrick. *Jonathan Swift: The Brave Desponder.* Carbondale: Southern Illinois University Press, 1982.

Rosenberg, Charles. "Framing Disease: Illness, Society, and History." Introduction to *Framing Disease: Studies in Cultural History*, edited by Charles E. Rosenberg and Janet Lynne Golden, xiii–xxvi. New Brunswick, NJ: Rutgers University Press, 1992.

Ross, John J. *Shakespeare's Tremor and Orwell's Cough: Diagnosing the Medical Groans and Last Gasps of Ten Great Writers.* New York: St. Martin's Griffin, 2012.

Rubin, Wallace. "The Natural History of the Vertigo Component of Meniere's Disease." In "Symposium on Meniere's Disease," edited by I. Kaufman Arenberg, 621–24. Special issue, *The Otolaryngologic Clinics of North America* 13, no. 4 (November 1980): 565–787.

Rushdy, Ashraf. "A New Emetics of Interpretation: Swift, His Critics and the Alimentary Canal." *Mosaic* 23, nos. 3–4 (June 1991): 1–32.

San Juan, E. "The Anti-Poetry of Jonathan Swift." *Philological Quarterly* 44, no. 3 (1 July 1965): 387–96.

Scott, Sir Walter. *Life of Swift.* Vol. 2 of *The Miscellaneous Prose Works of Sir Walter Scott, Bart.* Edinburgh: Robert Cadell, 1834.

Seidel, Michael. "*Gulliver's Travels* and the Contracts of Fiction." In *The Cambridge Companion to the Eighteenth-Century Novel*, edited by John Richetti, 72–89. Cambridge: Cambridge University Press, 1996.

Shackelford, Jole. Review of *"Divulging of Useful Truths in Physick": The Medical Agenda of Robert Boyle*, by Barbara Beigun Kaplan. *Journal of the History of the Behavioral Sciences* 32, no. 3 (July 1996): 256–58.

Shapiro, S. L. "The Medical History of Jonathan Swift." *Eye, Ear, Nose and Throat Monthly* 48, no. 8 (August 1969): 486–89.

Shinagel, Michael, ed. *A Concordance to the Poems of Jonathan Swift.* Ithaca, NY: Cornell University Press, 1972.

Shuttleton, David. *Smallpox and the Literary Imagination 1660–1820.* Cambridge: Cambridge University Press, 2007.

Siebers, Tobin. *Disability Theory.* Ann Arbor: University of Michigan Press, 2008.

Smith, Frederik N., ed. *The Genres of "Gulliver's Travels."* Newark: University of Delaware Press, 1990.

Spence, Joseph. *Observations, Anecdotes, and Characters of Books and Men.* Edited by James M. Osborn. 2 vols. Oxford: Clarendon Press, 1966.

Stolberg, Michael. "'You Have No Good Blood in Your Body': Oral Communication in Sixteenth-Century Physicians' Medical Practice." *Medical History* 59, no. 1 (January 2015): 63–82.

Stone, Edward. "Swift and the Horses: Misanthropy or Comedy?" *Modern Language Quarterly* 10, no. 3 (September 1949): 367–76.

Stubbs, John. *Jonathan Swift: The Reluctant Rebel*. New York: W. W. Norton & Company, 2016.

Takeda, Taizo, et al. "Decompression Effects of Erythritol on Endolymphatic Hydrops." *Auris Nasus Larynx* 36, no. 2 (April 2009): 146–51.

Temkin, Owsei. "The Scientific Approach to Disease: Specific Entity and Individual Sickness." In *Scientific Change: Historical Studies in the Intellectual, Social and Technical Conditions for Scientific Discovery and Technical Invention from Antiquity to the Present*, edited by A. C. Crombie, 629–47. New York: Basic Books, 1963.

Thackeray, William Makepeace. *The English Humourists of the Eighteenth Century: A Series of Lectures Delivered in England, Scotland, and the United States of America*. London: Smith, Elder, & Co., 1853.

Todd, Dennis. *Imagining Monsters: Miscreations of the Self in Eighteenth-Century England*. Chicago: University of Chicago Press, 1995.

Turner, David M. "Disability Humor and the Meanings of Impairment in Early Modern England." In *Recovering Disability in Early Modern England*, edited by Allison P. Hobgood and David Houston Wood, 57–72. Columbus: Ohio State University Press, 2013.

Turner, David M. *Disability in Eighteenth-Century England: Imagining Physical Impairment*. New York: Routledge, 2012.

Verwaal, Ruben E. "Fluid Deafness: Earwax and Hardness of Hearing in Early Modern Europe." *Medical History* 65, no. 4 (October 2021): 366–83.

Wagner, Darren Neil. "Sex, Spirits, and Sensibility: Human Generation in British Medicine, Anatomy, and Literature, 1660–1780." PhD diss., University of York, 2013.

Washington, Gene. "Swift's Ménière's Syndrome and *Gulliver's Travels*." *Swift Studies*, no. 10 (1995): 104–7.

Washington, Gene. "Swift's Struldbruggs and Alzheimer's Disease." *The Scriblerian*, no. 27 (1994): 92–93.

Watt, Nicholas. "Gulliver Described His Creator's Illness." *The Times*, 24 August 1993, 4.

Wear, Andrew. *Knowledge and Practice in English Medicine, 1550–1680*. Cambridge: Cambridge University Press, 2000.

Wear, Andrew. "Medical Practice in Late Seventeenth- and Early Eighteenth-Century England: Continuity and Union." In *The Medical Revolution of the Seventeenth Century*, edited by Roger French and Andrew Wear, 294–320. Cambridge: Cambridge University Press, 1989.

Weinbrot, Howard. *Menippean Satire Reconsidered: From Antiquity to the Eighteenth Century*. Baltimore, MD: Johns Hopkins University Press, 2005.

Weisser, Olivia. *Ill Composed: Sickness, Gender, and Belief in Early Modern England*. New Haven, CT: Yale University Press, 2015.

Whitley, E. M. "Contextual Analysis and Swift's Little Language of the *Journal to Stella*." In *In Memory of J. R. Firth*, edited by C. E. Bazell et al., 475–90. London: Longman, 1966.

Wilde, Sir William. *The Closing Years of Dean Swift's Life; with Remarks on Stella, and on Some of His Writings Hitherto Unnoticed*. 2nd rev. ed. Dublin: Hodges and Smith, 1849.

Williams, Harold. *Dean Swift's Library, with a Facsimile of the Original Sale Catalogue and Some Account of Two Manuscript Lists of His Books*. Cambridge: Cambridge University Press, 1932.

Williams, Henry. "Definition of Terms in Meniere's Disease." In "Symposium on Meniere's Disease," edited by Jack L. Pulec, 267–72. Special issue, *Otolaryngologic Clinics of North America* 1, no. 2 (January 1968): 265–715.

Wilson, T. G. "The Mental and Physical Health of Dean Swift." *Medical History* 2, no. 3 (July 1958): 175–90.

Wilson, T. G. "Swift's Deafness and His Last Illness." *Irish Journal of Medical Science*, 6th series, no. 162 (1939): 241–56.

Womersley, David. "'now deaf 1740': Entrapment, Foreboding, and Exorcism in Late Swift." In *Politics and Literature in the Age of Swift: English and Irish Perspectives*, edited by Claude Rawson, 162–84. Cambridge: Cambridge University Press, 2010.

Yunck, John A. "The Skeptical Faith of Jonathan Swift." *The Personalist*, no. 42 (1961): 533–54.

INDEX

Acheson, Lady Anne, 90, 93
Acheson, Sir Arthur, 90
acute disease, 9–10, 34, 35, 51, 55, 59, 75, 83–84, 158. *See also* Swift, Jonathan: shingles
Addison, Joseph, 57, 203n37, 225n82
Aesop, 143, 235n20
Alcock, Nathan, 190n30
Alcock, Thomas, 190n30
Allen, John, 197n59
Andersen, Hans Christian, 29
animal spirits, 40–41, 44–46, 47, 82, 196n51, 198n76
Anne, Queen of England, 9, 57, 65, 81, 87, 115, 167, 189n10, 202n29, 203n40, 220n19
Arbuthnot, John, xiv, 12, 15, 39–40, 42, 52, 54, 55, 57, 58, 60–63, 69, 76, 87, 88, 104, 106–7, 111, 120, 163, 177–80, 185n39, 187n56, 202n22, 202n29, 205n64, 205n66, 205n74, 209n16, 210n47, 215n23, 221n24, 223n51, 228n113, 244n12; *An Essay Concerning the Effects of Air on Human Bodies*, 15; *An Essay Concerning the Nature of Aliments, and the Choice of Them, According to the Different Constitutions of Human Bodies*, 15; *John Bull Still in His Senses*, 39–40, 221n24
Arikha, Noga, 13, 184n25, 188n63

Aristotle, 11, 47, 175
Armintor, Deborah, 233n97
Aronson, Jeffrey K., 189n6
Arrizabalaga, Jon, 193n67
Augustine of Hippo, 199n98
Austen, Jane, 29
autopathography, 18, 19–20, 35, 103, 189n6

Bacon, Francis, 216n39
Barber, John, 46, 75, 77, 80, 88, 90, 108, 110, 133, 237n5
Barber, Mary, 104, 110, 210n47
Barnard, Mrs., 217n50
Barton, Catherine, 85
Bathurst, Allen, First Earl Bathurst, 76
Beach, Mary, 112, 223n50
Beaumont, Joseph, 115
Beaumont, Sir George, 115
Beddoes, Thomas, 26, 27, 196n46
Behn, Aphra, 97
Beier, Lucinda McCray, 52
Benedict, Leah, 229n21
Berkeley, George, 44, 98
Bernard, Charles, 19, 189n10
Bickerton, G., 40, 41
Bindon, Francis, 25
Blachford, John, 58
Blankaart, Steven, 44–45, 80; *The Physical Dictionary*, 44, 80

Blayney, Seventh Lord (Cadwallader Blayney), 102–3
Boerhaave, Herman, 4–5, 52, 202n29
Bolingbroke, First Viscount (Henry St. John), 77, 87, 104, 106, 108–9, 111, 113, 114, 115, 169, 185n38, 204n51, 210n35, 210n47, 211n54, 220n19, 224n71
Bolingbroke, Viscountess (Marie-Claire Marcilly), 65, 111
Borman, Tracy, 227n104
Boswell, James, 159, 227n107
Boucé, Paul-Gabriel, 233n97
Boyle, John, Fifth Earl of Orrery. *See* Orrery, Fifth Earl of (John Boyle)
Boyle, Margaret, Lady Orrery, 117–18, 211n51
Boyle, Robert, 12, 16, 52
Brady, Frank, 160
Brent, Mrs. John (Swift's housekeeper), 80, 91
Brookes, Richard, 72, 244n17
Brown, Joseph, 197n54
Brown, Norman O., 236n36
Bucknill, John, 3, 4, 6, 28, 31, 32, 125, 192n53
Bulwer, John, 216n39; *Philocophus, or, The Deafe and Dumbe Mans Friend*, 216n39
Burns, Robert, 29
Burton, John, 208n8
Burton, Robert, 95, 159, 175, 239n54; *The Anatomy of Melancholy*, 239n54

Campbell, Archibald, Earl of Islay, 109
Campbell, Robert, 55; *The London Tradesman*, 55
Caroline of Ansbach, Queen of England, 121, 227n110
Carroll, Lewis, 29
Case, Arthur, 36–37, 194n23
Celsus (Aulus Cornelius Celsus), 53
Cervantes, Miguel de, 175

Chambers, Ephraim, 183n11, 188n74; *Cyclopædia*, 183n11, 188n74
Charles I, King of England, 163
Charles II, King of England, 46, 49, 162, 164
Chesterfield, Fourth Earl of (Philip Dormer Stanhope), 167
Chetwode, Knightley, 43, 59, 71, 83, 88, 89, 94, 106, 127, 215n19, 224n65
Cheyne, George, 9–10, 14–15, 17, 18, 47, 50, 51, 52, 53, 59, 67, 68–69, 74, 75, 84, 92, 185n29, 185n39, 188n68, 188n75, 189n6, 200n2, 209–10nn35–36, 217n56, 236n44; "The Case of the Author," 189n6; *The English Malady*, 68, 210n36; *An Essay of Health and Long Life*, 15, 68, 92, 217n56; *An Essay on Regimen*, 53, 68; *A New Theory of Continu'd Fevers*, 188n68, 188n75; *Philosophical Principles of Natural Religion*, 236n44
Child, Paul William, 182n4, 203n38, 236n40, 242n35
Chomel, Noel, 53; *Dictionary Oeconomique*, 53
Civil War, English, 163–64, 165, 170
Clark, Paul Odell, 231n58
clinical diagnosis, xi, xii, xiv, xv, 2, 3, 4–7, 25–33, 42, 124–25, 130, 161, 182n11, 185n41, 191n41, 192n53, 192n57, 193n67, 194n18, 228n3. *See also* Ménière's disease; retrospective diagnosis
Cockburn, William, 12, 19, 40–41, 52, 54, 57–58, 64, 82, 185n39, 187n56, 189n10, 203n43, 210n38
Compton, Sir Spencer, 109
Cook, Daniel, 190n16
Cook, Harold, 63, 206n81
Cook, John, 10
Cooper, Thomas, 11
Cope, Henry, 206n82
Cope, Robert, 244n10

corpuscular theory, 11, 12, 16
Couser, Thomas, 34, 35, 189n6; *Recovering Bodies*, 189n6
Creaser, Wanda, 182n4, 193n65
Cromwell, Oliver, 49
Culpeper, Nicholas, 71, 158, 207n90, 209n18; *The English Physician*, 209n18
Cunningham, Andrew, 4, 6, 193n67

Dale, Philip Marshall, 192n53
Daly ("Deally"), Charles, 58, 203n46
Damrosch, Leo, 3, 96, 213n71, 240n13
Deane, Seamus, 98, 143
Defoe, Daniel, 18, 97, 239n43; *Robinson Crusoe*, 18, 50, 239n43
deformity, 142–43, 155, 158, 162–63, 234n4, 234n6
Delany, Patrick, 23–24, 25, 37–38, 40, 73, 82, 83, 142–43, 149, 159, 165, 192n59, 205n66, 220n7, 230n24
DePorte, Michael, 155
Deutsch, Helen, 173, 191n33
Dickie, Simon, 143, 234n6
Dickinson, Emily, 29
digestion (coction, concoction), 8, 10–11, 12, 14, 15, 26–27, 37, 38, 39, 40, 41, 45–46, 63, 70, 71, 72, 73, 75–77, 80, 82, 162, 179, 180, 184n26, 184n28, 186nn46–47, 195n31, 205n78
Dingley, Rebecca, xvi, 19, 34, 37, 57, 62–63, 64, 65, 69, 71, 74, 77, 78, 79, 85, 87, 90, 94, 110, 115, 116, 118, 119–20, 168, 193n1, 203n40, 213n89, 226n93, 226n95, 227n109, 232n94, 244n17
Dioscorides (Pedanius Dioscorides), 53
disability, xiii–xiv, 29, 35, 91, 92, 111, 112, 115, 118, 142–43, 189n6, 193n70, 222n43, 234nn3–4, 234n6
Dorset, Duchess of (Elizabeth Sackville), 81
Dorset, Seventh Earl and First Duke of (Lionel Cranfield Sackville), 102, 205n66

Dryden, John, 162–63, 240n4, 241n30; *Absalom and Achitophel*, 162–63, 240n4, 241n30
Dublin Commission of Lunacy, 2, 221n21

Ehrenpreis, Irvin, 2, 89, 112, 125–26, 219n100, 229n11, 231n58
Elias, A. S., 190n16
Ettmüller, Michael, 197n59
Evans, John, Bishop of Meath, 106, 107
Exclusion Crisis, 162–63, 164

Fabricant, Carole, 48
Faulkner, George, 23, 168–69, 195n29, 242n36
Ferenczi, Sandor, 191n37, 229n19
Fernel, Jean, 182n11
Fielding, Henry, 97
Fissell, Mary, 53, 201n12
Flood, Frances, 189n6; *The Devonshire Woman*, 189n6
Floyer, Sir John, 196n43, 211n49
Flynn, Carol Houlihan, 78, 172, 173, 199n92, 212n71
Ford, Charles, 35, 52, 58, 63, 65, 77, 81–82, 87, 89, 92, 94, 103, 104, 105, 107, 110, 126, 137, 201n17, 202n19, 202n29, 210n47, 211n54, 221n27, 223n44
Forster, John, 36
Foucault, Michel, 5, 25, 183n11; *The Birth of the Clinic*, 183n11
Fountaine, Sir Andrew, 64, 115
Fox, Christopher, 155, 228n6, 229n19
Foxhall, Katherine, 193n67
Frank, Arthur, xv
Freedman, William, 191n37
Freind, John, 58
Freudian critics, 25, 152, 191n37, 229n19, 236n36
Fuller, Francis, 80; *Medicina Gymnastica*, 80

266   INDEX

Fuller, Thomas, 53, 201n17, 204n58; *Pharmacopoeia Extemporanea*, 53, 201n17, 204n58

Galen (and Galenic medicine), xi, 4–5, 7, 11, 12, 13, 14, 15, 26–27, 38, 54, 59, 67, 68, 69, 82, 124, 150, 179, 184nn25–26, 186n51, 187n60, 201n18, 204n57, 208n5, 208n8, 212n58, 228n3; *De Partium Usu*, 228n3; *De Sanitate Tuenda (On Hygiene)*, 208n5; "Notes on Hippocrates," 54; *Opera Omnia*, 54
Garth, Sir Samuel, 58, 189n10
Gay, John, 63, 81, 90, 91, 92, 104, 110, 111, 138, 174, 210n47
Gentleman's Magazine, 53
George I, King of England, 227n110
George II, King of England, 120, 121, 227n105, 227n110
Germain, Lady Elisabeth (Betty), 56, 81, 120
Gibson, Thomas, 53, 201n16; *The Anatomy of Humane Bodies Epitomized*, 201n16
Gillam, Stephen, 200n11
Glendinning, Victoria, 219n100
Glisson, Francis, 53, 201n16; *Anatomia Hepatis (Anatomy of the Liver)*, 53, 201n16
Glorious Revolution, 164
Goffman, Erving, 189n1
Goodall, Charles, 63, 206n80; *The Royal College of Physicians of London*, 63, 206n80
Gordin, Michael, 187n63
Gosse, Edmund, 24, 152, 155, 238n17
Gould, George, 192n53, 215n22
gout, 9, 10, 14, 76, 104, 226n95
Grattan, James, 82, 214n98
Grattan brothers, 89, 214n98
Green, Monica, 193n67
Greenacre, Phyllis, 191n37

Guerrini, Anita, 185n39
Guide to the Female Sex, 207n95
Gulliver's Travels (Swift), xii, xiv, xv–xvi, 1, 4, 5, 12, 16, 21, 23, 24, 26, 35, 41, 52, 57, 59–60, 84, 95, 107, 109, 112, 123, 124–41, 142–51, 152–60, 161, 163, 165, 171, 172–73, 175, 183n11, 187n61, 191n37, 225n74, 229nn18–19, 229n22, 230n24, 231n58, 231nn62–64, 232n70, 232n72, 232n91, 232n97, 235n30, 236–37nn43–45, 238n17, 238n41

Hammond, Brean, 96
Hammond, Eugene, 219n100
Handley, Sasha, 209n23
Harcourt, First Viscount (Simon Harcourt), 119
Harley, Edward, Second Earl of Oxford, 62, 81, 90, 92, 105, 114, 115, 116, 223n51
Harley, Henrietta Holles, Countess of Oxford, 81
Harley, Robert, First Earl of Oxford, 87, 104, 106, 114, 115–16, 220n19, 223n51, 224n71, 225n74
Harrison, Theophilus, 54, 201n18
Harvey, Gideon, 46
Harvey, William, 11, 13, 186n51
Hawkesworth, John, 4, 184n15
Hawkins, Anne Hunsaker, 18
Helmont, Jan Baptist van, 13, 52
Helsham, Richard, 12, 52, 54, 57, 58, 61, 82, 178, 187n56, 205n66, 206n82, 213n87
Hemingway, Ernest, 29
Hervey, John, Baron Hervey of Ickworth, 122, 227n105
Hippocrates (and Hippocratic medicine), xi, 7, 8, 11, 13, 54, 68, 69, 82, 150, 182n11, 184n25, 202n27, 208n5; *On Regimen*, 208n5; *On the Nature of Man*, 184n25

Hoadly, John, Archbishop of Dublin, 106
Hobart, Sir Henry, 226n101
Hospital for Incurables, 22–23, 95, 218n79
Howard, Charles, 122, 226n101
Howard, Henrietta, 36, 37, 44, 48, 109, 116, 118, 120–23, 127, 194n23, 226n101, 227nn104–5, 227n110, 227n112
Howard, Henry, Fifth Earl of Suffolk, 226n101
Howth, Earl of (William Howth), 103

iatrochemistry, 11–16, 26–27, 52, 54, 61, 204n57
iatromechanics (iatromathematics, iatrophysics), 11–16, 21–22, 26–27, 37, 40–41, 44, 47, 52, 54, 174, 177, 179, 186n51, 196n51, 209n34
Illich, Ivan, 101
Ingram, Allan, 1–2, 3, 4, 184n15, 200n6

Jacobitism, 87, 97, 164, 220n19
Jaffe, Nora Crow, 217n60
James II, King of England, 46, 164
Jersey, First Earl of (Edward Villiers), 9
Jervas, Charles, 185n29
Jewson, Nicholas D., 53, 200n11
Johnson, Esther (Stella), xvi, 19, 34, 37, 43–44, 57, 62–63, 64, 65, 71, 74, 77, 78, 79, 81, 85, 87, 90, 92–93, 94, 99, 104, 110, 111, 115, 116, 118–20, 135, 164, 168, 169, 193n1, 213n89, 217n60, 220nn8–9, 227n109, 231n63, 232n94, 240n13, 242n40, 244n17
Johnson, Samuel, 2, 24, 25, 26, 28, 29, 95, 108, 152, 154–55, 159, 164, 167–68, 182n7, 190n30, 218n77, 237n11, 239nn54–55
Johnston, Denis, 99
Jonston, John (Joannes Jonstonus), 41
Joyce, James, 29

Karenberg, Axel, 31, 193n67
Karpman, Ben, 191n37
Kelly, James, 226n97
Kerby-Miller, Charles, 229n10
Kerry, Lady Anne, 52, 64, 115, 118, 120
King, Helen, 184n25
King, Lester, 208n98
King, William, Archbishop of Dublin, 18–19, 79, 93, 105, 106
Koch, Julian, 191n36

labyrinthine vertigo. See Ménière's disease
LaCasce, Steward, 182n4, 203n38
Lane, Betty, 39
Larner, A. J., 193n67
Lecky, William, 25
Legg, J. Wickham, 27, 28
Leigh, James (Jemmey), 118, 225n87
Lémery, Louis, 38
Lewis, William, 66, 243n4; *The Edinburgh New Dispensatory*, 66, 179, 243n4
Leyden (medical school), 52, 64, 183n11
Lobb, Theophilus, 195n26
Locke, John, 23, 45, 155, 182n7
Long, Anne, 81
Lorch, Marjorie, 191n33, 193n67
Lower, Richard, 243n2
Lynall, Gregory, 174, 187n59
Lyon, John, 38, 195n29
Lyttelton, George, First Baron Lyttelton, 74, 209n35

Malcolm, Elizabeth, 218n79
Marcilly, Marie-Claire, Viscountess Bolingbroke, 65, 111
Marlborough, Duchess of (Sarah Churchill), 211n51
Marlborough, First Duke of (John Churchill), 154, 237n11
Mary II, Queen of England, 164

268 INDEX

Masham, Lady Abigail, 65, 115, 120, 224n71
McKeon, Michael, 98, 143
McMinn, Joseph, 167
Mead, Richard, 202n29
Melamed, Chaim, 191n37
Ménière, Prosper, 6, 27–28, 125, 181n2. *See also* Ménière's disease
Ménière's disease, xi, xii, xiv, 3, 4–6, 27–33, 42, 124–25, 130, 192n53, 193n65, 193n68, 193n70, 194n18, 228n3. *See also* clinical diagnosis; retrospective diagnosis
Milton, John, 29
Mitchell, Piers, 29
Motte, Benjamin, 95
Mounsey, Chris, 222n43
Moyle, John, 7, 8–9, 184n26
Muffett, Thomas, 38; *Healths Improvement*, 38
Muramoto, Osamu, 193n67

nerves, 11, 14, 21, 37, 40–41, 44–46, 47, 61, 82, 121, 177, 180, 190n30, 191n41, 195n26, 197n51, 197n54, 198n76, 198n80, 226n93, 228n3
Newtonian medicine, 14–15, 82
Nichols, John (editor and printer of Swift's works), 242n36
Nichols, John (surgeon), 206n82
Niebyl, Peter, 208n8
Nokes, David, 210n37, 220n8
non-naturals, 15, 52, 68–84, 110, 147, 150, 172, 208n8, 208n10

Ober, William, 28–29; *Boswell's Clap and Other Essays*, 28–29
O'Connor, Flannery, 29; "A Good Man Is Hard to Find," 29
original sin, 47, 48, 50, 55, 84, 110, 123
Orkney, Countess of (Elizabeth Villiers), 52, 65, 120, 240n13

Ormonde, Duchess of (Mary Butler), 120
Ormonde, Second Duke of (James Butler), 215n19
Orrery, Fifth Earl of (John Boyle), 2, 20–25, 36, 40, 41, 42, 43, 46, 89, 96, 97, 115, 145, 152, 154, 155, 166, 182n7, 190n22, 212n54, 214n24, 217n50, 218n77, 237n11, 241n24, 241n35
Orrery, Lady (Margaret Boyle), 117–18, 211n51
Orwell, George, 97, 165, 219n91
Oxford, First Earl of (Robert Harley). *See* Harley, Robert, First Earl of Oxford
Oxford, Second Earl of (Edward Harley). *See* Harley, Edward, Second Earl of Oxford

Paracelsus, 12, 13, 53, 61, 187n60; *Opera Omnia*, 187n60
Parnell, Thomas, 110
Parsons, Talcott, 101
Passmann, Dirk F., 201n19
Patrick (Swift's servant), 119
Paxton, Peter, 11, 14
Pearson, John, 186n42
Pelling, Margaret, 63
Pendarves, Mary, 36, 89, 90, 93, 103, 220n7, 240n13
Pepys, Samuel, 39
Phillips, Marmaduke, 220n14
Philosophical Transactions of the Royal Society, 146
phrenology, 24–25, 191n33
"Physician in London," 73
Pilkington, Lætitia, 20, 73, 79, 80, 93, 96, 127, 152, 153–54, 167, 169, 170–71, 190n16, 206n82, 212n62, 215n9, 217n56, 234n9, 241n30
Pilkington, Matthew, 20, 127, 190n16
Pinel, Philippe, 191n36
Plath, Sylvia, 29

Pope, Alexander, 1–2, 6, 29, 43, 46, 49, 62, 63, 72, 74, 76, 77, 80, 82, 90, 91–92, 93–94, 95, 97, 104, 107, 108, 110, 111–13, 114, 116, 117, 120, 121, 138, 142, 153, 175, 178, 185n29, 185n38, 200n6, 203n50, 204n51, 209n35, 211n49, 211n54, 212n63, 222n30, 223nn47–48, 223nn50–51, 223n53, 223n56, 237n5; "The Second Satire of the Second Book of Horace Paraphrased," 212n63
Pope, Edith, 111–12, 223n50
Porter, Dorothy, 53, 201n12
Porter, Roy, 44, 47, 53, 113, 198n75, 198n78, 200n1, 200n12
Primerose, James, 53
Prior, Matthew, 79, 87, 88, 110, 196n41, 213n87, 221n19
Probyn, Clive, 124, 182n4, 228n3
Providential explanation of disease, 18, 50
Ptolemy, 47
Pulteney, William, 54–55, 56, 63, 67–68, 81, 151

Queensberry, Duchess of (Catherine Douglas), 90, 116, 117, 120, 222n38
Queensberry, Second Duke of (James Douglas), 90
Quincy, John, 66

Rabelais, François, 123, 175, 229n19
Radcliffe, John, 9, 19, 52, 58, 64, 189n10
Rather, L. J., 208n8
Rawson, Claude, 96, 98, 126, 160, 166, 169, 171
Raymond, Anthony, 118, 225n87
Real, Hermann J., 201n19
regimen, xiv–xv, 14, 15, 51, 52, 53, 67–84, 98, 125, 136, 138, 148, 150–51, 170, 185n29, 208n5, 208n10. *See also* non-naturals

Regimen Sanitatis Salernitanum, 53, 68
Reilly, Patrick, 97
retrospective diagnosis, xi, 3, 4–7, 17–33, 42, 124–25, 130, 166, 191n33, 193n67, 216n22, 228n3. *See also* clinical diagnosis; Ménière's disease
Richardson, Katharine, 90, 105
Richardson, William, 30, 36, 90
Ridgeway, Anne, 217n50
Robinson, Nicholas, 82
Rolt, Martha (Patty), Mrs. Lancelot, 112
Rosenberg, Charles, 17, 189n1
Ross, John J., 29; *Shakespeare's Tremor and Orwell's Cough*, 29
Rousseau, G. S., 200n1
Royal College of Physicians of Edinburgh, 63–64
Royal College of Physicians of Ireland, 63–64, 187n56, 206n82
Royal College of Physicians of London, 63–64, 206nn80–81
Royal College of Surgeons in Ireland, 25
Royal Society, 146
Rubin, Wallace, 192n46
Rushdy, Ashraf, 242n46

Salmon, William, 53, 236n40, 243n2
Sanctorius of Padua (Santorio Santorio), 14, 72, 74, 209n24, 209n34; *Medicina Statica: Being the Aphorisms of Sanctorius*, 72, 209n24, 209n34
Scott, Walter, 25, 26, 28, 108, 152, 241n28
Scriblerians, 110, 126, 187n56, 222n40
Seidel, Michael, 155
Shadwell, Thomas, 29
Shaftesbury, First Earl of (Anthony Ashley Cooper), 162–63
Shakespeare, William, 29
Shaw, Peter, 39, 42, 180, 186n42, 212n58
Sheridan, Elizabeth, 90, 120

Sheridan, Thomas, xii, 35, 51–52, 59, 60, 69–70, 71, 78, 81, 86, 89–90, 98, 108, 109, 112, 120, 121, 159, 168, 189n13, 208n12, 216n39, 223n56, 234n3, 241n35
Sheridan, Thomas (biographer of Swift), 169, 234n3
Short, Thomas, 207n84
Siebers, Tobin, 222n43
Sloane, Sir Hans, 150
Smargins, Mary, 39, 196n44
Smith, Frederik N., 243n60
solids (and solidism), 11–12, 13–14, 16, 40, 82, 177, 179–80
Somers, John, Baron Somers of Evesham, 117, 154, 225n82
spiritual autobiography, 18, 175
Stannard, Eaton, 106, 221n21
Stella. *See* Johnson, Esther
Sterne, Laurence, 34–35, 97, 163; *Tristram Shandy*, 34–35, 163
St. John, Henry, First Viscount Bolingbroke. *See* Bolingbroke, First Viscount (Henry St. John)
Stolberg, Michael, 186n46
Stone, Edward, 155
Stopford, James, 227n109
Stubbs, John, 94, 192n54
Sunderland, Robert Spence, Second Earl of, 117, 225n82
Swieten, Gerard van, 76
Swift, Abigail (Swift's mother), 36–37, 99
Swift, Deane (Swift's cousin and biographer), 43, 49, 71, 79, 96–97, 154, 165–66, 217n50, 218n77, 219n100, 236n43
Swift, Godwin (Swift's uncle), 99
Swift, Jonathan (Swift's father), 48, 49, 99
Swift, Jonathan: ambivalence toward medical profession, 54–55, 57–58, 63–64, 69, 102, 150–51; autopsy, 37–38, 195n29, 201n18; cognitive functions, xiii, 6, 15–16, 19, 21–23, 27, 37, 41–47, 94–96, 108–9, 114, 127, 130, 131, 132, 144, 152–55, 156, 161, 170, 175, 237n5; diet, xiv, 38, 48, 70, 72, 73–78, 81, 88, 119, 147, 150; disability, 86, 89, 90, 91, 92, 104, 113, 118, 124–25, 134, 142, 161; "double consciousness," xiii, 97–100, 132, 143; "excremental vision," 4, 25, 148–49, 152, 171–74, 236n36, 242n46; exercise, xiv–xv, 69, 70, 72, 73–74, 77, 78–83, 84, 88, 91–92, 102–3, 136–39, 140; fruit, 48, 73–74, 77–78, 84, 119, 123, 154, 194n18, 228n3; genre, xvi, 174–75; identity, personal and social, xiii, xv, xvi, 3, 31, 32, 36, 48, 85–100, 104, 109–10, 113, 122, 125, 127, 130, 131–32, 134, 144–51, 160, 161, 166, 169, 170–71; infant "abduction," 96, 99, 231n64; Latino-Anglicus/Anglo-Latinus, 109, 168, 170, 241n35; "little language," xvi, 118, 134, 168, 213n89, 231n58; madness, xiv, xvi, 2–4, 5, 6, 21–25, 26, 37–38, 41, 43, 45, 46, 47, 95, 108, 125, 152–60, 161, 175, 182n7, 184n15, 190n20, 198n75, 198n78, 221n21, 238n17; medical interventions, xiv, 51–66, 72, 80, 83, 170; medical knowledge, 53–54; milk, 71, 75–76, 211n49, 211n51; monstrousness, 144–45, 146, 148, 155; prescriptions, 60–63, 177–80; psychopathy, 4, 25, 172, 236n36 (*see also* Freudian critics); regimen, xiv–xv, 15, 52, 67–84, 148, 150–51, 170; sexuality, 91–94, 96, 121, 122–23, 132, 134, 135, 136–41, 142, 145; shingles, 10, 14, 34, 38, 51, 56, 59, 62–63, 75, 83, 87, 93, 185nn41–42; in "sick role," xv, 91, 101–23, 125, 170; wine, 74, 76–77, 210n47, 211n54, 212n58, 212n62; wordplay, 109, 123, 131, 134, 147, 168, 170, 175
—, works: "The Answer," 40, 228n3; "An Argument against Abolishing Christianity," 169; autobiography,

96–100, 103, 152; *The Battel of the Books,* 13; "A Beautiful Young Nymph Going to Bed," 171–74; "Bec's Birthday," 9, 226n95; *The Bickerstaff Papers,* 169; "The Blunders, Deficiencies, Distresses, and Misfortunes of Quilca," 120; "Cassinus and Peter," 171–74, 198n67, 242n50; "A Character, Panegyric, and Description of the Legion Club," 22; "Dean of St. Patricks Petition to the H. of Lords, against the Lord Blaney," 102–3; "A Dialogue Between an Eminent Lawyer and Dr. Swift Dean of St. Patrick's, Being an Allusion to the First Satire of the Second Book of Horace," 107, 167; *A Discourse Concerning the Mechanical Operation of the Spirit,* 12; *The Drapier's Letters,* 76, 98, 166; "Family of Swift," 35–36, 37, 48, 49, 98–100, 194n23, 219n100, 231n64; *Hints Towards an Essay on Conversation,* 19; "Irel[an]d," 48; *Journal to Stella,* xvi, 9, 18, 34, 36, 38, 57, 60, 69, 79, 94, 110, 118, 134, 168, 185n41, 187n56, 193n1, 228n3, 240n13; "The Lady's Dressing Room," 171–74; *A Letter to a Young Gentleman, Lately Enter'd into Holy Orders,* 165; "The Life and Character of Dean Swift. Upon a Maxim in Rochefoucault," 105; "A Modest Proposal," 125, 126, 169, 171; "On His Own Deafness," 1, 96, 171; *Polite Conversation,* 105, 164–65; "The Progress of Beauty," 174; *A Proposal for Correcting, Improving and Ascertaining the English Tongue,* 165, 175, 236n30; "scatological" poems, xvi, 4, 25, 84, 126, 148, 152, 171–74; "In Sickness: Written Soon After the Author's Coming to Live in Ireland, upon the Queen's Death, October 1714," 88, 96, 171; "Strephon and Chloe," 171–74; *A Tale of a Tub,* 12, 45, 126, 165, 167, 171, 175; "To Quilca, a Country House in No Very Good Repair, Where the Supposed Author, and Some of His Friends, Spent a Summer, in the Year 1725," 189n13; "To Stella, Visting Me in My Sickness," 92–93; "To Stella ... Written on the Day of Her Birth, but Not on the Subject, When I Was Sick in Bed," 93, 111; *Verses on the Death of Dr. Swift, D.S.P.D. Occasioned by Reading a Maxim in Rochefoulcault,* 1, 35, 96, 107, 143, 153, 171, 182n1, 225n80; "When I Come to Be Old," 80, 93; "Written by the Reverend Dr. Swift. On His Own Deafness," 1, 96, 171. See also *Gulliver's Travels*

Swift, Thomas (Swift's grandfather), 47, 49, 50, 110, 163–64

Sydenham, Thomas, 4–5, 8, 53, 80, 236n40

Sylvius, Franciscus, 13, 52

Takeda, Taizo, 194n18

Temkin, Owsei, 184n20

Temple, Sir William, 13, 21, 36–37, 48, 54, 55–56, 58, 59, 67, 77, 79, 81, 87, 114, 164, 175, 194n23, 195n31, 203n37, 220n8, 223n48, 236n43; *An Essay upon Health and Long Life,* 13, 54, 55, 58, 195n31

Test Act, 164

Thackeray, William Makepeace, 24, 108, 152, 155

Tisdall, William, 169, 242n40

Tissot, Samuel, 196n46

Todd, Dennis, 144, 146

Turner, David, 91, 92, 217n57, 222n43

Valangin, François Joseph Pahud de, 208n8

Vanhomrigh, Esther (Vanessa), 43, 87–88, 93, 168, 220n8, 241n34

Vanhomrigh family, 74
Verwaal, Ruben E., 39

Wagner, Darren Neil, 198n76
Wainewright, Jeremiah, 208n8
Wallis, Thomas, 106
Walls, Thomas, 72, 106, 215n18
Walpole, Robert, 109
Walsh, Marcus, 187n62, 201n18
Waring, Jane, 104, 220n8
Washington, Gene, 182n4
Wear, Andrew, 13, 14, 208n10
Webster, Charles, 63
Weinbrot, Howard, 243n60
Weisser, Olivia, 109–10, 199n98
Wesley, John, 66; *Primitive Physick,* 66
Whiteway, John, 38, 195n29, 201n18
Whiteway, Martha, 19, 54, 70, 83, 89, 195n29, 208n12, 211n51, 217n56, 222n43
Whitley, E. M., 231n58
Whitworth, Viscount Charles, 228n113
Whole Duty of a Woman: or, A Guide to the Female Sex, The, 207n95

Wilde, Oscar, 191n39
Wilde, Sir William, 2, 3, 25–27, 28, 191n39; *The Closing Years of Dean Swift's Life,* 3
William III, King of England, 164
Williams, Abigail, 193n1, 209n18, 220n9, 228n3, 231n58
Williams, Harold, xvi, 204n58, 205n64, 222n37, 228n3
Williams, Henry, 193n68
Willis, Thomas, 52, 149–50, 198n80
Wilson, Benjamin, 196n44
Wilson, T. G., 25, 192n53
Womersley, David, 105, 228–29nn10–11, 229n18, 230n48, 236n30
Woodman, Philip, 243n2
Woolf, Virginia, 29
Woolley, David, xvi, 62, 181n1, 204n58, 225n82, 228n114 (chap. 7), 228n3 (chap. 8), 240n13
Wycherley, William, 185n29

Young, Edward, 46, 148, 225n82

PECULIAR BODIES: STORIES AND HISTORIES

The Importance of Being Different: Disability in Oscar Wilde's Fairy Tales
Chris Foss

They Run with Surprising Swiftness: The Woman Athletes of Early Modern Britain
Peter Radford

Melville's Other Lives: Bodies on Trial in "The Piazza Tales"
Christopher Sten

Lame Captains and Left-Handed Admirals: Amputee Officers in Nelson's Navy
Teresa Michals

Beyond the Moulin Rouge: The Life and Legacy of La Goulue
Will Visconti

Sapphic Crossings: Cross-Dressing Women in Eighteenth-Century British Literature
Ula Lukszo Klein

Sight Correction: Vision and Blindness in Eighteenth-Century Britain
Chris Mounsey

www.ingramcontent.com/pod-product-compliance
Lightning Source LLC
Chambersburg PA
CBHW021654230426
43668CB00008B/617